Novel Carriers for Drug Delivery

Novel Carriers for Drug Delivery

Manish K. Chourasia
M. Pharm, PhD
Sr. Scientist
Pharmaceutics Division,
CSIR-Central Drug Research Institute, Lucknow

Mohini Chaurasia
M. Pharm
Assistant Professor
Amity Institute of Pharmacy,
Amity University, Lucknow

Nitin K. Jain
M. Pharm, PhD
Scientist 'E'/Joint Director
Department of Biotechnology,
Ministry of Science & Technology,
Government of India, New Delhi

PharmaMed Press
An imprint of Pharma Book Syndicate
A Unit of BSP Books Pvt. Ltd.
4-4-309/316, Giriraj Lane,
Sultan Bazar, Hyderabad - 500 095.

Novel Carriers for Drug Delivery ***by M.K. Chourasia***

Published by

PharmaMed Press

An imprint of Pharma Book Syndicate

A unit of BSP Books Pvt. Ltd.

4-4-309/316, Giriraj Lane, Sultan Bazar, Hyderabad - 500 095.

Phone: 040-23445605, 23445688; Fax: 91+40-23445611

e-mail: info@pharmamedpress.com

ISBN: 978-93-85433-96-2 (HB)

Dedicated to

My Parents and My Children

Manish K. Chourasia

सी.एस.आई.आर.-केन्द्रीय औषधि अनुसंधान संस्थान, लखनऊ
(वैज्ञानिक तथा औद्योगिक अनुसंधान परिषद्)
सेक्टर 10, जानकीपुरम विस्तार, सीतापुर रोड, लखनऊ – 226 031 (भारत)
CSIR - Central Drug Research Institute
(Council of Scientific & Industrial Research)
Sector 10, Janakipuram Extension, Sitapur Road, Lucknow - 226 031 (India)

डॉ. एस. के. पुरी, एफएनएएससी
कार्यवाहक निर्देशक

Dr. SK Puri, FNASc
Acting Director

Foreword

It is a matter of great pleasure to learn that an extensive book covering the vast scope of novel drug delivery systems, targeted at both scientific and academic audience is being released in form of "Novel Carriers for Drug Delivery". I believe the book at hand encompasses almost every avenue associated with design and application of novel emerging carrier systems in an extremely compact manner. The text is lucidly written with evenly dispersed info graphics and easy to remember flow schemes.

Considering the boom in nanotechnology, and the relative dearth of quality opinion, the highlight of the compiled work seems to be the knowledge accumulated to deliver theoretically and experimentally viable information suited to requirements of students pursuing undergraduate, postgraduate or even doctoral programs. I anticipate the readers will extract maximum possible information, and utilize it for further strengthening of nanotechnology assisted healthcare modalities.

S.K. Puri

Preface

At the outset when we started working towards this book, the whole propaganda of pharmaceutical research seemed to have taken a leap of faith into far-fetched promise land: microparticles gave the impression of having replaced oral solid dosage forms; nanoparticles, liposomes, nanoemulsions had been sounded out as probable substitutes for parenteral solutions. The simplistic inference which we drew over the course of our continuous research, both as a scholars and as mentors was that general tendency of formulation scientists worldwide had shifted towards novel carrier based systems. This siege in mentality does not accurately reflect in the commercial aspect as of yet, and in no way undermines the importance as well as the future applicability of conventional drug delivery systems. But the future is very much 'nano' as far as drug delivery is concerned. With commercial launch of numerous formulations derived from novel carriers in the past decade, the scene is surely evolving and it is anticipated that this pharmaceutical advancement will play a prominent role in healthcare system in the very near future.

This discussion brings us to the real issue for compiling the current book. The accelerated innovations in pharmaceutics being laid bare in the laboratory or industry are not translated into the academic framework adapted for graduate and post-graduate students. We sincerely feel that the coursework implemented in specialization syllabi is contemporary to the times when tablets and capsules were at the forefront of pharmaceutical research. This implies that the student struggles to get a grasp of the theoretical and practical concepts dictating the behavior, applications and manufacturing technologies being actively employed to fabricate novel carriers. Although numerous reviews, books and articles are available, we do not feel they serve or match the purpose of a graduate or a post graduate student, often being written in a verbose form which is too intricate or simply inaccessible. It was therefore a genuine requirement to fill the knowledge pit which students of today, i.e., the researchers of tomorrow find themselves in. This book is therefore a small effort towards filling that void.

All the contributors have tried their best in presenting relevant text to the most prominent avenues of novel drug carriers and nanodiagnostics. It has also been our effort to include interactive flowcharts, representative schemes, generally practiced experimental protocols and explanatory diagrams wherever possible, so as to ease the reader into novel drug delivery systems. The chapters have been selected after careful consideration and have been presented in a manner so that each of them could be read independently without any dependency on the previous or following chapters. The body of each chapter is delineated into clearly headlined sections for direct reference. Finally, wherever necessary, descriptive examples have been provided to substantiate the applicability of theoretical and experimental portions described in the text. It is our belief that this book will provide distinctive knowledge to pharmacy students, bioengineers, and research scholars in related fields serving as a single point comprehensive guide and reference to their research and study.

Manish K. Chourasia
Mohini Chaurasia
Nitin K. Jain

Acknowledgement

What you have in your hands, is an end product of sustained efforts by many people. On the verge of releasing this book we would like to express our deepest gratitude to everyone involved in structuring of book, right from initial genesis to final completion. All the authors who provided quality verbatim input deserve praise, as it is their efforts which form the basic building blocks of the book. The matrix to these blocks was the encouragement and constructive suggestions by our peers in allowing the book to reach its final form. No words can aptly signify the efforts of our support team which assisted in designing, proof reading and facilitating miscellaneous background work and it would be unjustified if we do not mention their names. Special thanks are due to my research fellows Yuvraj, Jay, Vivek and Shalini who have imparted significant contribution in publication of the book.

The authors, apart from providing the content have also worked tremendously by performing proof reading and responded quickly to nay of the changes suggested by us. Thanks to BS Publications for bringing up the book from our minds to the market.

Manish K. Chourasia
Mohini Chaurasia
Nitin K. Jain

Contributors

Aviral Jain

Pharmaceutics Research Laboratory, Department of Pharmaceutics, Adina Institute of Pharmaceutical Sciences, Sagar-470 002, India.

D. Mishra

Department of Pharmaceutics, College of Pharmacy, IPS Academy, Indore-452 014, India.

Darshana Jain

Pharmaceutics Research Laboratory, Department of Pharmaceutics, Adina Institute of Pharmaceutical Sciences, Sagar-470 002, India.

J. G. Meher

Pharmaceutics Division, CSIR-Central Drug Research Institute, Lucknow-226 031, India.

M. Chaurasia

Amity Institute of Pharmacy, Amity University, Lucknow-226 028, India.

Manish K. Chourasia

Pharmaceutics Division, CSIR-Central Drug Research Institute, Lucknow-226 031, India.

Neha Gupta

Sagar Institute of Pharmaceutical Sciences, Sagar-470 003, India.

Nishi Mody

Pharmaceutics Research Laboratory, Department of Pharmaceutics, Adina Institute of Pharmaceutical Sciences, Sagar-470 002, India.

Nitin K. Jain

Department of Biotechnology, Ministry of Science & Technology, New Delhi-400 003, India.

P. Bhatnagar

Sri Aurobindo College of Pharmacy, SAIMS Campus, Indore-453 111, India.

P. Khare

Truba Institute of Pharmacy, Karond - Gandhi Nagar By Pass Road, Bhopal-462 038, India.

P.K. Mishra

Translational Research Lab, Department of Zoology, School of Biological Sciences, Dr. HS Gour Central University, Sagar-470 003, India.

Prem N. Gupta

Formulation & Drug Delivery Division, CSIR-Indian Institute of Integrative Medicine, Jammu-180 001, India.

Priyanka Jain

Pharmaceutics Research Laboratory, Department of Pharmaceutics, Adina Institute of Pharmaceutical Sciences, Sagar-470 002, India.

S. Asthana

Pharmaceutics Division, CSIR-Central Drug Research Institute, Lucknow-226 031, India.

Umesh Gupta

Department of Pharmacy, School of Chemical Sciences and Pharmacy, Central University of Rajasthan, Bandarsindri, Kishangarh, Ajmer-305 817, India.

V. Dhote

Truba Institute of Pharmacy, Karond - Gandhi Nagar By Pass Road, Bhopal-462 038, India.

V. K. Pawar

Pharmaceutics Division, CSIR-Central Drug Research Institute, Lucknow-226 031, India.

Varsha Tilwani

Pharmaceutics Research Laboratory, Department of Pharmaceutics, Adina Institute of Pharmaceutical Sciences, Sagar-470 002, India.

Y. Singh

Pharmaceutics Division, CSIR-Central Drug Research Institute, Lucknow-226 031, India.

CONTENTS

CHAPTER 12

Microparticles as Drug Delivery Systems

1

Drug Delivery using Polymeric and other Carrier Systems

Y. Singh[1], M. Chaurasia[2] and Manish K. Chourasia[1]
[1]Pharmaceutics Division, CSIR-Central Drug Research Institute, Lucknow-226031, India.
[2]Amity Institute of Pharmacy, Amity University, Lucknow-226028, India.

1.1 Introduction

Before advent of novel delivery systems, conventional delivery systems were mainstay in delivering drugs for treatment and prevention of diseases. The introduction of nanotechnology has revolutionized all scientific fields including medical, pharmaceutical and delivery systems. There are inherent problems associated with drug discovery including intricate and tedious research and in particular high cost associated in carrying such work. Further, the high cost is a strong deterrent especially for developing countries that cannot afford huge expenditure on such research. Nanotechnology has provided an excellent weapon to pharmaceutical scientist which is supportive in developing novel formulations of existing problematic drugs. Majority of drug used for treatment of dreaded diseases such as cancer and leishmaniasis have poor selectivity and profound toxicity towards normal body cells. The toxicity of such drugs can be substantially reduced by incorporation inside nano sized carrier systems. These polymeric nanoparticulate systems can deliver the entrapped therapeutic moiety in the vicinity of target area thereby reducing potential unwanted toxic effect with maximized efficacy. The prerequisite for polymeric carrier is biodegradability and biocompatibility, the qualities that are needed to get approval of regulatory agencies. The polymers belonging to synthetic and natural category including, poly lactic acid (PLA), poly(lactic-co-glycolic acid) (PLGA), poly(ε-caprolactone) (PCL), chitosan and bovine serum albumin (BSA) have been widely used for formulation and development of nanoparticles incorporating drugs having diverse physicochemical characteristics. Various methods for preparation of polymeric nanoparticles are available in literature and the choice depends on property of drug to be incorporated and nature of polymeric carrier. This chapter sketches out an overview of formulation and development of nano sized carriers including polymeric nanoparticles, nanocrystals, nanofibers and nanorods and their applicability in drug delivery and therapeutics.

1.2 Basic Methods of Polymeric Nanoparticle Production

Polymeric Nanoparticles (PNPs) can be prepared either by dispersing preformed polymers into nano sized particles or by inducing polymerization reactions in monomers during the process of nanoparticle manufacture itself (Fig. 1.1). Methods like solvent evaporation, nano-precipitation, salting out, dialysis, ionic gelation and supercritical fluid technology can be conveniently utilized to form PNPs out of preformed polymers. Polymerization techniques such as emulsion polymerization and its various sub techniques which employ a monomer and a suitable initiator are also used to form PNPs.

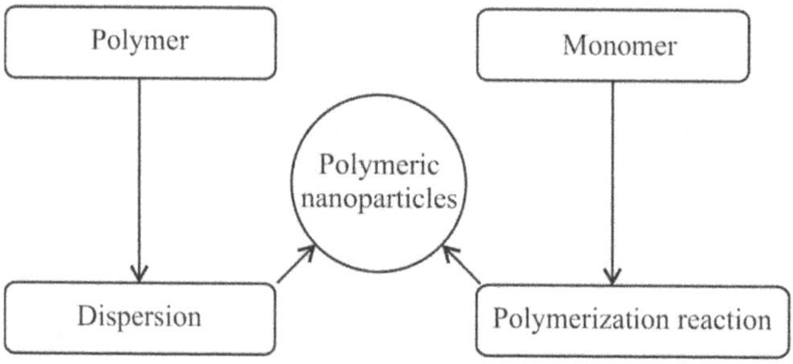

Fig. 1.1 Basic methods for production of polymeric nanoparticles.

The choice of preparation method is made on the basis of a number of factors such as type of polymeric system, area of application, size requirement, etc. For instance, a polymeric system developed for pharmaceutical field should be absolutely free of any organic solvents, and therefore would employ methods which either refrain altogether from organic solvents or utilize trace quantities. Another important factor which plays a vital role in method selection is the nature of drug molecule. For example solubility of the active molecule in different solvents, thermal and chemical stability of the active agent, reproducibility of the release kinetic profiles of drug (Natural polymers generally may not provide the batch-to-batch reproducibility), stability of the final product and residual impurities associated with the final product.

1.2.1 Dispersion of Preformed Polymers to Form PNPs

1.2.1.1 Emulsification/Solvent Evaporation

Emulsification-solvent evaporation involves two steps. The first step requires emulsification of the polymer solution into an aqueous phase. During the second step polymer solvent is evaporated, inducing polymer precipitation as nanospheres. A polymer organic solution containing the dissolved drug is dispersed into nanodroplets, in a non-solvent or suspension medium such as chloroform or ethyl acetate. The polymer precipitates in the form of nanospheres in which the drug is finely dispersed in the polymer matrix network. The solvent is subsequently evaporated by increasing the temperature under pressure or by continuous stirring. The size can be controlled by adjusting the stir rate, type and amount of dispersing agent, viscosity of organic and aqueous phases, and temperature.

Solvent evaporation is the most widely employed technique to prepare nanoparticles of polymers. In the conventional methods, two main strategies are used for the formation of emulsions: the preparation of single-emulsions, e.g., [oil-in-water (O/W)] to entrap lipophilic drugs or double-emulsions, for hydrophilic drugs e.g., [(water-in-oil)-in-water, (W/O)/W] (Fig. 1.2 and 1.3). The drug in this case may either be finely dispersed through the polymeric core or may be dissolved in the internal aqueous phase which is stored inside the polymeric shell, forming a nanocapsule.

These methods utilize high-speed homogenization or ultrasonication. Afterwards, the solidified nanoparticles can be collected by ultracentrifugation and washed with distilled water to remove additives such as surfactants. Finally, the product is lyophilized. Generally, a polymer dissolved in an organic solvent forms the oil phase, whereas the aqueous phase containing the stabilizer forms the water phase.

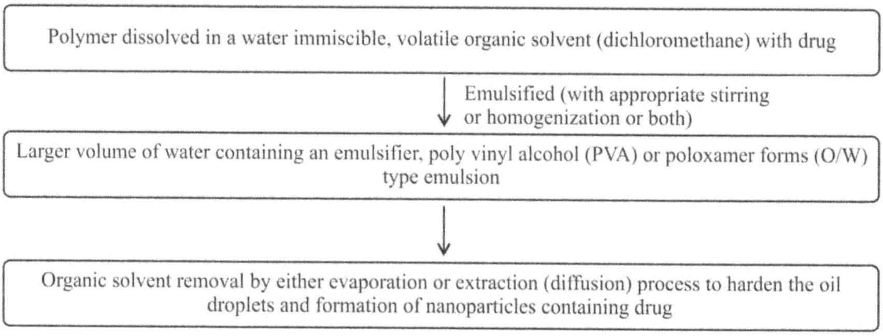

Fig. 1.2 Single emulsion method for lipophilic drugs.

Matsumoto *et al.,* (1999) described the preparation and the evaluation of biodegradable poly(L-lactide)-poly(ethylene glycol)-poly(L-lactide) copolymer (PLA-PEG-PLA) nanoparticles containing progesterone as a model drug by the above described single emulsion method. In another study, Ahlin *et al.,* (2002) reported the design and characterization of poly-(lactide-co-glycolide) (PLGA) and polymethylmethacrylate (PMMA) nanoparticles containing enalaprilat and evaluated the potential of these colloidal carriers for the transport of drugs through the intestinal mucosa. Nicoli *et al.,* (2001) prepared triptorelin loaded nanospheres for transdermal iontophoretic application using double emulsion method. In another study, nanoparticles were loaded with both a hydrophilic and a low molecular weight drug such as propranolol-HCl (Ubrich *et al.,* 2004).

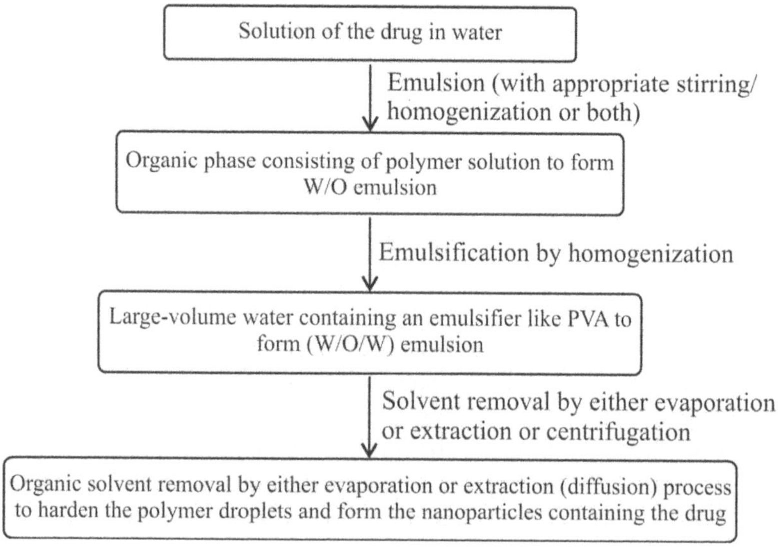

Fig. 1.3 Double emulsion process.

However, limitations are imposed by the scale-up of the high energy requirements in homogenization. Frequently used polymers are PLA, PLGA, ethylcellulose (EC), cellulose acetate phthalate, PCL, and poly (h-hydroxybutyrate) (PHB). Drugs or model drugs that have been encapsulated include albumin, tetanus toxoid, testosterone, loperamide, praziquantel, cyclosporin A, and indomethacin.

Major variables affecting the outcome of this process are the preparation temperature, solvent evaporation method, internal aqueous phase volume, surfactant concentration, and the influence of the molecular mass of the polymer on the particle size, the zeta potential, the residual surfactant percentage, and the polydispersity index. Because the process is governed by emulsification, utilizing a higher concentration of surfactant not only reduces the size of oil droplets, but also prevents their agglomeration. The concentrations of polymer and solvent used in the preparation of the emulsion also affect the final properties of the PNPs prepared by the solvent evaporation method. The mixing technique is also important in the preparation of PNPs by the solvent evaporation method. It was demonstrated that the duration of the second mixing step, which leads to the W/O/W emulsion, has a greater influence on the final mean particle size than the first step for the W/O emulsion.

1.2.1.2 Nanoprecipitation

The nanoprecipitation method was developed by Fessi *et al.,* (1989) for the preparation of PNPs. It is also called as solvent displacement method. The basic principle of this technique is based on the interfacial deposition of a polymer after displacement of a semipolar solvent, miscible with water, from a lipophilic solution acting as the oil phase for an infinitesimally small period of time. The basic difference from solvent evaporation lies with the fact that there is no apparent emulsification step, i.e., the formation of nanoparticles is instantaneous. Also it is a low energy method, i.e., moderate stirring is adequate, whereas high powered mechanized stirring is sometimes required in solvent evaporation to formulate the initial emulsion.

The process dynamics and the outcome are driven by the diffusion of solvent phase into the non-solvent water for most of the cases. Rapid diffusion of the solvent into non-solvent phase results in the decrease of interfacial tension between the two phases, which increases the surface area and leads to the formation of small droplets of organic solvent. The polymer and drug is consequently precipitated out in the non-solvent due to lack of solubility, forming a milky suspension of nano sized particles, however the overall colour of the suspension is dictated by the colour of drug and its percentage entrapment and can act as a crude visual indicator of its quality. A suspension of a coloured drug may turn out to be whitish if it is properly entrapped in the polymeric matrix. The drug as in solvent evaporation is dispersed throughout the polymeric matrix or adsorbed onto the surface; some amount of drug may also be dispersed throughout the solution in nano sized form, or may precipitate out (Fig. 1.4).

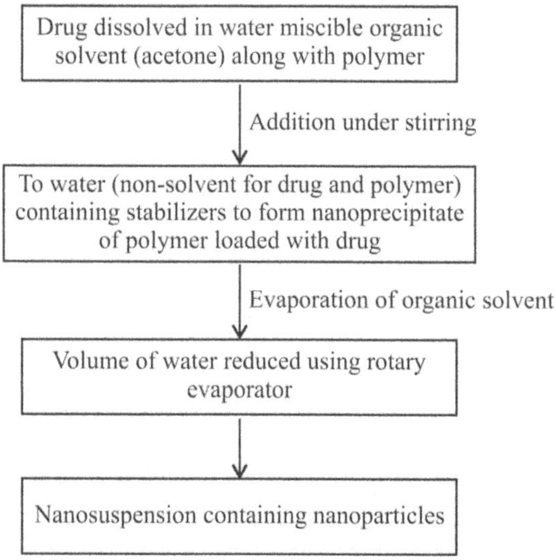

Fig. 1.4 Steps in nanoprecipitation method.

Nanoprecipitation system consists of four basic components: the polymer (synthetic, semi synthetic or natural), drug (to be entrapped), the polymer solvent and the non-solvent of the polymer with the optional presence of surfactants for example poloxamers, PVA, tweens, cetyl trimethyl ammonium bromide, Aerosol-AT etc. Organic solvent (i.e., ethanol, acetone, or dioxane) which is miscible in water and easy to remove by evaporation is chosen as polymer solvent. Due to this reason, acetone is the most frequently employed polymer solvent in this method. Sometimes, it consists of binary solvent blends, acetone with small amount of water, blends of acetone with ethanol and methanol. On the other hand, the non-solvent phase consisting of a non-solvent or a mixture of non-solvents is admixed with one or more naturally occurring or synthetic surfactants. Table 1.1 shows various examples of polymers, solvents, non-solvents and stabilizing agents used in the nanoprecipitation formulations and particle size achieved. Notice that, although an extensive range of polymers can be used theoretically, in practice only few are used regularly.

Table 1.1 Preparation of polymeric nanoparticles by nanoprecipitation method

Polymer	Solvent	Non-solvent	Stabilizing agent	Drug	Particle size (nm)	Ref.
PLGA	Acetone	Water	PVA	Curcumin	95-560	Yallapu *et al.*, 2010
Allylic starch	Acetone	Water	-	-	270	Tan *et al.*, 2009
PLA	Acetone	Water	Poloxamer 188	Muramyl-tripeptide cholesterol	250 ± 50	Seyler *et al.*, 1999
PLA	THF	Water	-	-	100-300	Legrand *et al.*, 2007
PCL	Acetone	Water	Span 20	Griseofulvin	741-924	Zili *et al.*, 2005
PCL	Acetone	Water	PVA		365 ± 5	Moinard-Checot *et al.*, 2008

The polymers commonly used are biodegradable polyesters, especially PCL, PLA and PLGA. Eudragit and polyalkylcyanoacrylate (PACA) have also been used for formulation of nanoparticles. PCL nanospheres of isradipine (Leroueil-Le Verger *et al.*, 1998) and nanocapsules of griseofulvin (Zili *et al.*, 2005) (poorly soluble drug) have been prepared by nanoprecipitation method. Chen *et al.*, prepared and characterized oleanolic acid (Chen *et al.*, 2005) (poorly soluble drug) nanosuspensions by the nanoprecipitation method to enhance the oral bioavailability by increasing dissolution rate and solubility. Nanoparticles of isradipine (Leroueil-Le Verger *et al.*, 1998) (poorly soluble drug), an antihypertensive agent, was encapsulated by the nanoprecipitation method using polymers including PCL, PLA and PLGA.

Natural polymers such as allylic starch, dextran ester can also be used; though synthetic polymers have higher purity and better reproducibility than natural polymers. Polymer modification or surface functionalization for example PEGylation can also be done in order to escape recognition from reticulo endothelial system and massive clearance. PNPs are produced by slow addition of the organic phase to the aqueous phase under moderate stirring. Reversing this order by adding the aqueous phase to the organic phase also leads to the formation of PNPs. The nanoparticles with a well-defined size are characterized by a narrow distribution formed instantaneously during the rapid diffusion of the polymer solution in the non-solvent phase. The presence of surfactant prevents agglomeration of these nanoparticles on standing by providing steric or electrostatic stabilization. The ratio of organic to aqueous phase and water solubility of the organic solvent has a strong effect on characteristics of PNPs.

The key variables determining the success of the method and affecting the physicochemical properties of PNPs include organic phase injection rate, aqueous phase agitation rate and the method of organic phase addition. Likewise, PNPs characteristics are influenced by the nature and concentration of their components for example drug to polymer ratio. Although, a surfactant is not required to ensure the formation of PNPs by nanoprecipitation, the particle size is influenced by the surfactant nature and concentration. Lince *et al.,* (2008) indicated that the process of particle formation in the nanoprecipitation method comprises three stages: nucleation, growth and aggregation. The rate of each step determines the particle size. The separation between the nucleation and the growth stages is the key factor for uniform particle formation. Ideally, operating conditions should allow a high nucleation rate so that a large number of evenly sized nanoparticles are formed. Even if growth stage cannot be retarded completely it should not fluctuate abruptly in certain areas of the suspension. Nanoprecipitation is a simple, fast and reproducible method which is widely used for the preparation of both nanospheres and nanocapsules. Till now it has been predominantly employed to entrap lipophilic drugs, with low entrapment efficiency obtained for hydrophilic drugs.

1.2.1.3 Salting-Out

The methods discussed in the previous sections require the use of organic solvents, which are hazardous to the environment as well as to physiological systems. As an alternative Ibrahim *et al.,* (1992) first developed a modified version of emulsion process that involves a salting-out process, which avoids surfactants and chlorinated solvents. The emulsion is formulated with a polymer solvent which is normally totally miscible with water, i.e., acetone, followed by emulsification of the polymer solution in the aqueous phase. This emulsification is a spontaneous no energy step and is achieved without employing any high-shear forces, by dissolving high concentration of salt or sucrose chosen for a strong salting-out effect in the aqueous phase. Magnesium chloride, calcium chloride and magnesium acetate are usually employed as the salting out agents. The miscibility properties of water with other solvents are modified as these components dissolve in the water. A reverse salting out effect, obtained by dilution of the emulsion with a large excess of water, leads to the precipitation of the polymer dissolved in the droplets of the emulsion. In fact, upon dilution, migration of the solvent for the polymer from the emulsion droplets is induced due to the reduction of the salt or sucrose concentration in the continuous phase of the emulsion (Fig. 1.5). PLA, Poly(alkylmethacrylate) (PMA) and EC have been used to produce nanoparticles in the size range of 1000 nm by the salting out method. A compilation of the polymer nanoparticles prepared by employing the salting-out method is given in (Table 1.2).

Table 1.2 Examples of polymer nanoparticles prepared by the salting-out method

Polymer	Salting-out agent	Organic solvent	Drug	Particle size (nm)	Ref.
EUDRAGIT L100-55	$MgCl_2 \cdot 6H_2O$	Acetone	Ibuprofen	174-557	Galindo-Rodriguez *et al.*, 2005
PMA	NaCl	Dilute HCl	Insulin	100-250	Fan *et al.*, 2006
PLGA	PVA	Acetone/ DCM	Dexamethasone	111.4 ± 2.3	Zhang *et al.*, 2006a
PLGA	$MgCl_2.6H_2O$	THF	Sunscreen agent	> 200	Perugini *et al.*, 2002
PLGA	PVA	Acetone/ DCM	Vincristine	60-120	Song *et al.*, 2008
PLA	PVA, $MgCl_2.6H_2O$	THF	Blank	< 200	Konan *et al.*, 2002
PLGA	PVA, $MgCl_2.6H_2O$	THF	Verteporfin	160-370	Konan-Kouakou *et al.*, 2005
DMAB* coated PLGA	$MgCl_2 \cdot 6H_2O$	DCM	Gene	180-237	Fay *et al.*, 2010
Poly (trimethylene carbonate)	PVA, $MgCl_2 \cdot 6H_2O$	THF	Dexamethasone	181 ± 1 - 214 ± 4	Zhang *et al.*, 2006b
PLGA,PEO	$MgCl_2 \cdot 6H_2O$	Acetone	-	139-250	Zweers *et al.*, 2004

*dimethyl didodecyl ammonium bromide

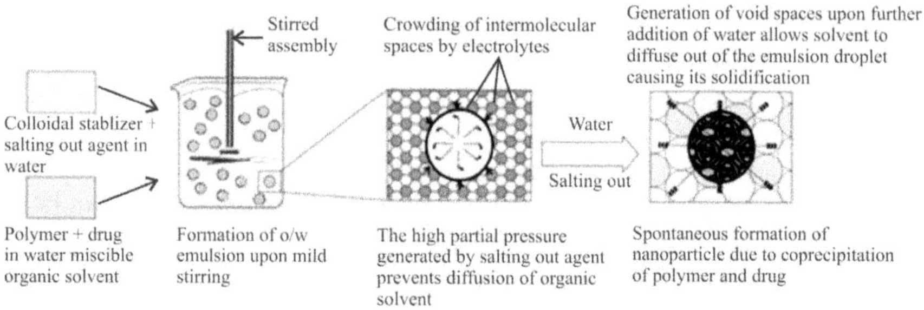

Fig. 1.5 Mechanism of salting out phenomenon in production of nanoparticles.

Salting-out procedure can be considered as a modification of the emulsification/solvent diffusion or nanoprecipitation method. Polymer and drug are initially dissolved in a solvent such as acetone, which is subsequently emulsified either spontaneously or upon mild agitation into an aqueous gel (so called due to its consistency because of high salt concentration) containing the salting-out agent and a colloidal stabilizer such as polyvinylpyrrolidone (PVP) or hydroxyethylcellulose (HEC). The system here exists in transition state as in nanoprecipitation for an extended period of time, only difference being that organic solvent cannot diffuse into bulk analogous to nanoprecipitation due to high concentration of salting out agent (Fig. 1.5). This oil/water emulsion is diluted with a sufficient volume of water or aqueous solution to enhance the diffusion of acetone into the aqueous phase, thus inducing the formation of nanospheres. The selection of the salting out agent is important, because it can play an important role in the encapsulation efficiency of the drug. Both the solvent and the salting-out agent are then eliminated by cross-flow filtration. Salting out does not require an increase of temperature and, therefore, may be useful when heat sensitive substances have to be processed. The greatest disadvantages are exclusive application to lipophilic drugs and the extensive nanoparticles washing steps.

1.2.1.4 Dialysis

Dialysis offers a simple and effective method for the preparation of small, narrow-distributed PNPs. Polymer and drug are dissolved in an organic solvent and the organic solution is placed inside a dialysis tube with proper molecular weight cut off (MWCO). Dialysis is performed against a non-solvent (for the polymer and drug); for example water which is freely miscible with the organic solvent present inside the dialysis tube (Fig. 1.6). The displacement of the solvent inside the membrane which moves towards the bulk to attain overall equilibrium is followed by the progressive aggregation of polymer due to a loss of solubility in the non-solvent and the formation of homogeneous suspensions of nanoparticles which are loaded with the drug. The mechanism of PNPs formation by dialysis method is not fully understood at present. It is thought that it may be based on a mechanism similar to that of nanoprecipitation as solvent displacement is followed by instantaneous precipitation of PNPs.

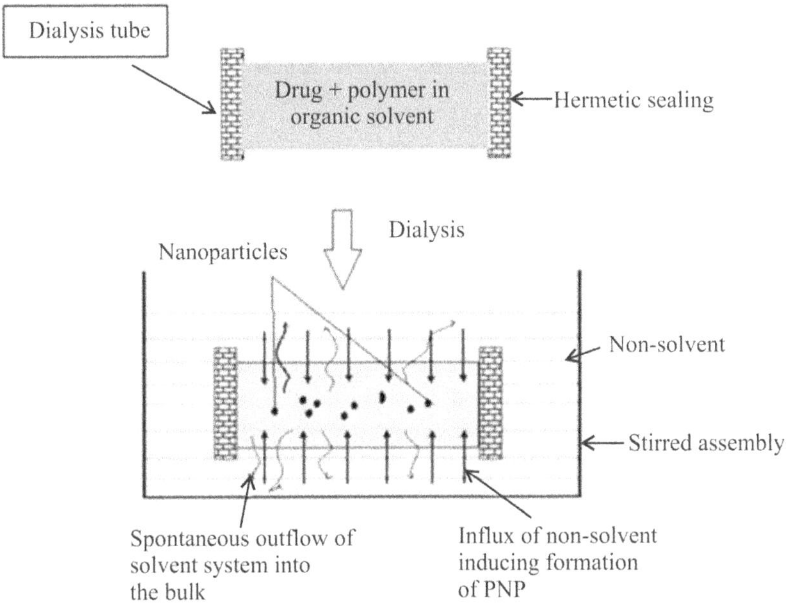

Fig. 1.6 Production of nanoparticles using dialysis method.

A number of polymer and copolymer nanoparticles have been obtained in this system. Careful selection of the lower MWCO membrane plays an important role in determining the size range of the PNPs. For example a low MWCO will exclude any loss of PNPs above that MWCO. Due to progressive dilution of solvent the washing step is simultaneously carried out. The time duration for which dialysis is carried out has a bearing on the process. Usually a period of 24 hours is sufficient to ensure complete diffusion of solvent system. Table 1.3 depicts the summary of the ingredients used and the results obtained with dialysis method.

Table 1.3 Examples of nanoparticles developed by dialysis method

Polymer	Solvent	MWCO (kg/mol)	Dialysis time (hr)	Drug	Particle size (nm)	Ref.
PBG-PEO	DMF	-	24	Norfloxacin	250-362	Jeon *et al.*, 2000b
PLGA	DMSO	12-14	48	Retionic acid	635 ± 102	Errico *et al.*, 2009
PCL-PVA	DMSO	03.5	96	Technitium^{99}	87	Park *et al.*, 2007
PLA	DMSO	15	6	HIV-1 p 24 antigen	300-600	Ataman-Önal *et al.*, 2006
PLGA	DMSO	12	24	Norfloxacin	248.9 ± 3.9	Jeon *et al.*, 2000a
PGA*	DMF	50	72	Ovalbumin	152 ± 44	Akagi *et al.*, 2005
PEG–PLGA	DMF	6-8	12	Estrogen	43.5 ± 2.3	Choi and Kim, 2007
PBG-PEO	DMF	-	24	Adriamycin	250-362	Oh *et al.*, 1999
PEG-PTMC**-PEG	DMF	-	24	Methotrexate	51.0-158.9	Zhang and Zhuo, 2005
Starch	DMSO	12	12	-	300-500	Namazi *et al.*, 2011

*Poly glutamic acid **Poly trimethylene carbonate

1.2.1.5 Ionic Gelation Method

This method utilizes the polycondensation reaction between oppositely charged cations and polyanions leading to formation of neutral particles which are insoluble in reaction media and can be separated by simple filtration methods. It is conceived that drug is also simultaneously fixated or trapped in the condensing polymeric matrix. The reaction is carried out in such a way that there is an associated loss of solubility (induced by change in pH of drug environment) of drug at the very instance this condensation reaction takes place. This method can be utilized for both hydrophilic as well as lipophilic drugs. Hydrophilic drugs are dissolved in any one of the electrolyte solutions whereas entrapment of lipophilic drug requires its dispersion in an oil emulsion or co-solublization in water miscible organic solvent. For example a solution of sodium aliginate (possessing aliginate anion) when injected drop wise into calcium chloride solution leads to cross linking of aliginate by calcium forming calcium alginate beads. This crude experiment can be suitably modulated to obtain particles of micro and nano size. There have been instances where more than one polyelectrolyte has been utilized in the same reaction to obtain reinforced nanoparticles or to impart suitable functionalization properties on the PNPs.

The ionic gelation method is principally employed for production of chitosan nanoparticles (Fig. 1.7). Chitosan nanoparticles have been developed to encapsulate proteins such as bovine serum albumin, tetanus and diphtheria toxoid, vaccines, anticancer agents, insulin and nucleic acids. Chitosan considerably enhances the absorption of peptides such as insulin and calcitonin across the nasal epithelium. Chitosan nanoparticles obtained by formation of a spontaneous complex between chitosan and polyanions such as tripolyphosphate (TPP) have small diameters (200-500 nm). The principal factors affecting characters of formed PNPs include those associated with addition of one ionic phase into other such as dropping rate, stirring rate, the viscosity of solution and also pH of the solution which dictates the state of ionization of participating polyelectrolytes and the drug.

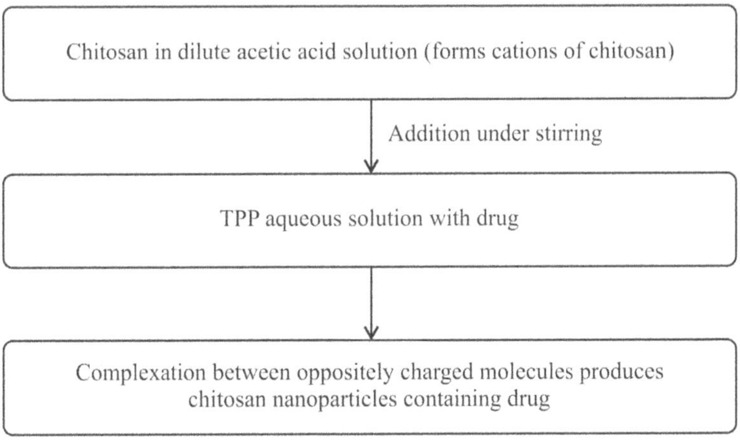

Fig. 1.7 Steps involved in ionic gelation method.

1.2.1.6 Preparation of Nanoparticles with a Membrane Contactor

Despite the numerous methods available to produce nanoparticles on a lab scale, there are still problems in establishment of large scale production methods. This is considered to be one of the major stumbling blocks in successful introduction of the nanoparticles to the clinic and the pharmaceutical market. Charcosset and Fessi (2005) have developed a method for mass production of nanoparticles using a specialized device known as membrane contactor shown in the Fig. 1.8. The organic phase is pressed through the membrane pores allowing the formation of small droplets. The reaction occurs between the droplets of the organic phase and the aqueous phase flowing tangentially to the membrane surface. Large scale industrial pumps, membrane contactor and automated process control can be employed to obtain massive yields with fairly uniform properties.

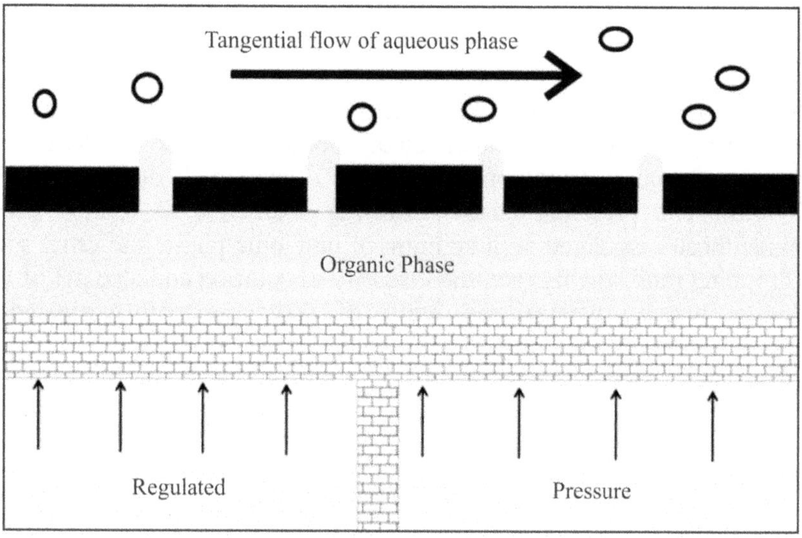

Fig. 1.8 Membrane reactor assembly.

This process may be compared to the membrane emulsification or the dialysis process, where the oil (or the water phase) permeates through the membrane pores to form droplets in water (or oil phase) for the preparation of O/W or W/O emulsions, respectively. The tangentially flowing aqueous phase sweeps along the formed nanostructures and is collected in a compartment where nanoparticles can be washed, purified and collected. The two main parameters of the process are the aqueous phase cross-flow velocity and the organic phase pressure. Another advantage of this membrane reactor is its versatility for the preparation of either nanocapsules or nanospheres, by methods involving a polymerization of dispersed monomers or a dispersion of preformed polymers, and the control of the average nanoparticles size by an appropriate choice of the membrane.

1.2.1.7 New Techniques based on Supercritical or Compressed Fluids

Some of the techniques described above are complex, and the products may often be characterized by high residual solvent content, low drug loading, drug degradation or denaturation, ineffective drug release, or unsuitable physical properties. Techniques based on supercritical or compressed fluid have come up as suitable alternatives which have huge potential to be exploited industrially. Supercritical fluid is any substance at a temperature and pressure above its critical point, where distinct liquid and gas phases do not exist. It can diffuse through solids like a gas, and dissolve materials like a liquid. In addition, close to the critical point, small changes in pressure or temperature results in large changes in density, allowing many properties of a supercritical fluid to be fabricated as per requirement. Supercritical fluids are suitable as a substitute for organic solvents in a range of industrial and laboratory processes. Carbon dioxide and water are the most commonly used supercritical fluids. Supercritical fluids provide a number of ways of achieving this by rapidly exceeding the saturation point of a solute by dilution, depressurization or a combination of these. These processes occur faster in supercritical fluids than in liquids, promoting nucleation over crystal growth and yielding very small and regularly sized particles.

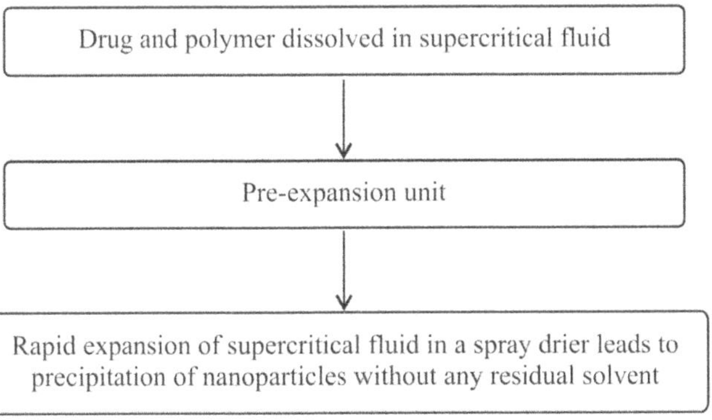

Fig. 1.9 Flowchart illustrating the basic steps in supercritical fluid expansion producing nanoparticles.

Recent supercritical fluids have shown the capability to reduce particles up to a range of 5-2000 nm. In this technique, the drug and the polymer are solubilized in a supercritical fluid and the solution is expanded through a nozzle either into ambient air or an aqueous non solvent system with additional colloidal stabilizers (Fig. 1.9). The supercritical fluid is evaporated in the spraying process, and the solute particles eventually precipitate. The polymer concentration in the pre-expansion supercritical solution plays a vital role in determining the product morphology. This technique is clean, because the precipitated solute is free of solvent. It also provides advantages such as suitable technological and biopharmaceutical properties and high quality. It has been demonstrated for numerous applications involving protein drug delivery systems. Protein drugs such as insulin (Elvassore *et al.,* 2001) has been encapsulated in (PEG/PLA) nanoparticles by this technique. Other drugs whose nanoparticles have been prepared using this technique include Coenzyme Q-10, curcumin, fluorouracil, atorvastatin, methotrexate, etc. However, this new process requires a high initial capital investment for equipment, and elevated operating pressures requiring high pressure equipment. In addition, compressed supercritical fluids require elaborate recycling measures to reduce energy costs. Finally, it is very difficult to dissolve strong polar substances in supercritical CO_2. In fact, supercritical CO_2 has solvating properties characteristic of both fluorocarbons and hydrocarbons. However, the use of co-solvents and/or surfactants to form microemulsions makes it possible to dissolve polar and ionic species.

1.2.2 Polymerization of Monomers

The techniques discussed previously involve the production of PNPs from preformed polymers and did not involve any polymerization processes. To attain the desired properties for a particular application, suitable polymer nanoparticles must be designed, which can be done during the polymerization of monomers. The point here is that sometimes the properties of preformed polymers are too robust to be modified or manipulated; consequently they do not yield PNPs suited for the desired purpose. In this particular process polymerization starts from a monomer and can be processed to obtain the properties as per our requirements. Additionally, the advantage of obtaining nanoparticles by this method is that the polymer is formed *in situ,* allowing the polymer membrane to follow the contours of the inner phase of an oil/water or water/oil emulsion. But like every coin there is a flip side to this technique as well, wherein batch to batch reproducibility in the polymerization process is a difficult task. The polymer so synthesized can be difficult to characterize sometimes, and in these conditions, using commercially standardized preformed polymers is a better option.

1.2.2.1 Emulsion Polymerization

Emulsion polymerization is the most common method used for the production of a wide range of polymers which in turn form PNPs. Emulsion polymerization is one of the fastest methods for nanoparticles preparation and is readily scalable. In the conventional system, the ingredients like any polymerization reaction consists of a monomer of low water solubility, water-soluble initiator along with added drug molecule, surfactant and the most suited reaction media water. At the end of these actions, PNPs are typically nanosized, each containing many polymer chains which entangle amongst each other encapsulating the drug. The procedure is visualized in Fig. 1.10. As is evident from figure the small emulsion droplets formed initially on dispersion of oil phase into water function as minute nanoreactors and it is inside these the basic polymerization reaction takes place. So the sizes of nanoreactors directly determine the particle size of the eventual PNPs formed. The surfactant molecule ensures that the nanoreactor assemblies do not coalesce whilst the reaction is still taking place or before the oil droplets have hardened into PNPs. Colloidal stabilizers may be electrostatic, steric or electrosteric, displaying both stabilizing mechanisms. Initiation occurs when a monomer molecule dissolved in the aqueous phase collides with an initiator molecule. The monomer might also function as an auto initiator, when induced by photostimulation or λ-radiation, colliding with further monomer molecules carrying on the polymerization to its completion. Phase separation and formation of solid particles can take place before or after the termination of the polymerization reaction as shown in the figure. Polystyrene (PS), poly(methylmethacrylate) (PMMA), poly(vinyl-carbazole), poly(ethylcyanoacrylate) (PECA) and poly(butylcyanoacrylate) nanoparticles have been produced by dispersion *via* surfactants into solvents, such as cyclohexane, n-pentane, and toluene. These polymers have been used to entrap variety of drugs for example doxorubicin, ampicillin, dexamethasone, triamcinolone, insulin, vinblastine, etc.

Conventional emulsion polymerization systems require surfactants that need to be eliminated from the final product. But even after sustained efforts their complete removal cannot be guaranteed. In order to circumvent this drawback emulsion polymerization has been performed in the absence of any added emulsifier. The reagents used in an emulsifier free system include deionized water, a water-soluble initiator (i.e., KPS, potassium persulfate) and monomers, more commonly vinyl or acryl monomers. In such polymerization systems, stabilization of PNPs occurs through the use of ionizable initiators or ionic co-monomers. In such

PNPs the initiator molecule preferentially deposits on the surface and prevents agglomeration due to electrostatic repulsion.

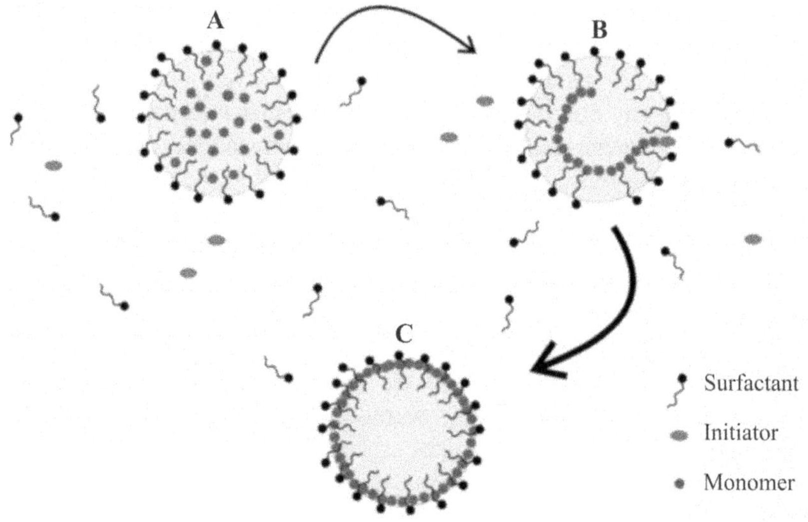

Fig. 1.10 Basic steps taking place in emulsion polymerization ultimately leading to formation of PNPs. A: Oil droplet with solubilized drug and monomer, dispersed randomly in aqueous phase consisting of surfactant and water. B: The initiator makes contact with monomer at oil-water interface to initiate polymerization reaction. C: Polymerization continues until a solid interfacial polymeric film is deposited, containing trapped drug.

1.3 Nanocrystals

The number of poorly soluble drugs is constantly on an upswing. With the pharmaceutical industry having already exhausted most of the simple molecules as potential drug candidates it has to look into complex bulky structures which are usually poorly water soluble and consequently have a very low bioavailability. The oral route is the most preferred for administration of drugs. However poor aqueous solubility of drugs with consequent low bioavailability makes oral administration unviable. The need of the hour requires the pharmaceutical scientist to work around these severe limitations and come up with ideas to overcome the low bioavailability of these new drug candidates as well as other existing BCS class II and class IV drugs.

Solubility is the property of a solid, liquid, or gaseous chemical substance called solute to dissolve in a solid, liquid, or gaseous solvent to form a homogeneous solution of the solute in the solvent. The solubility of a substance fundamentally depends on the used solvent as well as on temperature and pressure. The extent of the solubility of a substance in a specific solvent is measured as the saturation solubility at that defined condition of temperature and pressure, where adding more solute does not increase the concentration of the solution. Solubility of a drug substance in water tends to dictate its bioavailability as drugs are available for absorption in systemic circulation only in solution form. Therefore any method which increases the solubility of drug substance will tend to increase its bioavailability.

One such universal approach to enhance the solubility and in turn the bioavailability of drugs is reduction of particle size such as micronization. Reduction in particle size increases the surface area exponentially, yielding higher dissolution rates according to Noyes-Whitney's equation. This technique has worked well for a few drugs such as griseofulvin whose bioavailability has been considerably enhanced, but has failed on most other drugs which are either more poorly water soluble or are very hydrophobic. The next obvious step to enhance the solubility of these insoluble drugs is to further reduce the particle size so as to move from micronization to nanoniztion of drug powder. Below a certain critical size, around 1 μm, saturation solubility becomes dependent on particle size, i.e., smaller particles have a higher solubility than larger ones. Such a state when the particle size of the drug powder is reduced to nanometer scale that is below 1000 nm, it is said to have assumed a nanocrystal structure. Thus nanocrystals are nanoparticles of drug molecules in crystalline form without any associated coating or dispersion of any form. They are composed totally of drug and do not possess any carrier moiety such as polymeric matrix or lipoidal structure.

Dispersion of nanocrystals in liquid media yields nanosuspension. Generally nanosuspensions need to be stabilized by surfactants, colloidal stabilizers or viscosity enhancers, so as to prevent any flocculation, clumping, gradual coalescence, particle size growth and ultimately phase separation. The dispersion media could be aqueous, or non-aqueous such as low viscosity poly-ethylene glycol. The nanocrystals display properties in between those of crystals and amorphous structures. They have higher solubility compared to their crystalline counterparts but also show extended stability which is non-existent in their amorphous analogues, amalgamating advantages of the two states.

1.3.1 Approaches to Formulating Nanocrystals

Nanocrystals can be obtained directly through 'bottom up' by modified crystallization/antisolvent precipitation or indirectly 'top down' by mechanical breakage/attrition of a crystalline powder. The production of nanosized particle by direct crystallization/precipitation can be carried out using extreme super saturation conditions in order to favor nucleation over growth. The stability upon agglomeration during rapid crystallization needs to be assessed for developmental feasibility. Another way to generate nanocrystals is to limit the amount of material available for crystallization by reducing the working volume. Microfluidics set-up or emulsion crystallization can be the method of choice to generate microcrystalline material, but the scalability and the energy input is a major limiting factor.

1.3.1.1 Precipitation Method

The intellectual property of this technique is owned by pharmaceutical giant Novartis. It is basically similar to the classical nanoprecipitation method utilizing solvent non-solvent interaction. The drug is dissolved in a solvent and the solution is poured into a non-solvent system for the drug but having affinity for the drug solvent. The solvent immediately diffuses throughout the non-solvent system leaving back minute nanoprecipitates of drug.

Problem arises in maintaining the particle size in nano range and preventing further aggregation. This requires introduction of a suitable steric, electronic or colloidal stabilizer. Viscosity enhancing agent can also be used which impedes any sedimentation or brownian motion of suspended nanocrystals and reduces the probability of particle-particle contact which can bring about growth. Additionally drug should be soluble in some solvent which in turn should have affinity for a non-solvent for drug. The probability of these conditions happening together is extremely low for modern day drugs which have solubility issues both in aqueous and non-aqueous media.

1.3.1.2 Homogenization Method

1.3.1.2.1 Drug Nanocrystals Produced by High-Pressure Homogenization

The Microfluidizer (Microfluidics^{TM} Inc., U.S.A.) is based on the jet-stream principle (Fig. 1.11); seen in regular fluid energy mills. Two streams of liquid collide, diminution of droplets or crystals is achieved mainly by particle collision, but occurrence of cavitation is also considered.

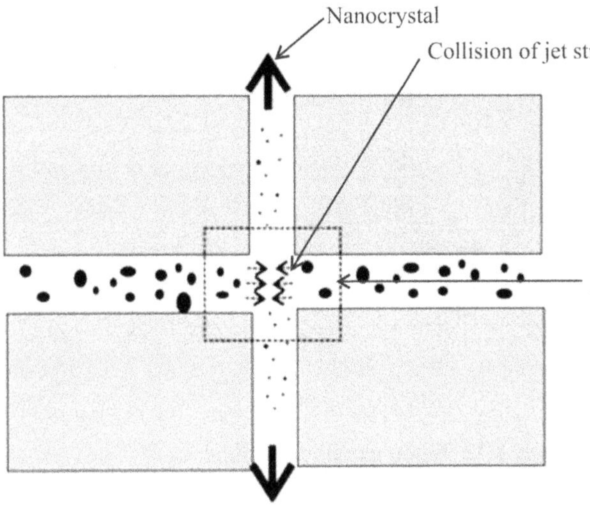

Fig. 1.11 Jet stream homogenization

Typical pressures for the production of drug nanosuspensions are 1000-1500 bar (corresponding to 100-150 Mpa, 14504-21756 psi); the number of required homogenization cycles varies from 10 to 20 depending on the properties of the drug i.e., its crystal strength. Sometimes upto 100 cycles might be required to induce desired particle size reduction. The particles breakdown due to high energy of impaction which also dissipates in form of heat requires cooling. The heating problem is also reduced to some extent by using water as the dispersion medium. The biggest advantage of this highly efficient process apart from scalability is zero contamination of feed material as the reduction is being effected by the particles themselves.

1.3.1.2.2 Piston Gap Homogenizer

The piston gap homogenizers work on the principle of colloid mills. The drug is made to pass through a narrow gap (of dimension less than 10 μm) between a fixed stator and a rapidly moving rotor. Size reduction is caused due to high shear, stress and grinding forces generated between rotor and stator. The upper ceiling of particle size can be ascertained by fixing the dissipation gap to required size. This means that yield will not be obtained unless and until the particles are ground down to a size which is equal or lower to that of the gap between rotor and stator. A basic visualization is displayed in Fig. 1.12.

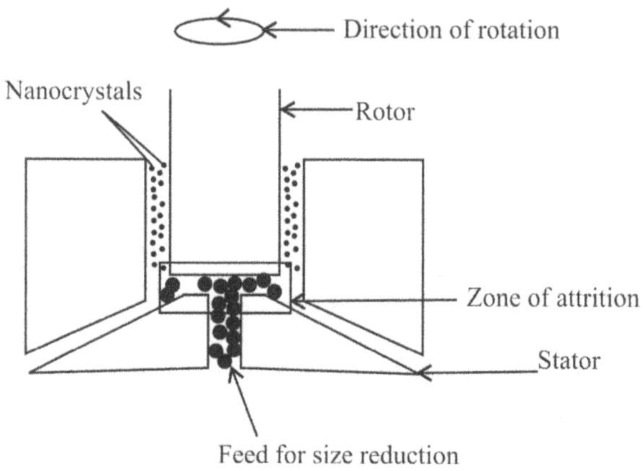

Fig. 1.12 Piston gap homogenizer.

1.3.1.3 Pearl/Ball-Milling Technology for the Production of Drug Nanocrystals

These mills consist of a milling container filled with fine milling pearls or larger-sized balls. The container can be static and the milling material is moved by a stirrer; alternatively, the complete container is moved in a complex movement leading to movement of the milling pearls. The basic difference between a ball and a pearl mill is related to the size of the grinding material, larger in case of ball mill. The principle of size reduction is combined impact and attrition. Since there are more dead spaces in a ball mill, the particle size distribution is broader. There are different milling materials available, traditionally steel, glass, and zircon oxide are used. New materials are special polymers, i.e., hard polystyrene. A problem associated with the pearl milling technology is the erosion from the milling material during the milling process introducing a chance of contamination. Apart from the milling material, the erosion from the container also needs to be considered. These factors play an important role in selection of milling material and type of mill. Normally, product containers are made of steel and can be covered with various materials to fulfill the required quality specifications of the formulation. Surfactants or stabilizers have to be added for the physical stability of the produced nanosuspensions. In the production process the coarse drug powder is dispersed by high-speed stirring in a surfactant/stabilizer solution to yield a macrosuspension which then is subjected to milling operations.

1.3.1.4 Production of Drug Nanocrystal Compounds by Spray-Drying

Spray drying is an excellent technique which has industrial feasibility. Starting from an aqueous macrosuspension containing the original coarse drug powder, surfactant, and water-soluble excipient, the homogenization process can be performed in an easy one step yielding a fine aqueous nanosuspension. In a subsequent step the water has to be removed from the suspension to obtain a dry powder. One method of removing the water from the formulation is freeze drying, but it is complex and cost-intensive leading to increase in the cost of the product. An alternative method for the industrial production is spray drying. The drug nanosuspension can directly be produced by high-pressure homogenization in aqueous solutions of water-soluble matrix materials, e.g., polymers [PVP, PVA or long chained PEG, sugars (saccharose, lactose), or sugar alcohols (mannitol, sorbitol)]. Afterward the aqueous drug nanosuspension can be spray dried under adequate conditions; the resulting dry powder is composed of drug nanocrystals embedded in a water-soluble matrix of drug nanocrystal-loaded spray-dried compounds.

1.4 Nanocapsules

Theoretically, polymeric nanocapsules are vesicular particles smaller than 1 μm composed of an oily core surrounded by an ultrathin polymeric wall. These devices are stabilized by surfactants and/or steric agents (Fig. 1.13).

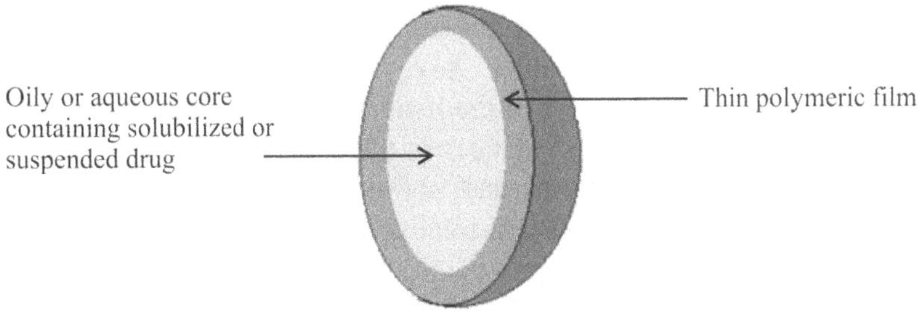

Fig. 1.13 Cross section of a polymeric nanocapsule

The structure differs from a nanoparticle or nanosphere in the way represented in Fig. 1.14. Nanospheres are matrix systems in which the drug is dispersed within the polymeric network throughout the particle. Contrarily, nanocapsules are vesicular or "reservoir" (heterogeneous) systems, in which the drug is essentially confined to a cavity surrounded by a tiny polymeric membrane. The most advantageous feature of developing a nanocapsule has been the high payload or entrapment efficiency especially for lipophilic drug obtained in these systems expending extremely low polymer content, when compared to nanoparticles.

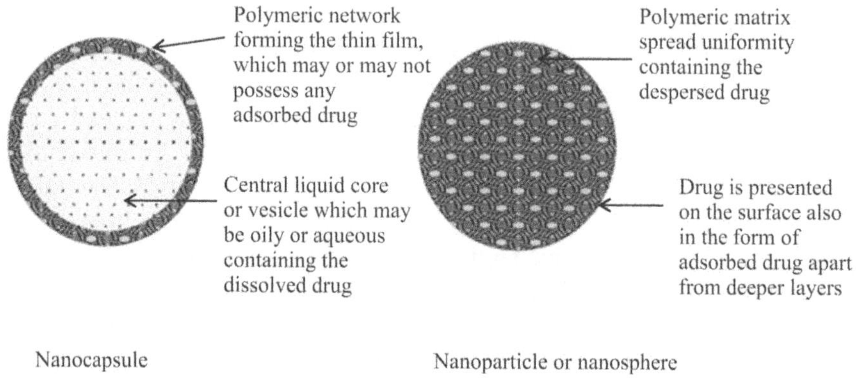

Fig. 1.14 Basic difference between a nanoparticle and nanocapsule.

The chances of burst effect are reduced since there is little or no surface adsorbed drug. Moreover any irritation reaction produced by drug at the site of administration is also absent due to avoidance of direct contact.

As far as formulation of nanocapsules is concerned, it is composed of polymer which forms the film, a solubilizing material such as oil, water or an organic solvent along with drug, a dispersion media (might be aqueous or non-aqueous) and stabilizer to prevent capsule growth. In general, polymeric nanocapsules have an oily core composed of triglycerides, the liquid active ingredient and, in addition, some cases have a mixture of chemical substances as the core, such as capric/caprylic triglycerides or vegetable oils and sorbitan monostearate. The basic strategies of production remain similar to that of nanoparticles, due to structural similarity, the only prerequisite being the hardening of the thin polymeric film, and the utilization of a solvent to dissolve the drug. The polymer utilized to encapsulate should not have any tendency to dissolve into the core solvent.

Nanocapsules can either be obtained by interfacial polymerization of monomers or from preformed polymers. In the former, the molar mass of the coating polymer will depend on the preparation conditions and even on the drug used, whereas in the later, it is determined at the outset.

Polymerization of monomers may lead to a covalent linkage between the polymer and the drug. To date, all the methodologies described for preparing nanocapsules involve the preparation of emulsions. (O/W) emulsions lead to the formation of nanocapsules with an oily core, suspended in water whereas (W/O) emulsions lead to nanocapsules with an aqueous core, suspended in oil.

1.4.1 Preparation

1.4.1.1 Nanocapsules Formulation by Interfacial Polymerization

The technique of obtaining nanocapsules by interfacial polymerization allows the polymer membrane to follow the contours of the internal phase of an O/W or W/O emulsion, minimizing drug escape by ensuring proper trapping, although there is always a slight chance of drug also undergoing some sort of chemical transformation. For a polymerization reaction to qualify as a fabrication tool for nanocapsules, it should be rapid and proceed preferentially along the interface. Alkylcyanoacrylates are excellent candidates for undergoing rapid polymerization within seconds, and have consequently been heavily utilized for the preparation of both oil- and water-containing nanocapsules.

1.4.1.1.1 Oil-Containing Nanocapsules

Nanocapsules which harbor oil in their core are adept at encapsulating lipophilic drugs. Most routine method of fabrication is interfacial polymerization of alkylcyanoacrylates. Initially O/W emulsion is prepared in an aqueous solution supplemented with ethanol/acetone and surfactant. Ethanol/acetone is necessary to disperse oil droplets uniformly in the aqueous phase. To initiate polymerization specific initiator, viz. ion or free radical is added to water. In typical method (Fig. 1.15) oil, monomer, and drug are dissolved to form a homogenous organic phase. Organic phase is then injected into aqueous phase under stirring. After formation of nanocapsules the residual organic phase is removed under reduced pressure. The excipient profile of nanocapsules, includes vegetable, mineral oils and derived compounds such as ethyl oleate and benzyl benzoate, Miglyol®, Lipiodol® (al Khouri *et al.,* 1986), benzyl benzoate Poloxamers, Triton X-100 and Tween 80. The only drawback of his method is that, simultaneous formation of small amount of nanospheres cannot be precluded. Solvents such as acetone, ethanol, n-butanol and acetonitrile lead to high-quality nanocapsule formation.

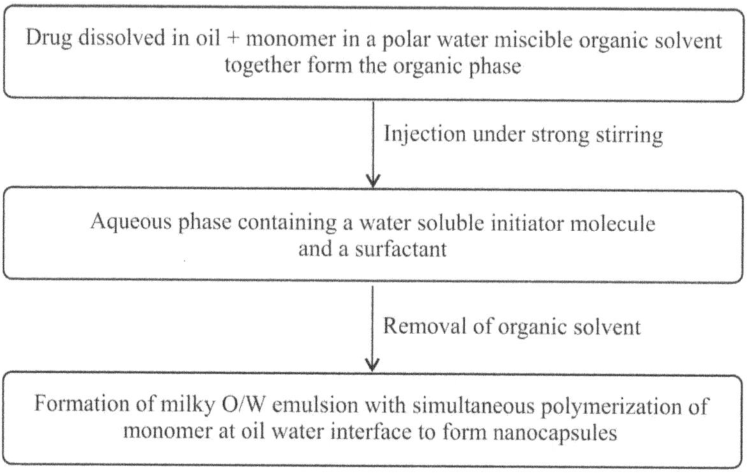

Fig. 1.15 General sequence of steps leading up to formation of oil containing nanocapsules.

1.4.1.1.2 Nanocapsules Containing an Aqueous Core

Considering the mechanism of nanocapsule formation explained above, it is difficult to comprehend the inclusion of water soluble compounds, like proteins, peptides within nanocapsules. Yet water soluble compounds have been captured in aqueous core. Interfacial polymerization, is the predominant pathway here too and the alkylcyanoacrylates monomers are added to external phase of a W/O emulsion. Polymerization of the monomer in the oily phase is initiated at the interface by initiators such as hydroxyl ions in the aqueous phase, leading to the formation of nanocapsules with an aqueous core. In a sample procedure, an aqueous phase consisting of ethanol and water is prepared. This solution is emulsified in an organic phase made up of Miglyol® or Montane® 80. Following this the monomer is slowly added to the external medium under stirring, leading to formation of aqueous nanocapsules. These nanocapsules are very useful for the encapsulation of hydrophilic compounds such as oligonucleotides and peptides. A basic illustration of the steps involved in formation of these nanocapsules is depicted in Fig. 1.16.

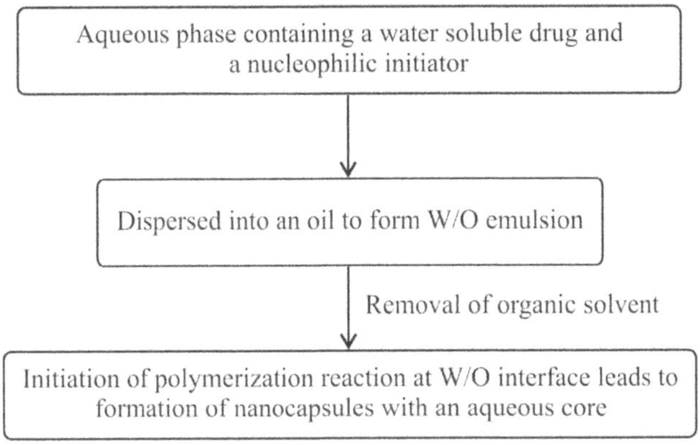

Fig. 1.16 Steps leading up to formation of aqueous core containing nanocapsules.

1.4.1.2 Nanocapsules Obtained from Preformed Polymers

Nanocapsules from preformed polymers are preferred in cases where the batch to batch variability of, interfacial polymerization is a cause of concern. The lack of control on polymeric mass, non-uniformity of size distribution and presence of trace amount of residual monomers all drawbacks, which can be circumvented by using pre formed polymers with standardized physic-chemical properties. Polymers are usually in soluble in both oil and water and consequently require an organic solvent to undergo solubilization in oil phase. Once formed this homogenous organic phase is added to aqueous phase. Due to the tremendous amount of turbulent forces generated, by the fluctuation in surface free energy of the system, the polymer diffuses with organic solvent towards the aqueous phase, only to be precipitated at the interface of oil and water. This leads to surrounding of oil phase with polymeric shell, forming a nanocapsule. If the organic solvent is not soluble in water as is the case with dichloromethane, an emulsion is formed upon stirring, in which the solvent droplets are distributed throughout the aqueous media. In such cases evaporation of the organic solvent under reduced pressure or otherwise is responsible for precipitation of polymer around the oily core. The basic outline of nanocapsule formation is described in Fig. 1.17. Synthetic polymers such as PLA, PLGA, PCL and poly (alkylcyano-acrylate) are most frequently employed. The size of nanocapsules is usually found between 100 and 500 nm, and depends on several factors, namely, the chemical nature and the concentration of the polymer and the encapsulated drug, the amount of surfactants, the ratio of organic solvent to water, the concentration of oil in the organic solution, and the speed of diffusion of the organic phase in the aqueous phase.

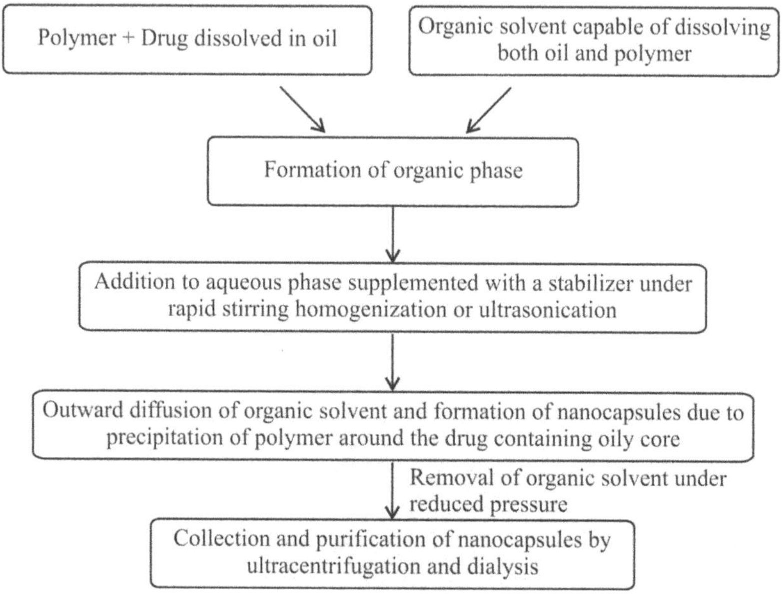

Fig. 1.17 Basic steps involved in formation of nanocapsules from preformed polymer.

1.5 Nanofibers

Nanofibers are porous polymeric thread like structures, entangled with each other, each individual fiber having a diameter in the range of 2 nm to several micrometers. These are classified as fibers due to their structural similarity to the fibrous structures such as silk found naturally or those synthesized, only difference being the size. The special nanometric size of these fibers accords them several specialized properties non-existent in their parent materials normally. Nanofibers have a very large surface-area-to-volume ratio, as large as 1000 times that of a microfiber. High porosity, interconnectivity, micro scale interstitial space, and a high aspect ratio means that nanofiber meshes are an excellent material for biomembrane replication, especially in biotechnology and environmental engineering applications. Nanofibers can form an effective size exclusion membrane for particulate removal from waste water.

Nanofibers can entrap drugs both within their polymeric structures and within the minute interstitial spaces due to surface adsorption or drug locking. The drug so dispersed in the nanofibrous structure is consequently even smaller in size, and becomes faster dissolving. The dispersion of drug in the nanomeric fibers controls drug release like all polymeric network structures either by producing a rate controlling barrier, or by providing a tortuous pathway, limiting entry and exit of dissolving media. Polymers which hydrate or swell but are insoluble can also be used to create sustained-release nanofibers. Xiao-Mei Wu *et al.,* (2011) prepared core-shell PAN nanofibers encapsulated α-tocopherol acetate and ascorbic acid 2-phosphate for photoprotection. The results showed that core-shell nanofibers alleviated the initial burst release and gave better sustainability. Maedeh Zamani *et al.,* (2010) have developed biodegradable PCL nanofibers of metronidazole benzoate for treatment of periodontal infections prolonging drug release upto 19 days. These examples just elucidate the capability of nanofibres to modulate release rate of trapped drug as per requirement.

Dissolution rate can be accelerated by dispersing the drug in a nanofiber made out of water soluble polymer such as polyethylene glycol. The fiber instantaneously dissolves when in contact with water leaving behind nanomerized drug subject to rapid dissolution as in case of nanocrystals. Fibers have high encapsulation efficiency as there is no loss during the preparation. Nanofibres could pave the way for the development of a 'smart' polymeric drug delivery system. For example, a drug-loaded, pH-sensitive polymer is targeted to diseased cells through cell receptor binding of a ligand. It is subsequently endocytosed. In the low pH environment of the endosome, the polymer backbone detaches from the drug, disrupting the endosomal membrane, and releases the drug into the cytoplasmic compartment of the cells. One of the outstanding features of nanofibers is that they mimic the extracellular matrix developed by variety of proteins present in the human body to such an extent that they even stimulate cell proliferation when placed inside the body. This proves to be doorstep of huge possibilities of utilizing nanofibers in field of organ-transplant, tissue regeneration and bone reconstruction.

1.5.1 Polymers used for Development of Nanofibers

There are a wide range of polymers that are used in electrospinning and are able to form fine nanofibers within the submicron range. Nanofibers can be prepared from various materials including synthetic polymers, natural polymers or a blend including proteins, nucleic acids and even polysaccharides. Typical natural polymers include collagen, chitosan, gelatin, casein, cellulose acetate, silk protein, chitin and fibrinogen. Scaffolds fabricated from natural polymers promise better clinical functionality. Over the years, more than 200 polymers have been used. Enteric-release nanofibers can be created by enteric polymers such as methacrylic acid copolymers, and sustained-release nanofibers can be created by PLA, PLGA or any other suitable polymers. Currently, there are three techniques available for the synthesis of nanofibers: electrospinning, self-assembly, and phase separation and out of these, electrospinning is the most widely studied technique.

1.5.2 Electrospinning

Electrospinning, an electrostatic fiber fabrication technique is most popular technique used for development of nanofibers. Electrospinning uses an electrical charge to draw very fine (typically on the micro or nano scale) fibres from a liquid. Electrospinning from molten precursors is also practised; this method ensures that no solvent can be carried over into the final product. Currently, there are two standard electrospinning setups, vertical and horizontal. Electrospinning is conducted at room temperature with atmosphere conditions. The typical set up of electrospinning apparatus is shown in Fig. 1.18. Basically, an electrospinning system consists of three major components: a high voltage power supply, an injector (usually a hypodermic syringe) and a grounded collector and utilizes a high voltage source to inject charge of a certain polarity into a polymer solution or melt, which is then accelerated towards a collector of opposite polarity. Most of the polymers are dissolved in some solvents before electrospinning, and when it completely dissolves, forms polymer solution. The polymer fluid is then introduced into the capillary tube for electrospinning.

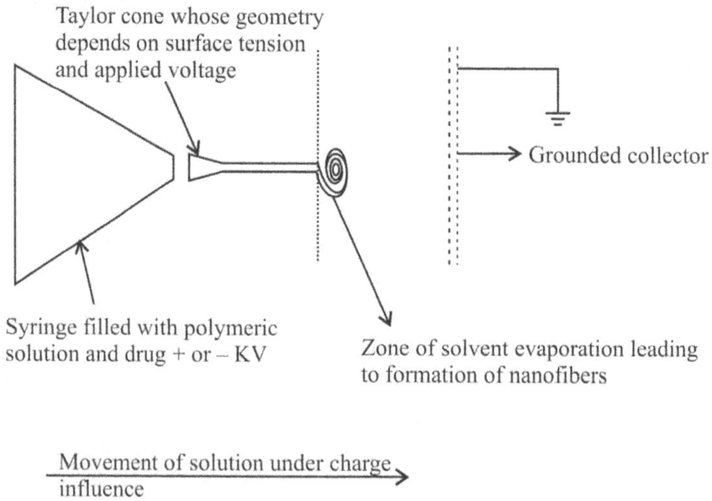

Fig. 1.18 Horizontal set up of electrospinning apparatus.

When a sufficiently high voltage is applied to a liquid droplet, the body of the liquid becomes charged. This charge creates an electrostatic repulsion within the solution which starts opposing the surface tension acting on the liquid and consequently causes surface disruptions and stretching of the polymeric solution; at a critical voltage, stream of liquid erupts from the surface. This point of eruption is known as the Taylor cone as the shape acquired by the liquid is that of a cone. If the molecular cohesion of the liquid is sufficiently high, stream does not breakup into tiny droplets (if it does, droplets are said to be electrosprayed instead of electrospinning) and a charged liquid jet is formed. As the jet of polymeric solution dries in flight due to evaporation of volatile solvent it is also elongated by a whipping process caused by electrostatic repulsion initiated at small bends in the fiber, until it is finally deposited on the grounded collector. Elongation of the fiber resulting from this bending instability leads to the formation of uniform fibers with nanometer-scale diameters. A stable jet is formed when the charge is increased above a critical voltage, and there is a balance between the surface tension of the fluid and the repulsive nature of the charge. The presence of molecular entanglements in the polymer solution prevents the jet from breaking into droplets. When more volatile solvents are used, solvent-rich regions begin to form during electrospinning that transform into pores (Bognitzki *et al.,* 2001). Drugs which are not thermolabile can be directly woven into fibers by employing polymeric melts. This avoids use of any organic solvents, which are always a concern. The electrospinning process is affected by many parameters, classified roughly into solution parameters, process parameters, and ambient parameters. Solution parameters include concentration, viscosity, conductivity, molecular weight, and surface tension, process parameters include applied electric field, tip to collector distance and feeding or flow rate. Orifice diameter, flow rate of polymer, and electric potential are influences fiber diameter. Process parameters such as distance between capillary and metal collector determine the extent of evaporation of solvent from the nanofibers, and deposition on the collector, whereas motion of collector determines the pattern formation during fiber deposition. The above stated parameters thus affect the fibers morphology obtained as a result of electrospinning, and by proper manipulation of these parameters we can get nanofibers of desired morphology and diameters (Chong *et al.,* 2007). In addition to these variables, working parameters such as the humidity and temperature of the surroundings also play a significant role in determining the morphology and diameter of electrospun nanofibers (Li and Xia, 2004).

1.5.3 Spontaneous Assembly

It is also known as molecular assembly. It is the spontaneous organization of individual molecules into structurally-defined stable arrangements through preprogrammed non-covalent interactions, such as hydrogen bonds, van der Waals forces, hydrophobic interactions, London forces, dipole-dipole interaction, dipole induced dipole interaction and other electrostatic interactions. Self-assembly is a bottom up technique utilizing small building blocks such as peptides, small chain amino acids, polymeric segments and even monomers. A special class of compounds known as polymeric amphiphiles have been utilized in fabrication of nanofibers used to mimic bioactive structures such as collagen. In such cases the lipophilic tail much like as in micelles undergo spontaneous association (Fig. 1.19) due to hydrophobic bonding. The association is brought about by a triggering stimulus such as pH change, temperature fluctuation, introduction of a catalyst, or a bivalent cation such as calcium which neutralize the electrostatic repulsion between molecules to allow clustering of the hydrophobic tails in the core.

Under similar principles, synthetic diblock/triblock polypeptides and dendrimers can also self-assemble into nanofibrous structures. Ionic self-complementary oligopeptides (consisting of repeating ionic hydrophilic and hydrophobic amino acids) can also serve as building blocks to self-assemble into nanofibers.

The advantages of self-assembly for nanofiber fabrication include the simple fabrication process and easy drug encapsulation. It also paves the way for development of injectable form of nanofibers which undergo *in situ* scaffold formation in response to a triggering stimulus like temperature fluctuation, pH change, etc. Although the mechanical properties of nanofibers formed by self-assembly can be adjusted to some extent, they are often insufficient to provide a stable structure. There are also other shortcomings such as the limited choice of self-assembly molecules.

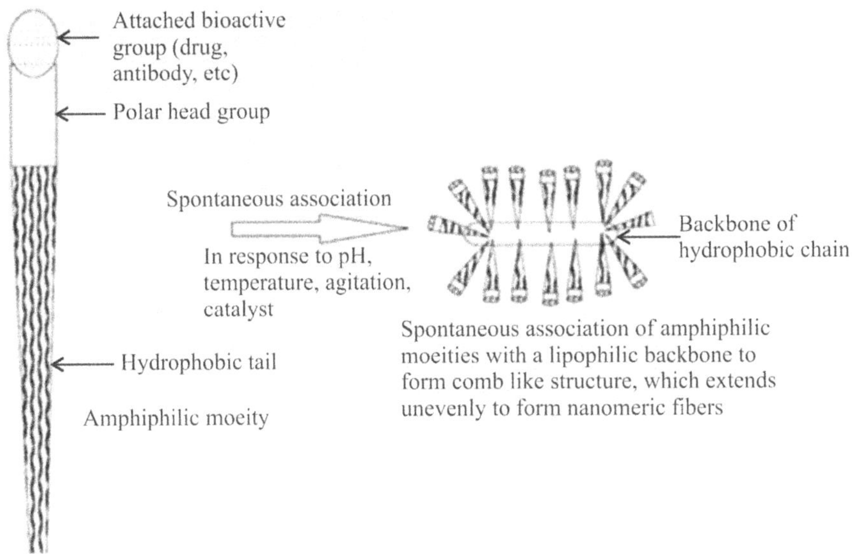

Fig. 1.19 Self-assembly for fabrication of nanomeric fibers.

1.5.4 Temperature Induced Phase Separation

In order to mimic the structure of collagen present in natural extra cellular matrix, developed a new technique called thermally induced liquid-liquid phase separation for the formation of nanofibrous foam materials has been developed (Ma and Zhang, 1999). Nano-fibrous matrices are prepared from the polymer solutions (such as PLA, PCL & PLGA) by a procedure involving thermally induced gelation, solvent exchange, and freeze-drying.The five basic steps of this method include:

1. Dissolution of polymer.
2. Liquid-liquid phase separation.
3. Polymer gelation (controls the porosity of nanoscale scaffolds at low temperature).
4. Extraction of solvent from the gel with water.
5. Freezing and freeze-drying under vacuum.

Gelation is the most critical step that controls the porous morphology of the nanofibrous foams. Other steps that can control the outcome include operating parameters such as duration and temperature of cooling, each and every step involved in process of freeze drying, etc. The duration of gelation varies with polymer concentration, solvent behaviour, gelation temperature and nature of drug molecule. The procedure needs to be evaluated carefully since the system has to undergo freeze drying, which leads to very sensitive products and raises the operating cost aswell. A typical procedure is depicted in Fig. 1.20.

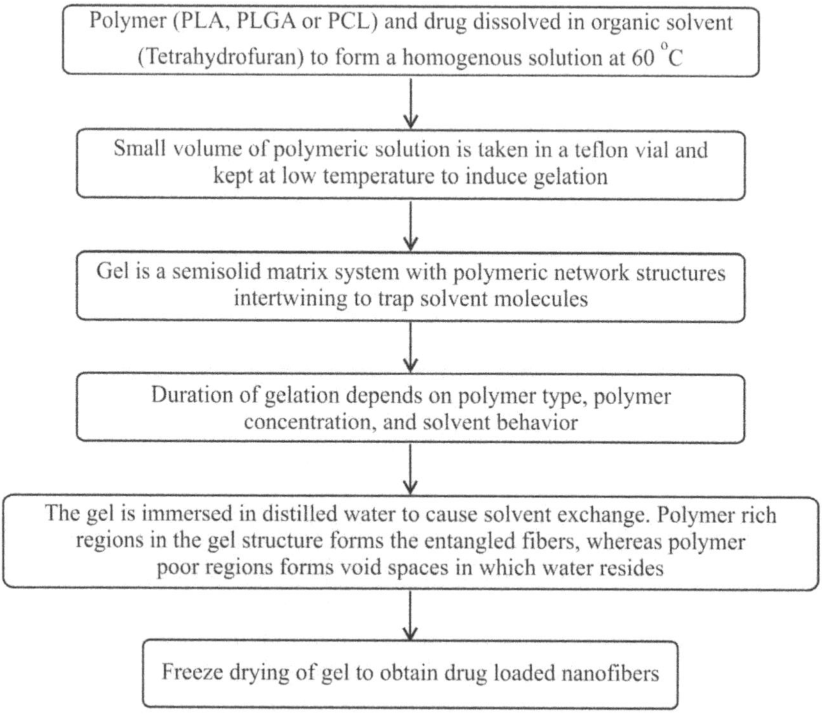

Fig. 1.20 Temperature induced phase separation/gelation causes formation of nanofibers.

1.6 Nanorods

In nanotechnology, nanorods are one class of nanoscale objects. They differ from the structures discussed above as each of their dimensions range from 1-100 nm which might not be the case in nanofibers. They may be synthesized from metals or semiconducting materials. Thus nanorods may be defined as shape anisotropic nanoparticles whose standard aspect ratios (length divided by width) are 3-25. Nanorods are produced by direct chemical synthesis. A large number of ligands act as shape control agents and bond to different facets of the nanorods with different strengths. Ligands provide:

(i) Control over nanorods shape during their synthesis,

(ii) The enhancement of colloidal stability of nanorods in solutions, and

(iii) The realization of specific properties and functions of nanorods.

This allows different faces of the nanorods to grow at different rates, producing an elongated object. In comparison to spherical particles, asymmetric particles offer addition of freedom in self-assembly due to their inherent shape anisotropy. Furthermore, the ability to synthesize nanorods with different sections provides the opportunity to introduce multiple chemical functionalities by exploiting the selective binding of different ligands to the different portions (Sun *et al.,* 2002). This facility to engineer nanorods with multiple functionalities in spatially defined region offers the potential for increased efficacy for drug and gene delivery systems.

1.6.1 Synthesis of Nanorods

1.6.1.1 Seed-Mediated Growth

Seed-mediated synthesis is the most frequently used method for producing metal nanorods such as gold (Au), silver (Ag), palladium (Pd), or copper (Cu). In order to synthesize rods with a narrow size distribution, the formation of seeds and their growth from these seeds has to be separated into two distinct stages, so that only growth of these seeds takes place in the second step and no new seeds are formed. For example, in the case of the synthesis of Au nanorods, seeds with dimensions in the range from 1 to 5 nm are prepared by reducing Au (III) to Au (0) with a strong reducing agent (sodium borohydride), while further formation of seeds in the second stage is inhibited by using a weak reducing agent (ascorbic acid) that can only reduce Au (III) to Au (I) in the presence of surfactant cetyltrimethylammonium bromide (CTAB) and silver ions. Longer nanorods (up to an aspect ratio of 25) can be obtained in the absence of silver nitrate by use of a three-step addition procedure. Elemental silver, has a lower reduction potential (less negative) than gold i.e., it has a higher affinity for electron and undergoes reduction more rapidly than gold; silver gets more rapidly deposited on the crystal structure than gold, thereby retarding the growth rate of specific crystal facets, allowing for one-directional growth and rod formation. The formation of Au nanorods from the Au seeds is achieved by the selective binding of CTAB to distinct Au crystal facets, which controls the growth rates of the different facets of the particles (Pérez-Juste *et al.,* 2005).

1.6.1.2 Synthesis of Nanorods at High Temperatures in Organic Solvents

Thermal decomposition of organometallic precursors and metal-surfactant complexes in high-boiling-point organic solvents is used to synthesize semiconductor, metal oxide, and metal nanorods with a diameter of 3-50 nm and the length 9-200 nm. The synthesis is performed *via* kinetically controlled anisotropic growth of inorganic crystals using various capping agents such as alkylamines, alkyl acids, alkylphosphonic acids, or trioctylphosphine oxide (TOPO). Generally, this method yields nanorods with a high crystallinity and a narrow size distribution. The method enables the synthesis of nanorods with a reduced number of internal defects and a uniform surface reconstruction. Both features lead to well defined physical properties of the nanorods.

1.6.1.3 Template Method

The template method for the synthesis of gold nanorods was first introduced by Martin and co-workers (Foss *et al.,* 1992); the method is based on the electrochemical deposition of gold within the pores of nanoporous polycarbonate or alumina template membranes. The method can be explained as follows: initially a small amount of silver or copper is sputtered onto the alumina template membrane to provide a conductive film for electrode position. This is then used as a foundation onto which the gold nanoparticles can be electrochemically grown. Subsequently, gold is electrodeposited within the nanopores of alumina (stage II). The next stage involves the selective dissolution of both the alumina membrane and the copper or silver film, in the presence of a polymeric stabilizer such as PVP. In the last stage, the rods are dispersed either in water or in organic solvents by means of sonication or agitation. The diameter of the gold nanoparticles thus synthesized coincides with the pore diameter of the alumina membrane. This means, that the gold nanorods with different diameters can be prepared by controlling the pore diameter of the template. The length of the nanorods can be controlled through the amount of gold deposited within the pores of the membrane.

1.6.1.4 Electrochemical Method

This method was demonstrated by Wang (1997). The synthesis is conducted within a simple two-electrode type electrochemical cell. Gold metal plate (typically 3.0 cm × 1.0 cm × 0.05 cm) is used as anode while the cathode is a platinum plate with similar dimensions. Both electrodes are immersed in an electrolytic solution containing a cationic surfactant, CTAB. CTAB not only functions as a stabilizer but also as a co-electrolyte. During the synthesis, the bulk gold metal anode is initially consumed, forming $AuBr_4^-$. These anions are complexed to the cationic surfactants and migrate to the cathode where reduction occurs. Sonication is needed to shear the resultant rods as they form away from the surface or possibly to break the rod off the cathode surface.

1.6.1.5 Zinc Oxide (ZnO) Nanorods

In the thermal evaporation method, commercial ZnO powder is mixed with SnO_2 and evaporated by heating the mixture at elevated temperature. In the chemical reduction method, zinc vapor, generated by the reduction of ZnO, is transferred to the growth zone, followed by reoxidation to ZnO. ZnO nanorods can be prepared by following procedure reported by Xiaowang *et al.,* (Liu *et al.,* 2009). Aligned ZnO nanorod films on ITO (Indium tin oxide) glass are synthesized *via* a two-step solution approach. First, a layer of ZnO nanoparticles is formed on the surface of ITO glass by thermally decomposing of zinc acetate at 320 °C for 20 min. Then the treated ITO glass is suspended in an aqueous solution containing zinc nitrate hydrate (0.025M) and methenamine (0.025M) at 90 °C for 3 hr. On completion of the reaction, the ITO glass is removed from the solution and rinsed with deionized water.

References

Ahlin P, Kristl J, Kristl A, and Vrecer F (2002). Investigation of polymeric nanoparticles as carriers of enalaprilat for oral administration. *International Journal of Pharmaceutics* **239:** 113-120.

Akagi T, Kaneko T, Kida T, and Akashi M (2005). Preparation and characterization of biodegradable nanoparticles based on poly(γ-glutamic acid) with l-phenylalanine as a protein carrier. *Journal of Controlled Release* **108:** 226-236.

al Khouri N, Fessi H, Roblot-Treupel L, Devissaguet J.P, and Puisieux F (1986). [An original procedure for preparing nanocapsules of polyalkylcyanoacrylates for interfacial polymerization]. *Pharmaceutica Acta Helvetiae* **61:** 274-281.

Ataman-Önal Y, Munier S, Ganée A, Terrat C, Durand P.Y, Battail N, Martinon F, Le Grand R, Charles M.H, Delair T, *et al.,* (2006). Surfactant-free anionic PLA nanoparticles coated with HIV-1 p24 protein induced enhanced cellular and humoral immune responses in various animal models. *Journal of Controlled Release* **112:** 175-185.

Bognitzki M, Frese T, Steinhart M, Greiner A, Wendorff J.H, Schaper A, and Hellwig M (2001). Preparation of fibers with nanoscaled morphologies: Electrospinning of polymer blends. *Polymer Engineering & Science* **41:** 982-989.

Charcosset C, and Fessi H (2005). Preparation of nanoparticles with a membrane contactor. *Journal of Membrane Science* **266:** 115-120.

Chen Y, Liu J, Yang X, Zhao X, and Xu H (2005). Oleanolic acid nanosuspensions: preparation, *in-vitro* characterization and enhanced hepatoprotective effect. *Journal of Pharmacy and Pharmacology* **57:** 259-264.

Choi S.W, and Kim J.H (2007). Design of surface-modified poly(d,l-lactide-co-glycolide) nanoparticles for targeted drug delivery to bone. *Journal of Controlled Release* **122:** 24-30.

Chong E.J, Phan T.T, Lim I.J, Zhang Y.Z, Bay B.H, Ramakrishna S, and Lim C.T (2007). Evaluation of electrospun PCL/gelatin nanofibrous scaffold for wound healing and layered dermal reconstitution. *Acta Biomaterialia* **3:** 321-330.

Elvassore N, Bertucco A, and Caliceti P (2001). Production of insulin-loaded poly(ethylene glycol)/poly(l-lactide) (PEG/PLA) nanoparticles by gas antisolvent techniques. *Journal of Pharmaceutical Sciences* **90:** 1628-1636.

Errico C, Bartoli C, Chiellini F, and Chiellini E (2009). Poly(hydroxyalkanoates)-based polymeric nanoparticles for drug delivery. *Journal of Biomedicine & Biotechnology* **2009:** 571-702.

Fan Y.F, Wang Y.N, Fan Y.G, and Ma J.B (2006). Preparation of insulin nanoparticles and their encapsulation with biodegradable polyelectrolytes *via* the layer-by-layer adsorption. *International Journal of Pharmaceutics* **324:** 158-167.

Fay F, Quinn D.J, Gilmore B.F, McCarron P.A, and Scott C.J (2010). Gene delivery using dimethyldidodecylammonium bromide-coated PLGA nanoparticles. *Biomaterials* **31:** 4214-4222.

Fessi H, Puisieux F, Devissaguet J.P, Ammoury N, and Benita S (1989). Nanocapsule formation by interfacial polymer deposition following solvent displacement. *International Journal of Pharmaceutics* **55:** R1-R4.

Foss C.A, Hornyak G.L, Stockert J.A, and Martin C.R (1992). Optical properties of composite membranes containing arrays of nanoscopic gold cylinders. *The Journal of Physical Chemistry* **96:** 7497-7499.

Galindo-Rodriguez S.A, Puel F, Briancon S, Allemann E, Doelker E, and Fessi H (2005). Comparative scale-up of three methods for producing ibuprofen-loaded nanoparticles. *European Journal of Pharmaceutical Sciences : Official Journal of the European Federation for Pharmaceutical Sciences* **25:** 357-367.

Ibrahim H, Bindschaedler C, Doelker E, Buri P, and Gurny R (1992). Aqueous nanodispersions prepared by a salting-out process. *International Journal of Pharmaceutics* **87:** 239-246.

Jeon H.J, Jeong Y.I, Jang M.K, Park Y.H, and Nah J.W (2000a). Effect of solvent on the preparation of surfactant-free poly(dl-lactide-co-glycolide) nanoparticles and norfloxacin release characteristics. *International Journal of Pharmaceutics* **207:** 99-108.

Jeon H.J, Jeong Y.I, Jang M.K, Park Y.H, and Nah J.W (2000b). Effect of solvent on the preparation of surfactant-free poly(DL-lactide-co-glycolide) nanoparticles and norfloxacin release characteristics. *International Journal of Pharmaceutics* **207:** 99-108.

Konan-Kouakou Y.N, Boch R, Gurny R, and Allémann E (2005). *In vitro* and *in vivo* activities of verteporfin-loaded nanoparticles. *Journal of Controlled Release* **103:** 83-91.

Konan Y.N, Gurny R, and Allémann E (2002). Preparation and characterization of sterile and freeze-dried sub-200 nm nanoparticles. *International Journal of Pharmaceutics* **233:** 239-252.

Legrand P, Lesieur S, Bochot A, Gref R, Raatjes W, Barratt G, and Vauthier C (2007). Influence of polymer behaviour in organic solution on the production of polylactide nanoparticles by nanoprecipitation. *International Journal of Pharmaceutics* **344:** 33-43.

Leroueil-Le Verger M, Fluckiger L, Kim Y.I, Hoffman M, and Maincent P (1998). Preparation and characterization of nanoparticles containing an antihypertensive agent. *European Journal of Pharmaceutics and Biopharmaceutics : Official Journal of Arbeitsgemeinschaft fur Pharmazeutische Verfahrenstechnik eV* **46:** 137-143.

Li D, and Xia Y (2004). Electrospinning of Nanofibers: Reinventing the Wheel? *Advanced Materials* **16:** 1151-1170.

Lince F, Marchisio D.L, and Barresi A.A (2008). Strategies to control the particle size distribution of poly-epsilon-caprolactone nanoparticles for pharmaceutical applications. *Journal of Colloid and Interface Science* **322:** 505-515.

Liu X, Hu Q, Wu Q, Zhang W, Fang Z, and Xie Q (2009). Aligned ZnO nanorods: A useful Film to Fabricate Amperometric Glucose Biosensor. *Colloids and Surfaces B, Biointerfaces* **74:** 154-158.

Ma P.X, and Zhang R (1999). Synthetic nano-scale fibrous extracellular matrix. *Journal of Biomedical Materials Research* **46:** 60-72.

Matsumoto J, Nakada Y, Sakurai K, Nakamura T, and Takahashi Y (1999). Preparation of nanoparticles consisted of poly(L-lactide)-poly(ethylene glycol)-poly(L-lactide) and their evaluation *in vitro*. *International Journal of Pharmaceutics* **185:** 93-101.

Moinard-Checot D, Chevalier Y, Briancon S, Beney L, and Fessi H (2008). Mechanism of nanocapsules formation by the emulsion-diffusion process. *Journal of Colloid and Interface Science* **317:** 458-468.

Namazi H, Fathi F, and Dadkhah A (2011). Hydrophobically modified starch using long-chain fatty acids for preparation of nanosized starch particles. *Scientia Iranica* **18:** 439-445.

Nicoli S, Santi P, Couvreur P, Couarraze G, Colombo P, and Fattal E (2001). Design of triptorelin loaded nanospheres for transdermal iontophoretic administration. *International Journal of Pharmaceutics* **214:** 31-35.

Oh I, Lee K, Kwon H.Y, Lee Y.B, Shin S.C, Cho C.S, and Kim C.K (1999). Release of adriamycin from poly(γ-benzyl-l-glutamate)/ poly(ethylene oxide) nanoparticles. *International Journal of Pharmaceutics* **181:** 107-115.

Park K.H, Song H.C, Na K, Bom H.S, Lee K.H, Kim S, Kang D, and Lee D.H (2007). Ionic strength-sensitive pullulan acetate nanoparticles (PAN) for intratumoral administration of radioisotope: ionic strength-dependent aggregation behavior and (99m) Technetium retention property. *Colloids and Surfaces B, Biointerfaces* **59:** 16-23.

Pérez-Juste J, Pastoriza-Santos I, Liz-Marzán L.M, and Mulvaney P (2005). Gold nanorods: Synthesis, characterization and applications. *Coordination Chemistry Reviews* **249:** 1870-1901.

Perugini P, Simeoni S, Scalia S, Genta I, Modena T, Conti B, and Pavanetto F (2002). Effect of nanoparticle encapsulation on the photostability of the sunscreen agent, 2-ethylhexyl-p-methoxycinnamate. *International Journal of Pharmaceutics* **246:** 37-45.

Seyler I, Appel M, Devissaguet J.P, Legrand P, and Barratt G (1999). Macrophage Activation by a Lipophilic Derivative of Muramyldipeptide within Nanocapsules: Investigation of the Mechanism of Drug Delivery. *Journal of Nanoparticle Research* **1:** 91-97.

Song X, Zhao Y, Wu W, Bi Y, Cai Z, Chen Q, Li Y, and Hou S (2008). PLGA nanoparticles simultaneously loaded with vincristine sulfate and verapamil hydrochloride: Systematic study of particle size and drug entrapment efficiency. *International Journal of Pharmaceutics* **350:** 320-329.

Sun Y.P, Fu K, Lin Y, and Huang W (2002). Functionalized Carbon Nanotubes: Properties and Applications. *Accounts of Chemical Research* **35:** 1096-1104.

Tan Y, Wang P, Xu K, Li W, An H, Li L, Liu C, and Dong L (2009). Designing Starch-Based Nanospheres to Make Hydrogels with High Mechanical Strength. *Macromolecular Materials and Engineering* **294:** 855-859.

Ubrich N, Bouillot P, Pellerin C, Hoffman M, and Maincent P (2004). Preparation and characterization of propranolol hydrochloride nanoparticles: a comparative study. *Journal of Controlled Release : Official Journal of the Controlled Release Society* **97:** 291-300.

Wu X.M, Branford-White C.J, Yu D.G, Chatterton N.P, and Zhu L.M (2011). Preparation of core-shell PAN nanofibers encapsulated alpha-tocopherol acetate and ascorbic acid 2-phosphate for photoprotection. *Colloids and Surfaces B, Biointerfaces* **82:** 247-252.

Yallapu M.M, Gupta B.K, Jaggi M, and Chauhan S.C (2010). Fabrication of curcumin encapsulated PLGA nanoparticles for improved therapeutic effects in metastatic cancer cells. *Journal of Colloid and Interface Science* **351:** 19-29.

Yu Chang S.S, Lee C.L, and Wang C.R.C (1997). Gold Nanorods: Electrochemical Synthesis and Optical Properties. *The Journal of Physical Chemistry B* **101:** 6661-6664.

Zamani M, Morshed M, Varshosaz J, and Jannesari M (2010). Controlled release of metronidazole benzoate from poly epsilon-caprolactone electrospun nanofibers for periodontal diseases. *European Journal of Pharmaceutics and Biopharmaceutics : Official Journal of Arbeitsgemeinschaft fur Pharmazeutische Verfahrenstechnik eV* **75:** 179-185.

Zhang Y, and Zhuo R.X (2005). Synthesis and drug release behavior of poly (trimethylene carbonate)–poly (ethylene glycol)–poly (trimethylene carbonate) nanoparticles. *Biomaterials* **26:** 2089-2094.

Zhang Z, Grijpma D.W, and Feijen J (2006a). Poly(trimethylene carbonate) and monomethoxy poly(ethylene glycol)-block-poly(trimethylene carbonate) nanoparticles for the controlled release of dexamethasone. *Journal of Controlled Release : Official Journal of the Controlled Release Society* **111:** 263-270.

Zhang Z, Grijpma D.W, and Feijen J (2006b). Poly(trimethylene carbonate) and monomethoxy poly(ethylene glycol)-block-poly(trimethylene carbonate) nanoparticles for the controlled release of dexamethasone. *Journal of Controlled Release* **111:** 263-270.

Zili Z, Sfar S, and Fessi H (2005). Preparation and characterization of poly-epsilon-caprolactone nanoparticles containing griseofulvin. *International Journal of Pharmaceutics* **294:** 261-267.

Zweers M.L.T, Engbers G.H.M, Grijpma D.W, and Feijen J (2004). *In vitro* degradation of nanoparticles prepared from polymers based on dl-lactide, glycolide and poly(ethylene oxide). *Journal of Controlled Release* **100:** 347-356.

2

Dendrimers in Drug Delivery

Umesh Gupta
Department of Pharmacy, School of Chemical Sciences and Pharmacy,Central University of Rajasthan, Bandarsindri, Kishangarh, Ajmer – 305817, India.

2.1 Background and Introduction

Last three decades of pharmaceutical research have attracted scientific community enormously towards capabilities of the novel drug delivery systems in the benefit of human health. Novel drug delivery systems including liposomes, nanoparticles, microspheres, dendrimers and nano-emulsions have given beneficial results in the treatment of complex diseases like AIDS, cancer, tuberculosis and leishmaniasis etc. Though vast research has taken place related to novel carriers, the commercialization of these drug delivery systems is itself a big challenge. The present chapter highlights about the properties, chemistry and applications of one of the novel drug carriers, "dendrimers" in drug delivery. In couple of years, dendrimers have emerged as one of the most promising nano-particulate carrier systems that has greatly attracted the scientific community. Dendrimer chemistry was first reported by Vogtle and co-workers in 1978 (Buhleier *et al.,* 1978). However, dendrimer were discovered in the early 1980's by Donald A. Tomalia and co-workers and for the first time these hyper-branched molecules were called as 'dendrimers'. The term *dendrimers* originates from Greek ('*dendrons*' meaning tree or branch and '*meros*' meaning part) and refers to class of structurally hyper-branched polymers (Tomalia *et al.,* 1985). At the same time in early 1980's, Newkome's group independently reported synthesis of similar macromolecules (Newkome *et al.,* 1985). They called them 'arborols' from the Latin word 'arbor' also meaning a tree. The other synonym for dendrimers include *cascade molecules*; however, among all dendrimer is the most popular.

Dendrimers are defined as three dimensional, unimolecular, highly branched mono-dispersed macromolecules, which are obtained by an iterative sequence of reaction steps producing a precise, unique branching structure like tree. Dendrimers consist of three characteristic scaffolds (Fig. 2.1):

(i) multi-functional initiator core,

(ii) inner generations (branches), which consist of repeating branched units or branches; and

(iii) exterior or terminal surface groups, attached to the outermost generation.

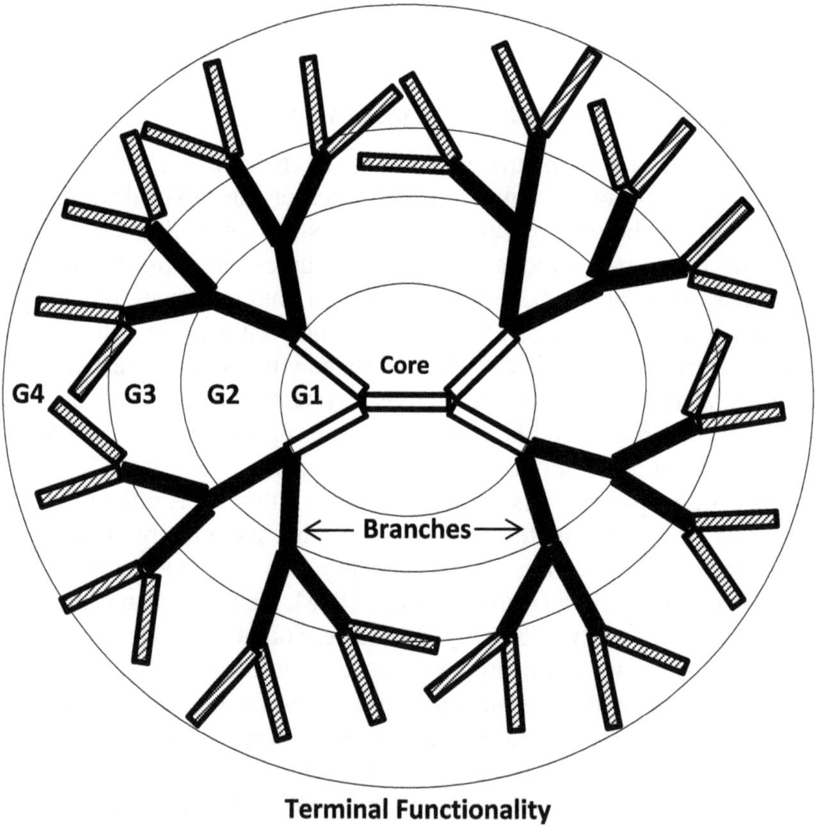

Fig. 2.1 Typical dendrimer skeleton with core, branches and; terminal functional groups. Each circle represents a generation (G1 to G4).

Number of molecules has been reported so far which can act as a dendrimer core e.g., ammonia, ethylene diamine (EDA), diaminobutane (DAB), triazine, polyethylene glycol (PEG), bis(4-fluorophenyl)sulfone, carbosilane etc. The branches emanate from the core and the synthetic growth follows the pattern like a branch of tree. Based on different type of core, repeating units and surface functionalities; different types of dendrimers such as poly amidoamine (PAMAM), poly propylene imine (PPI), peptide dendrimers, citric acid dendrimers and triazine dendrimers has been reported.

Dendrimer size is represented by 'generation' number. Each layer of the branching units constitutes a 'generation'. Unlike traditional linear polymer synthesis that produces a mixture of materials ranging in molecular weight, dendrimers are the product of multi-step organic synthesis. At the same time their synthesis can be so optimized as to control their size, shape, molecular mass, composition and reactivity. One of the most appealing feature of dendrimers is the existence of a high number of functional groups at the periphery, by which the properties of these macromolecules can be modulated. This tailor made functionality makes dendrimers a versatile polymer with immense potential in different biomedical applications.

Many novel drug carriers are in pipeline today waiting for commercialization, in future. Some of them are still in initial phase of research, however, only few of them have proven their capability in market as established formulation, either for the diagnostic purposes or therapeutically for the treatment of diseases like cancer, psoriasis and others. Dendrimers are among one of those novel carriers which have proven there commercial reality in the market. The very first product based on dendrimers was VivaGel™ which was introduced by Starpharma™. After VivaGel™ several other dendrimer based products e.g., Stratus CS™, SuperFect™ and Alert Ticket™ are commercial today (Table 2.1). Some of the dendrimers e.g., PAMAM, PPI and polylysine are available commercially in different functionality and generations. In the present chapter we will discuss the properties, synthetic strategies, characterization approaches and applications of dendrimers in pharmaceutical sciences and drug delivery. The chapter is designed mainly to emphasize on the drug delivery possibilities with dendrimers.

Table 2.1 Marketed preparations based on dendrimers.

Product	Application	Manufacturer
VivaGel™	Vaginal gel for preventing HIV infection	Starpharma, Australia
Stratus CS™	Cardiac marker	Dade Behring, USA
SuperFect™	Gene transfection	Qiagen, USA
PrioFect™	siRNA transfection reagent	Starpharma, Australia
Alert Ticket™	Anthrax detection	US Army Research Laboratory, USA

2.2 Dendrimer Synthesis

Dendrimers can be synthesized using either divergent or convergent approach. Both the methods can be precisely controlled at each step of the propagation unlike traditional polymers which often have poorly defined molecular structures. Convergent and divergent approaches have a fundamental difference in the growth and propagation of dendrimers during synthesis. There are several other methods has also been reported to synthesize dendrimers however they are not so popular compared to divergent and convergent methods. Other than convergent and divergent methods we also come across the methods like double exponential growth, click chemistry approach, lego chemistry approach for the synthesis of dendrimers (Jain and Khopade, 2001).

2.2.1 Divergent Approach

In the divergent approach, first reported by Newkome and Tomalia, the growth of dendrimers starts from core (Newkome *et al.,* 1985; Tomalia *et al.,* 1985). The core gradually combines with the emanating/repeating groups (called branches) and forms newer generation of dendrimer with a specific terminal functional group (Fig. 2.2). So typically, when the core binds with branches in first step the whole structure is referred to as first generation. For the synthesis of second generation the functional groups on the surface of first generation reacts further with newer building blocks or branches. Each repetition cycle leads to the addition of one more layer of branches (called a "generation") to the dendrimer framework. Therefore, the generation number of the dendrimer is equal to the number of repetition cycles performed, and may be easily determined by counting the number of branch points as one proceeds from the core to the periphery. This repetition is continued up to the desired degree of branching is achieved. The divergent synthetic approach is effective in synthesizing higher generation dendrimers.

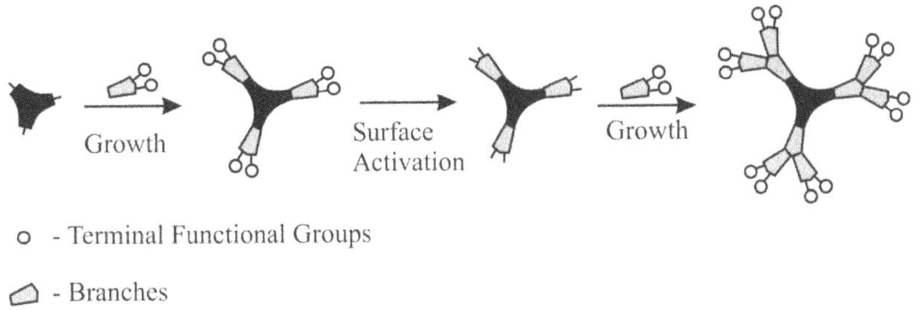

Fig. 2.2 Divergent synthetic approach.

First synthesized dendrimers using divergent approach were PAMAM, also called as "starburst" dendrimers (Tomalia *et al.,* 1985). The term starburst is the trademark of the DOW Chemicals Company. PAMAM dendrimers are available commercially manufactured today by Dendritech Inc. USA. The commercial dendrimers are available with different terminal groups like -OH, -NH_2 or mixed with different core e.g., ethylene diamine (EDA) as well as ammonia. PPI dendrimers are also available commercially and are synthesized by divergent approach using di-amino butane (DAB) or EDA as core. These dendrimers are available for purchase under the trade name Astramol™ by DSM, Netherlands. Other classes of dendrimers were synthesized by divergent approach includes polylysine, triazine, peptide etc.

Conceptually this synthetic strategy seems quite interesting and flawless, however practically it is not the case. As the generation number increases the number of functional groups increases exponentially on the same molecule. However it is sometimes difficult to achieve the desired degree of purity and number of functional groups even though the reaction is efficient enough. So it is always better to purify and separate the structurally similar byproducts having similar structure during synthesis (Jain and Khopade, 2001).

2.2.2 Convergent Approach

Convergent as the word meaning says, it is the method which is opposite in approach than divergent. In this method the dendrimer synthesis starts from terminal surface towards dendrimer core (Fig. 2.3). First reported by Hawker and Fréchet in 1990 the synthesis proceeds from what will become the dendron molecular surface (periphery) inward to a central core (focal point). This method offer the advantage of synthesis of more homogenous and pure dendrimers compared to divergent approach. Additionally, very few reaction steps are involved and since only two reactions are carried out at given point of time formation of structurally flawed product is less likely. Also the mass difference between any byproduct and desired product is so large that it is easy to separate and purify. On the other hand, the convergent strategy is often limited to synthesis of lower generation dendrimers. Also the steric crowding slows the reaction steps (Hawker and Frechet, 1990).

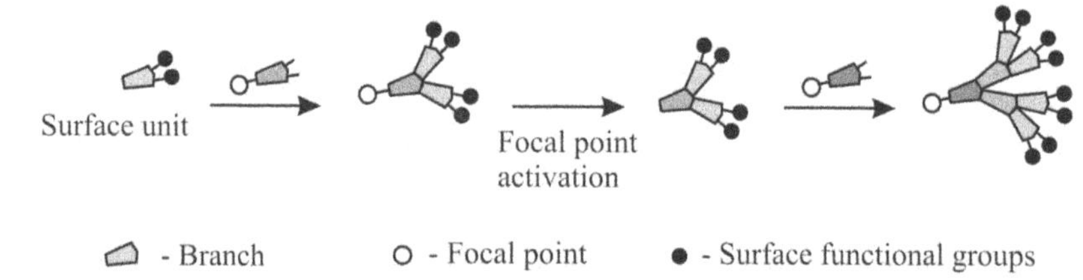

Fig. 2.3 Convergent synthetic approach.

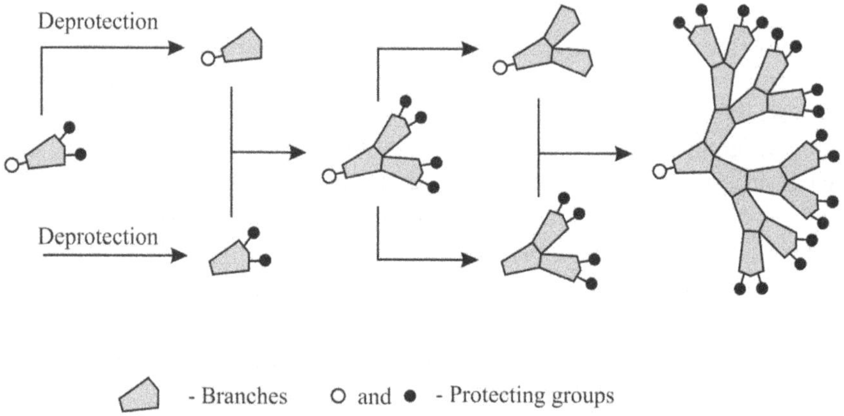

Fig. 2.4 Double exponential synthetic approach.

2.2.3 Double Exponential Growth

This approach allows the preparation of monomers for both divergent and convergent growth from a single starting material (Fig. 2.4). It is quite similar to the rapid growth technique for linear polymers. Then resulted two products are reacted to give an orthogonally protected trimer, which can be used to repeat the growth again. The advantage of double exponential growth method is fast synthesis and desirable extension of synthesis with either divergent or convergent growth easily (Kawaguchi *et al.,* 1995).

2.2.4 'Click' Chemistry Approach

The method was reported for some specialized dendrimer classes. By this approach dendrimers with various surface groups in high purity and excellent yield can be obtained. All generation 2 and some generation 3 Cu(I)-catalyzed dendrimers have been isolated with only sodium chloride as the major byproduct (Svenson and Tomalia, 2005).

2.3 Molecular Structure and Properties

Dendrimer has hyperbranched architecture which leads to some of the unique molecular properties. As the generation number grows the properties changes. Lower generation dendrimers poses open structure and are highly asymmetric in shape as compared to higher generation. As the generation number grows the structure becomes more and more globular and compact (up to 4 or higher generations) and as they extend out to the periphery they forms a closed membrane-like structure (Caminati *et al.,* 1990). When a critical stage is reached dendrimers cannot grow because of lack of space. This is sometimes referred to as 'starburst effect'. In case of PAMAM dendrimers the starburst effect can be observed after generation 10. The other changes which are observed in higher generation of dendrimers due to increased branches density is the development of internal cavities in dendrimer structure. These internal cavities along with terminal functional groups play important role in controlling the properties of encapsulated or complexed (Fig. 2.5) therapeutic moieties (Jain and Khopade, 2001).

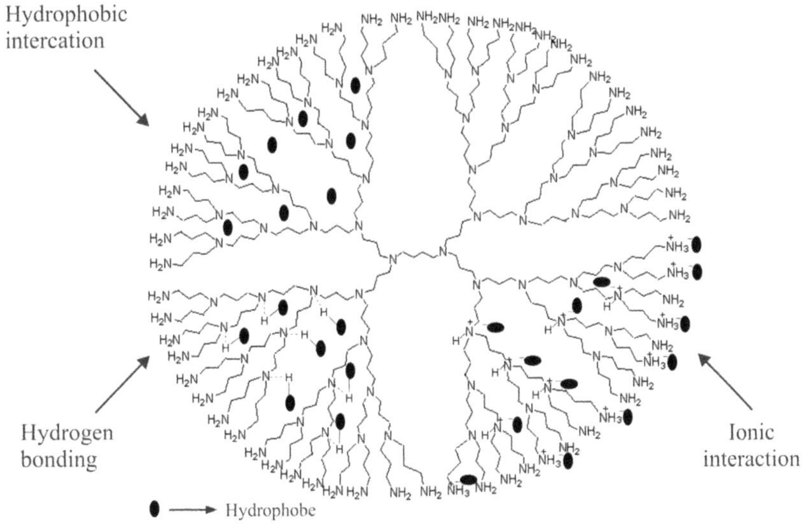

Fig. 2.5 Mechanisms of dendrimer-drug complexation (possible mechanism behind solubilization and drug encapsulation).

Dendrimers are truly nanoscale molecules ranging from 10 Å to 130 Å in diameter for generation 0 (G0) through generation 10 (G10). The size range of dendrimers makes them an important carrier system. Other distinguished properties of dendrimers are its mono-disperse nature, globular shape and highly controlled architecture, making them efficient carrier system for drugs (Jain and Gupta, 2008). Because of their molecular architecture, dendrimers show some significantly improved physical and chemical properties when compared to traditional linear polymers. In linear polymers the polymerization is usually random in nature and produces molecules of different sizes, whereas size and molecular mass of dendrimers can be specifically controlled during synthesis. Also, various linear polymers and other hyper branched structures have randomly distributed functional groups, polydispersive nature, no characteristic shape and lack uniform molecular weight distribution, which is not the case with dendrimers. Dendrimers in solution have lower viscosity than linear polymers. Also the intrinsic viscosity of dendrimers increases with increase in generation upto level fourth and thereafter the viscosity declines. While in case of linear polymers the intrinsic viscosity increases as the molecular weight increases. The decline in viscosity of dendrimer is one of the important factors responsible for the uni-molecular miceller nature of dendrimers.

The chemical reactivity and solubility of dendrimers is quite higher compared to their linear counterpart proved in a study of polyester dendrimers. The higher solubility of dendrimers is because of the presence of many terminal functional groups at dendrimer surface. Dendrimers with hydrophilic surface groups are more soluble in polar solvents while dendrimers having hydrophobic end groups are soluble in nonpolar solvents (Frechet, 1994).

The early reports that dendrimers can encapsulate some bioactive or chemical moieties were based on encapsulation of pyrene dye (Hawker *et al.,* 1993). Later, Meijer and coworkers reported the concept of "dendritic boxes". In this study authors trapped small molecules like rose bengal or p-nitrobenzoic acid inside the 'dendritic box' of PPI dendrimer with 64 branches on the periphery. Then a shell was formed on the surface of the dendrimer by reacting the terminal amines with an amino acid (L-phenylalanine) and guest molecules were stably encapsulated inside the box. Hydrolysing the outer shell could liberate the guest molecules. The shape of the guest and the architecture of the box and its cavities determine the number of guest molecules that can be entrapped. The research group described experiments in which they had trapped four molecules of rose bengal or eight to ten molecules of p-nitrobenzoic acid in dendrimer (Meijer *et al.,* 1994). So far many drugs have been successfully encapsulated and solubilized using dendrimers. The encapsulation efficiency increases as the generation number and concentration of dendrimer increases (Gupta *et al.,* 2006).

Another important property of dendrimers is tailor-made functionality and surface charge. The property to develop dendrimers of desired functional groups provides versatility in conjugation of bioactive agents like ligand, drug and antibodies to the dendrimers' surface. In general dendrimer's cationic charge is responsible for the membrane toxicity in biological tissues. "Cationic" dendrimers (e.g., amine terminated PAMAM and PPI) that form cationic groups at low pH, are generally hemolytic and cytotoxic. Their toxicity is generation-dependent and increases with the number of surface groups. PAMAM dendrimers (generation 2, 3 and 4) interact with erythrocyte membrane proteins causing changes in protein conformation. These changes increase with generation number and the concentration of dendrimers. However these interactions are weaker in case of anionic dendrimers (hydroxyl or carboxylic terminated PAMAM dendrimers). Anionic dendrimers, bearing a carboxylate or hydroxyl groups, are not cytotoxic over a broad concentration range (Duncan and Izzo, 2005).

Current research focuses to reduce the cationic toxicity by surface engineering of dendrimers. Number of molecules has been conjugated to the dendritic surface like carbohydrates, peptides, biocompatible ligands to reduce the associated cationic toxicity of the dendrimers.

2.4 Characterization

Dendrimers are just in between molecular chemistry and polymer chemistry. They pertain to the molecular chemistry world by virtue of their step by step controlled synthesis, and they pertain to the polymer world because of their repetitive structure made of monomers. Thus, they should benefit from analytical techniques derived from both worlds. There are several techniques by which dendrimers can be characterized. In the spectroscopic and spectrometric methods FTIR and NMR spectroscopy exhibit important role in elucidation of structure while MALDI-TOF is used for the determination of mass of higher as well as lower generation of dendrimers. The other methods used in this category are UV-Vis spectroscopy, Fluorescence, Chirality, Optical rotation, Circular dichroism and X-ray diffraction. These methods give an idea about the chemical structure of dendrimers. The internal structure and radius of gyration of the dendrimers can be determined by the scattering techniques like small angle X-ray scattering, small angle neutron scattering, and laser light scattering (LLS). In some of the studies LLS has also been used for the determination of molecular weight of the dendrimers.

Microscopic techniques can be used for observing the surface morphology of the dendrimers. Two types of microscopy, very different in principle, have been used for imaging dendrimers. In transmission microscopy, electrons or light produce images that amplify the original, with a resolution ultimately limited by the wavelength of the source. In scanning microscopy, such as atomic force microscopy, the images are produced by touch contact at a few angstroms of a sensitive cantilever arm with the sample. Size exclusion chromatography has been used in the purification and separation of the dendrimers from by products during synthesis. Rheological and other properties can be determined by differential scanning calorimetry, and dielectric spectroscopy (Caminade *et al.,* 2005).

In last few years of dendrimers research, many techniques have been used and reported for the characterization of dendrimers. Now it is quite possible to well characterize and purify dendrimer at each synthetic step.

2.5 Major Classes of Dendrimers

2.5.1 Polyamidoamine (PAMAM) Dendrimers

PAMAM is the most researched and popular class of dendrimers. PAMAM is also the first synthesized class of dendrimer reported by Tomalia *et al.,* in early 80's (Fig. 2.6 and Table 2.2). These are commercially supplied by Dendritech Inc. USA. PAMAM dendrimers are available with different terminal functionalities like amine; hydroxyl and carboxylic terminated as well as with mixed functional groups up to generation 10 either as methanolic or aqueous solution. PAMAM dendrimers have several pharmaceutical and biological applications e.g., in drug delivery, gene delivery, drug targeting, solubilization, photo therapy, transdermal drug delivery and as diagnostic tool. Many surface modified PAMAM dendrimers are non-immunogenic, water-soluble and possess terminal-modifiable amine functional groups for binding various targeting or guest molecules. PAMAM dendrimers generally display concentration-dependent toxicity and hemolysis. PAMAM dendrimers are hydrolytically degradable only under harsh conditions because of their amide backbones, and hydrolysis proceeds slowly at physiological temperatures.

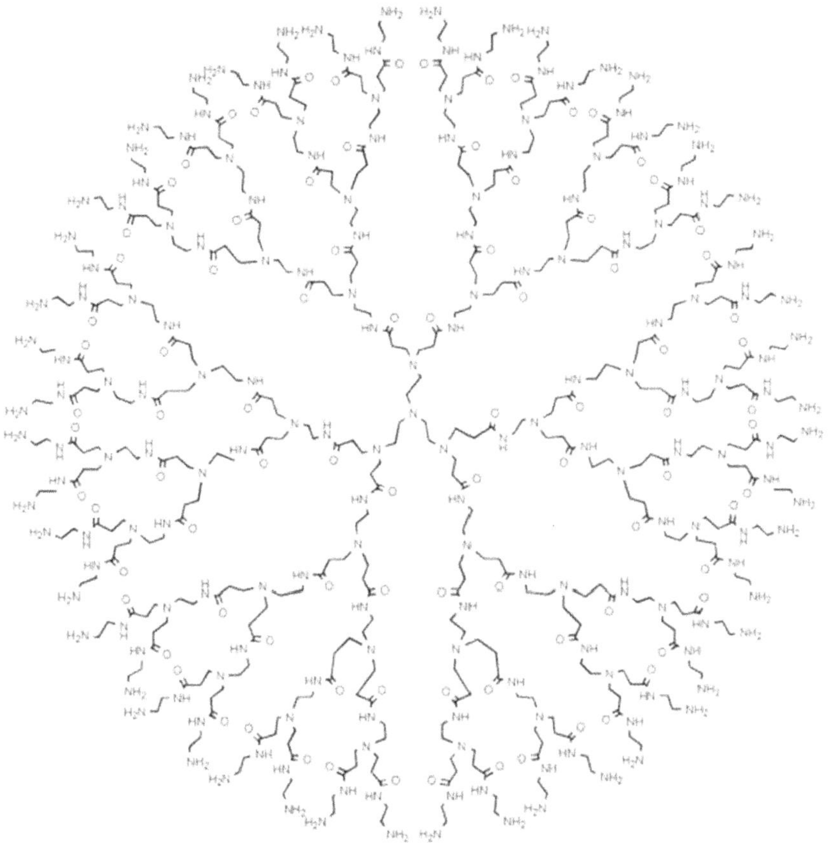

Fig. 2.6 PAMAM (polyamido amine) dendrimer.

2.5.2 Polypropylene(imine) (PPI) Dendrimers

Firstly reported by Vogtle, PPI dendrimers closely resembles PAMAM dendrimers except repeating units (Fig. 2.7). Alkyl chains in PPI dendrimers make the internal microenvironment less polar compared to PAMAM dendrimers, which have alkyl chains with amido groups as repeating units. More feasible synthesis of PPI dendrimers was reported by de Brabander-van den Berg and Meijer in 1993. PPI dendrimers can be synthesized using EDA or DAB as core (Table 2.2). These dendrimers are commercially available as Astramol™ by DSM Netherlands up to generation 5 (de Brabander-van den Berg and Meijer, 1993).

Table 2.2 Theoretical properties of PAMAM and PPI dendrimers.

Generation	PAMAM Dendrimer				PPI Dendrimer			
	Ammonia core		EDA core		EDA core		DAB core	
	Molecular weight	No. of terminal groups	Molecular weight	No. of terminal groups	Molecular weight	No. of terminal groups	Molecular weight	No. of terminal groups
0	359	3	516	4	60	2	88	2
1	1043	6	1428	8	288	4	316	4
2	2411	12	3252	16	746	8	774	8
3	5147	24	6900	32	1658	16	1686	16
4	10619	48	14196	64	3486	32	3510	32
5	21563	96	28788	128	7140	64	7168	64

EDA - Ethylenediamine; DAB - Diaminobutane; PPI - Polypropyleneimine; PAMAM - Polyamidoamine

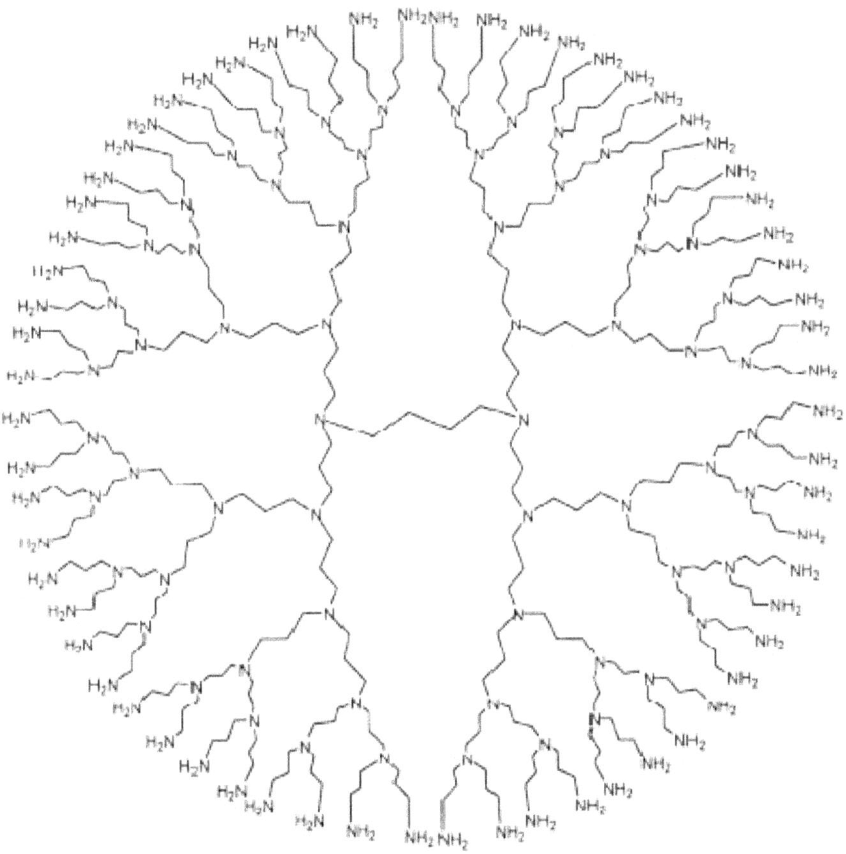

Fig. 2.7 PPI (polypropylene imine) dendrimer.

2.5.3 Peptide Dendrimers

Continuously the research has been carried out in the search of dendrimers based on biocompatible components. Peptide dendrimers are among the one which represents this property. Dendrimers having peptides/peptide linkages on the surface of the traditional dendrimer framework and dendrimers incorporating amino acids as branching or core units are both defined as 'peptide dendrimers'. As mentioned earlier, advantage of these dendrimers is bio-compatibility. Because of biological and therapeutic relevance of peptide molecules, peptide dendrimers play an important role in diverse areas including cancer, antimicrobials, antiviral, central nervous system, analgesia, asthma, allergy and Ca^{+2} metabolism. On the basis of their ability to be taken up by cells, peptide dendrimers are very useful for drug delivery. One more interesting application of peptide dendrimers is that they can be used as contrast agents for magnetic resonance imaging (MRI), magnetic resonance angiography (MRA), fluorogenic imaging and serodiagnosis (Crespo *et al.,* 2005).

2.5.4 Triazine Dendrimers

This is the class of the dendrimer which utilizes triazine trichloride as core. Triazine dendrimers have been reported for a variety of applications including drug delivery with an emphasis on cancer, non-viral DNA and RNA delivery systems, in sensing applications, and as bioactive materials. Triazine trichloride offers several advantages including its ability to diversify the chemical functionality without using protecting groups and the nucleophilic aromatic substitution on its ring occurs sequentially in temperature dependent manner excluding the need of functional groups manipulation.

2.5.5 Glyco or Carbohydrate Dendrimers

Glycodendrimers is the class of dendrimers which is either composed of or surface engineered with the carbohydrates. These are either carbohydrate-coated, carbohydrate centered or fully carbohydrate-based. Glycodendrimers have been used for a variety of biologically relevant applications such as, glycodendrimers with surface carbohydrate units have been used to study the protein-carbohydrate interactions (Turnbull and Stoddart, 2002). Several surface modified dendrimers with different sugars e.g., mannose, galactose etc., has been reported in drug targeting to liver and other tissues (Bhadra *et al.,* 2005). The accessibility of the sugars is an important consideration for glycodendrimers used effectively to evaluate protein-carbohydrate interactions. Like this, incorporation into analytical devices, formulation of gels, targeting of MRI contrast agents, drugs and gene delivery systems are some of the areas where glycodendrimers are likely to be beneficial.

2.5.6 Tecto Dendrimers

Tecto dendrimers are actually a composite dendrimer which is surrounded by other dendrimers. Tecto-dendrimers are composed of a core dendrimer, which may or may not contain the therapeutic agent. The surrounding dendrimers can be of several types, each type designed to perform a function necessary to a smart therapeutic nano-device. Tecto dendrimers may be designed to perform the functions like diseased cell recognition, diagnosis of disease state, drug delivery, reporting location and reporting outcome of therapy (Betley *et al.,* 2002).

2.5.7 Chiral Dendrimers

The chirality in these dendrimers is based upon the construction of constitutionally different but chemically similar branches to chiral core. Chiral, non-racemic dendrimer with well-defined stereochemistry is particularly interesting subclass, with potential applications in asymmetric catalysis and chiral molecular recognition.

2.5.8 Miscellaneous

There are several other types of dendrimers reported in literature e.g., amphiphilic, hybrid, poly(amidoamine-organosilicon) (PAMAMOS) and liquid crystalline dendrimers. These classes have their own properties e.g., liquid crystalline dendrimers are composed of mesogenic (liquid crystalline) monomers, e.g., mesogen functionalized carbosilane dendrimers, whereas PAMAMOS are inverted unimolecular micelles that consist of hydrophilic, nucleophilic PAMAM interiors and hydrophobic organosilicon exteriors. Hybrid dendrimers are kind of graft copolymers in which the whole dendrimer is composed of both linear as well as dendritic polymers (Jain and Khopade, 2001).

2.6 Biomedical Applications

2.6.1 Solubilization of Insoluble Drugs

Dendrimers with hydrophobic core and hydrophilic periphery have shown to exhibit micelle-like behavior and have container properties in solution. The use of dendrimers as unimolecular micelles was proposed by Newkome in 1985 (Newkome *et al.,* 1985). This analogy highlighted the utility of dendrimers as solubilizing agents. Dendrimer mediated solubilization depends on several factors such as generation size, dendrimer concentration, pH, core, temperature, and terminal functionality (Gupta *et al.,* 2006). More than 50 insoluble drugs/bioactive(s) has been successfully solubilized and reported using dendrimers (Table 2.3). Dendrimers have unique structure which is responsible for the solubilization and encapsulation of hydrophobic drugs. Usually the interior of dendrimers (e.g., PAMAM, PPI) is hydrophobic while the exterior or terminal functionality of the dendrimers is hydrophilic in nature. The hydrophobic interior is responsible for encapsulation of hydrophobes and in turn solubilization.

Ionic interaction, hydrogen bonding, and hydrophobic interactions are the possible mechanisms by which a dendrimer exerts its solubilizing property to the hydrophobic drugs (Fig. 2.5).

Table 2.3 Some of the drugs solubilized using different types of dendrimers.

Dendrimer	Drug solubilized	Reference
PEGylated PAMAM	5 Fluorouracil	Bhadra *et al.*, 2003
PEGylated polyether	Indomethacin	Kwon *et al.*, 1997
Hydroxyl and amine terminated PAMAM	Indomethacin	Chauhan *et al.*, 2003
PPI	Indomethacin, Famotidine and Amphotericin B	Gupta *et al.*, 2007
PAMAM	Flurbiprofen	Asthana *et al.*, 2005
Polyglycerol	Paclitaxel	Ooya *et al.*, 2003
Ester and amine terminated PAMAM	Nifedipine	Devarakonda *et al.*, 2004
PAMAM and lauroyl conjugated PAMAM	Propranolol	D'Emanuele *et al.*, 2004
PAMAM and PEGylated PAMAM	Methotrexate	Khopade *et al.*, 2002; Kojima *et al.*, 2000
PAMAM	Ibuprofen	Milhem *et al.*, 2000
PEGylated lysine	Artemether	Bhadra *et al.*, 2005
PAMAM	Niclosamide	Devarakonda *et al.*, 2004
PAMAM	Naproxen, Ketoprofen, Ibuprofen, Diflunisal	Yiyun and Tongwen, 2005

2.6.2 Drug Delivery Applications

Dendrimers' unique properties like polyvalency, hydrophobic interior, monodispersity and nanometric size make them suitable carrier for drug delivery. Nano-metric size plays a major role as it is responsible for enhanced permeation and retention effect in the diseases like cancer where the passive targeting can be achieved due to leaky vasculature in tumor tissues. Dendrimers property to encapsulate higher amount of drug molecule due to hydrophobic interior makes it a promising carrier for drug delivery and solubilization. Polyvalency of the dendrimers can be utilized in the conjugation of targeting ligand e.g., antibodies in order to achieve targeted drug delivery.

2.6.2.1 Controlled and Targeted Drug Delivery

In the last two decades much attention has been given to the targeted drug delivery research. Targeting of drugs is specifically advantageous in the diseases like cancer because of the nonselective action of highly potent drugs, resulting in dose limiting side effects. Targeting of drugs to the tumor offer dual advantage of increased therapeutic index at tumor and reduced chances of drug resistance. Dendrimers have ideal properties of targeting carrier. Number of ligands e.g., folic acid, dextran and hyaluronic acid has been conjugated to the surface of dendrimers for the targeted delivery of anticancer drugs to the tumors. Membrane associated receptors for these ligands are generally overexpressed in tumor tissues. These receptors are responsible for the uptake of the ligand conjugated dendrimers and in turn the release of anticancer drugs in the tumor vicinity (Fig. 2.8).

PAMAM dendrimers have been conjugated with the folic acid and fluorescein isothiocyanate for the purpose of targeting the tumor cells and imaging, respectively (Choi *et al.,* 2005). Antibody has also been conjugated to the dendritic surface for targeting. It was found that the dendrimer-antibody conjugate bound specifically to the antigen-expressing cells in a time- and dose- dependent fashion with an affinity similar to that of the free antibody. Further results indicated that cellular internalization of the dendrimer conjugate did take place (Thomas and Finnin, 2004). During another study, folic acid was conjugated to dendrimers as targeting agent and then coupled with a model drug Methotrexate (MTX). These conjugates were injected to immunodeficient mice bearing Human KB tumors and evaluated. Bio-distribution study shows that percentage of the injected dose particularly in tumor cells after one day was around three times higher with targeted polymer conjugates (with folic acid) compared to non-targeted polymer conjugates (without folic acid) (Kukowska-Latallo *et al.,* 2005). Patri and co-workers have investigated that complexing a drug with dendrimer as an inclusion complex improves its solubility in water. A cleavable, while covalently linked dendrimer conjugate is better for targeted drug delivery because it does not release the drug prematurely in biological conditions. They reported less cytotoxic effect with the covalently linked dendrimer (Patri *et al.,* 2005).

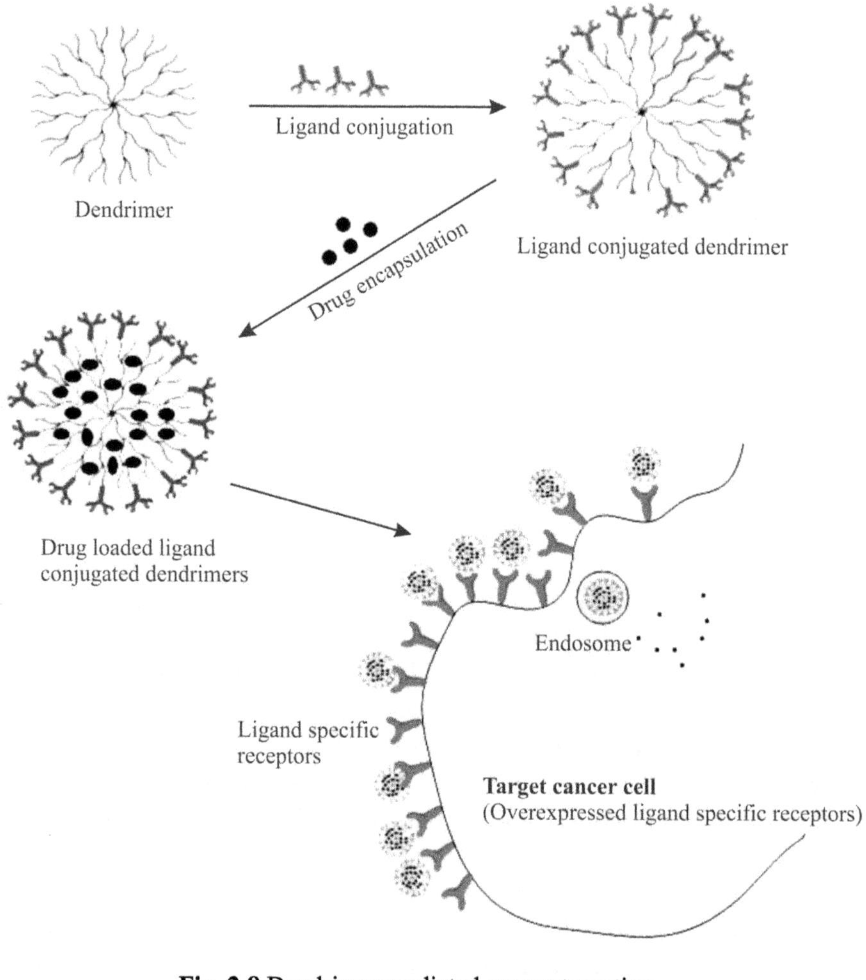

Fig. 2.8 Dendrimer mediated cancer targeting.

Dendrimers have the capacity to encapsulate drugs in a higher dose. In the early studies Jansen *et al.,* reported that dendritic boxes can retard the release of Rose Bengal because of close packing of the dendritic shell with amino acids leading to physical locking of the guest molecules. Surface engineering of dendrimers can lead to the sustained release of entrapped drug. In another study (Kojima *et al.,* 2000) found that MTX loaded MPEG-PAMAM dendrimers released the drug slowly because the drug was thought to be tightly bound with the interior of dendrimers *via* electrostatic interactions. (Kumar *et al.,* 2006) also found the slow release of rifampicin from mannosylated and Pegylated PPI dendrimers at physiological pH (7.4). (Dutta and Jain, 2007) reported the prolonged release rate up to 144 hr from lamivudine-loaded mannosylated PPI dendrimer. Similarly, (Agrawal *et al.,* 2007) demonstrated sustained release of drug from galactose anchored 4G poly-L-lysine dendrimers which might be due to their possible larger, compact and peripherally sealed structure. In the same study, researchers reported *in vivo* drug release in a similar fashion as compared to *in vitro* drug release. Several other reports have demonstrated the controlled and sustained drug delivery potential of dendrimers.

2.6.2.2 Oral Drug Delivery

Oral route of drug administration is most preferred due to its several significant advantages mainly convenience and patient compliance. Some reports are available demonstrating the ability of dendrimers to cross gastrointestinal GI membrane. Caco 2 cells were used in most of the studies to prove the oral delivery potential of the dendrimers. In the early studies (Wiwattanapatapee *et al.,* 2000) investigated transport of cationic PAMAM (3G and 4G) and anionic PAMAM dendrimers across the intestine of adult rats. Investigations suggested that transport of dendrimers across the intestinal membrane was charge dependent. Another group of researchers (Jevprasesphant *et al.,* 2003) investigated the effect of dendrimer generation and conjugation on the cytotoxicity, permeation and transport of PAMAM and surface-modified PAMAM dendrimer using monolayers of the human colon adenocarcinoma cell line, Caco-2 and found improved permeation. (Thiagarajan *et al.,* 2013) reported recently the toxicity issues with the oral delivery of different dendrimers as it is one of the important issues which need consideration before designing dendrimers for the oral drug delivery. (D'Emanuele *et al.,* 2004) synthesized propranolol–PAMAM dendrimers conjugate and investigated transport of the conjugate across Caco-2 cell monolayers. The results showed that propranolol–dendrimer conjugate was able to bypass the P-gp efflux transporter. Investigators have lastly concluded that dendrimers conjugate with drug could reduce the effect of intestinal P-gp on drug absorption of propranolol and many other orally administered drugs.

2.6.2.3 Transdermal Drug Delivery

Alternative route of drug delivery is always full of challenges as well as advantages. Considerable research has been reported about the dendrimer skin interactions and it has been found that dendrimers possess the potential of transdermal drug delivery. Venuganti and Perumal, 2009, studied the effect of dendrimer generation, charge and concentration on the skin permeability of dendrimers using 5-FU as model drug. The results showed that cationic dendrimers with lower generations were more permeable to skin. The transdermal studies were performed on porcine skin. In another study by (Venuganti and Perumal, 2009) effect of iontophoresis was studied on the skin permeation of dendrimers. The authors found that cationic dendrimers showed higher penetration. The localization of dendrimers in the skin can be achieved using iontophoresis.

As mentioned earlier the dendrimers have solubilizing capacity of insoluble drugs. This property was utilized by some of the researchers to encapsulate insoluble drugs belonging to the category of non-steroidal anti-inflammatory drugs (NSAIDs) like indomethacin, diflunisal and ketoprofen in order to achieve the enhanced solubility in water and drug delivery by transdermal route. NSAIDs are very effective in the treatment of acute and chronic rheumatoid and osteoarthritis, however, clinical use of NSAIDs is often limited by adverse events such as gastrointestinal side effects (dyspepsia, gastrointestinal bleeding) and renal side effects when given orally. Transdermal drug delivery can overcome these adverse effects; however transdermal delivery suffers poor rates of transcutaneous delivery due to barrier function of the skin. PAMAM dendrimer complex with NSAIDs could improve the drug permeation through the skin as penetration enhancer (Chauhan *et al.,* 2003; Cheng *et al.,* 2007). Enhanced *in vitro* permeation was observed with dendrimer-NSAIDs complex. In case of indomethacin when tested against rat model, the indomethacin concentration was significantly higher with PAMAM dendrimers when compared to the pure drug suspension. The results showed that effective concentration could be maintained for 24 hr in the blood with the G4 dendrimer–indomethacin formulation. Tamsulosin has also been delivered transdermally through dendrimers (Wang *et al.,* 2003).

2.6.2.4 Ocular and Pulmonary Drug Delivery

There are few reports that dendrimers could have applicability *via* other delivery routes such as ocular, pulmonary and topical. Ocular delivery is preferred route of administration in eye related disorders. However residence time of the topically applied drugs is very less due to drainage by nasolachrymal duct and tears. The ideal ocular drug-delivery systems should be nonirritating, sterile, isotonic, biocompatible, does not run out from the eye and biodegradable. Some of the research groups have attempted to achieve the desired properties of ocular drug delivery systems using dendrimers. Pilocarpine nitrate and tropicamide bioavailability has been found to be enhanced using dendrimers (Vandamme and Brobeck, 2005). Results of a miotic activity test on albino rabbits indicated that PAMAM dendrimers improved bioavailability of pilocarpine nitrate compared to control and also prolonged the miotic effect, indicating increased precorneal residence time. Precluding 4G PAMAM dendrimers, in case of mydriatic activity test of tropicamide, all the dendrimer generations enhanced pharmacological activity compared with controls. In a study the ocular absorption of the puerarin and gatifloxacin has been found to be enhanced using dendrimers.

Dendrimers has not been studied much for the pulmonary delivery of the drugs. However researchers have attempted to deliver dendrimers based formulations using pulmonary route (Bai *et al.,* 2007). In a recent study pulmonary absorption of low molecular weight heparin (LMWH) was found to be enhanced using PEGylated PAMAM dendrimers. The authors concluded that PEGylated PAMAM dendrimer could potentially be used as a carrier for pulmonary delivery of LMWH for the long-term management of deep vein thrombosis as studied in rat model. In another study, efficacy of PAMAM dendrimers in enhancing pulmonary absorption of enoxaparin was also studied by measuring plasma anti-factor Xa activity, and by observing prevention efficacy of deep vein thrombosis in a rodent model. PAMAM dendrimers increased the relative bioavailability of enoxaparin by 40%, while half generation dendrimers had no effect. Formulations did not adversely affect mucociliary transport rate or produce extensive damage to the lungs demonstrating that positively charged dendrimers are suitable carrier for enoxaparin pulmonary delivery (Bai *et al.,* 2007).

2.6.3 Applications in Gene Delivery

The first human clinical trials of gene transfection were initiated in 1990, but so far success has been limited by a shortage of methods for delivering the genetic material. The development of efficient and nontoxic vectors that can transport exogenous DNA into cells is required to complement the original viral vectors. Dendrimers can act as non-viral vectors, in gene therapy (Tang *et al.,* 1996). Vectors transfer genes through the cell membrane into the nucleus. PAMAM dendrimers due to their cationic charge have been tested as genetic material carriers. Terminal amino groups present on the dendrimer surface interact with phosphate groups of nucleic acids. This ensures consistent formation of transfection complexes (Fig. 2.9). A transfection reagent called SuperFect™ consisting of activated dendrimers is commercially available. Activated dendrimers can carry a larger amount of genetic material than viruses. SuperFect–DNA complexes are characterized by high stability and provide more efficient transport of DNA into the nucleus than liposomes. The other most common class of dendrimers used for gene delivery is PPI. The use of dendrimers as gene transfection agents and drug-delivery devices have been extensively reviewed (Boas and Heegaard, 2004).

2.6.4 Applications as MRI Contrast Agent

Dendrimers were found to act as MRI contrast agents in early 1990 (Wiener *et al.,* 1994). Magnetic resonance imaging (MRI) is a technique of diagnosis which gives anatomical images of organs and blood vessels of patient in the effect of a generated, defined magnetic field. The photograph is the result of the nuclear resonance signal of water, which is assigned to its place of origin. Addition of contrast agents (paramagnetic metal cations) improves sensitivity and specificity of the method. Gadolinium salt of diethylene triamine pentaacetic acid (DTPA) is used clinically. Dendrimers due to their properties are highly suited for use as image contrast media. Several groups have prepared dendrimers containing gadolinium ions chelated on the surface. Preliminary tests show that such dendrimers are stronger contrast agents than conventional ones. They also improve visualisation of vascular structures in MRA of the body.

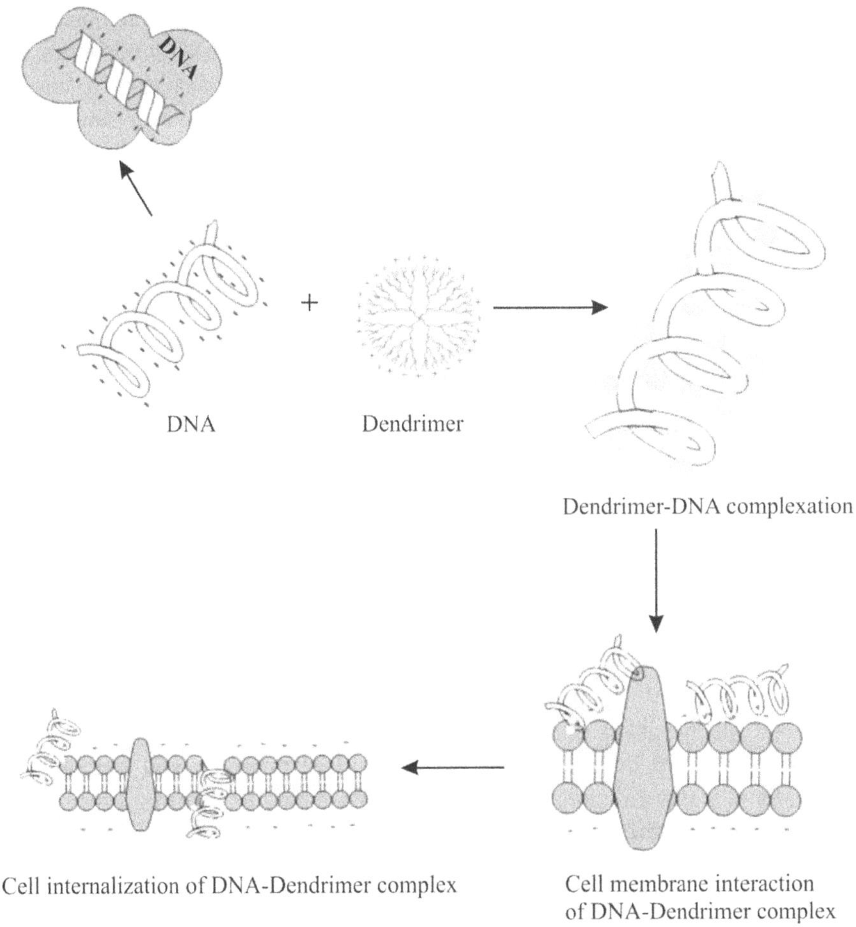

Fig. 2.9 Dendrimer's role in gene delivery.

2.6.5 Applications in Boron Neutron Capture Therapy (BNCT)

BNCT is a radiation therapy that brings together two components that when kept separate have only minor effects on cells. The first component is a stable isotope of boron (boron-10) that can be concentrated in tumor cells by attaching it to tumor seeking compounds. The second is a beam of low-energy neutrons. Boron-10 in or adjacent to the tumor cells disintegrates after capturing a neutron and the high energy heavy charged particles produced destroy only the cells in close proximity to it, primarily cancer cells, leaving adjacent normal cells largely unaffected. The use of dendrimers as boron carriers for antibody conjugation has been reported due to the well-defined structure and polyvalency. In initial studies, (Barth *et al.,* 1994) conjugated isocyanato polyhedral borane to the periphery of second- and fourth-generation PAMAM dendrimers. In another study, boronated PAMAM dendrimers were designed to target the epidermal growth factor (EGF) receptor, a cell surface receptor that is frequently overexpressed in brain tumors. In this study [G-5] PAMAM dendrimer carrying 1100 boron atoms was conjugated to cetuximab, a monoclonal antibody specific for the EGF receptor. *In vivo* studies showed that, after intratumoral injection, the conjugates were present at an almost tenfold greater concentration in brain tumors than in normal brain tissues (Wu *et al.,* 2004).

2.6.6 Applications in Photodynamic Therapy (PDT)

PDT is one of the novel therapies for the treatment of cancer. Dendrimers have been reported to have applications in PDT. This cancer treatment involves the administration of a light activated photosensitizing drug that selectively concentrates in diseased tissue (Dougherty *et al.,* 1998). Subsequent activation of the photosensitizer leads to the generation of reactive oxygen species, primarily singlet oxygen, that damage intracellular species such as lipids and amino acid residues through oxidation, ultimately leading to cell death. The possibility of improving the properties of dendrimers through appropriate functionalization of their periphery makes dendrimers promising carriers for photosensitizers. 5-aminolevulinic acid has been used in dendrimers based studies for PDT. It is a natural precursor of the photosensitizer protoporphyrin IX, and its administration is known to increase cellular concentrations of protoporphyrin. Some of poly aryl ether dendrimers have been reported applications in the field of PDT (Nishiyama *et al.,* 2003).

References

Agrawal P, Gupta U, and Jain N.K (2007). Glycoconjugated peptide dendrimers-based nanoparticulate system for the delivery of chloroquine phosphate. *Biomaterials* **28:** 3349-3359.

Asthana A, Chauhan A.S, Diwan P.V, and Jain N.K (2005). Poly(amidoamine) (PAMAM) dendritic nanostructures for controlled site-specific delivery of acidic anti-inflammatory active ingredient. *AAPS PharmSciTech* **6:** E536-542.

Bai S, Thomas C, and Ahsan F (2007). Dendrimers as a carrier for pulmonary delivery of enoxaparin, a low-molecular weight heparin. *Journal of Pharmaceutical Sciences* **96:** 2090-2106.

Barth R.F, Adams D.M, Soloway A.H, Alam F, and Darby M.V (1994). Boronated starburst dendrimer-monoclonal antibody immuno-conjugates: evaluation as a potential delivery system for neutron capture therapy. *Bioconjugate Chemistry* **5:** 58-66.

Betley T.A, Hessler J.A, Mecke A, Banaszak Holl M.M, Orr B.G, Uppuluri S, Tomalia D.A, and Baker J.R (2002). Tapping Mode Atomic Force Microscopy Investigation of Poly(amidoamine) Core−Shell Tecto(dendrimers) Using Carbon Nanoprobes. *Langmuir : the ACS Journal of Surfaces and Colloids* **18:** 3127-3133.

Bhadra D, Bhadra S, Jain S, and Jain N.K (2003). A PEGylated dendritic nanoparticulate carrier of fluorouracil. *International Journal of Pharmaceutics* **257:** 111-124.

Bhadra D, Yadav A.K, Bhadra S, and Jain N.K (2005). Glycodendrimeric nanoparticulate carriers of primaquine phosphate for liver targeting. *International Journal of Pharmaceutics* **295:** 221-233.

Boas U, and Heegaard P.M (2004). Dendrimers in drug research. *Chemical Society Reviews* **33:** 43-63.

Buhleier E, Wehner W, and Vögtle F (1978). Cascade and nonskid-chain-like synthesis of molecular cavity topologies. *Synthesis* **2:** 155-158.

Caminade A.M, Laurent R, and Majoral J.P (2005). Characterization of dendrimers. *Advanced Drug Delivery Reviews* **57:** 2130-2146.

Caminati G, Turro N.J, and Tomalia D.A (1990). Photophysical investigation of starburst dendrimers and their interactions with anionic and cationic surfactants. *Journal of the American Chemical Society* **112:** 8515-8522.

Chauhan A.S, Sridevi S, Chalasani K.B, Jain A.K, Jain S.K, Jain N.K, and Diwan P.V (2003). Dendrimer-mediated transdermal delivery: enhanced bioavailability of indomethacin. *Journal of Controlled Release : Official Journal of the Controlled Release Society* **90:** 335-343.

Cheng Y, Man N, Xu T, Fu R, Wang X, Wang X, and Wen L (2007). Transdermal delivery of nonsteroidal anti-inflammatory drugs mediated by polyamidoamine (PAMAM) dendrimers. *Journal of Pharmaceutical Sciences* **96:** 595-602.

Choi Y, Thomas T, Kotlyar A, Islam M.T, and Baker J.R, Jr. (2005). Synthesis and functional evaluation of DNA-assembled polyamidoamine dendrimer clusters for cancer cell-specific targeting. *Chemistry & Biology* **12:** 35-43.

Crespo L, Sanclimens G, Pons M, Giralt E, Royo M, and Albericio F (2005). Peptide and amide bond-containing dendrimers. *Chemical Reviews* **105:** 1663-1681.

D'Emanuele A, Jevprasesphant R, Penny J, and Attwood D (2004). The use of a dendrimer-propranolol prodrug to bypass efflux transporters and enhance oral bioavailability. *Journal of Controlled Release : Official Journal of the Controlled Release Society* **95:** 447-453.

de Brabander-van den Berg E.M.M, and Meijer E.W (1993). Poly(propylene imine) Dendrimers: Large-Scale Synthesis by Hetereogeneously Catalyzed Hydrogenations. *Angewandte Chemie International Edition in English* **32:** 1308-1311.

Devarakonda B, Hill R.A, and de Villiers M.M (2004). The effect of PAMAM dendrimer generation size and surface functional group on the aqueous solubility of nifedipine. *International Journal of Pharmaceutics* **284:** 133-140.

Dougherty T.J, Gomer C.J, Henderson B.W, Jori G, Kessel D, Korbelik M, Moan J, and Peng Q (1998). Photodynamic therapy. *Journal of National Cancer Institute* **90:** 889-905.

Duncan R, and Izzo L (2005). Dendrimer biocompatibility and toxicity. *Advanced Drug Delivery Reviews* **57:** 2215-2237.

Dutta T, and Jain N.K (2007). Targeting potential and anti-HIV activity of lamivudine loaded mannosylated poly (propyleneimine) dendrimer. *Biochimica et Biophysica Acta* **1770:** 681-686.

Frechet J.M (1994). Functional polymers and dendrimers: reactivity, molecular architecture, and interfacial energy. *Science* **263:** 1710-1715.

Gupta U, Agashe H.B, Asthana A, and Jain N.K. (2006). Dendrimers: novel polymeric nanoarchitectures for solubility enhancement. *Biomacromolecules* **7:** 649-658.

Gupta U, Agashe H.B, and Jain N.K (2007). Polypropylene imine dendrimer mediated solubility enhancement: effect of pH and functional groups of hydrophobes. *Journal of Pharmacy & Pharmaceutical Sciences : A Publication of the Canadian Society for Pharmaceutical Sciences, Societe Canadienne des Sciences Pharmaceutiques* **10:** 358-367.

Hawker C.J, and Frechet J.M (1990). Preparation of polymers with controlled molecular architecture. A new convergent approach to dendritic macromolecules. *Journal of the American Chemical Society* **112:** 7638-7647.

Hawker C.J, Wooley K.L, and Fréchet J.M (1993). Unimolecular micelles and globular amphiphiles: dendritic macromolecules as novel recyclable solubilization agents. *Journal of the Chemical Society, Perkin Transactions* **1:** 1287-1297.

Jain N.K, and Gupta U (2008). Application of dendrimer-drug complexation in the enhancement of drug solubility and bioavailability. *Expert Opinion on Drug Metabolism & Toxicology* **4:** 1035-1052.

Jain N.K, and Khopade A.J (2001). Dendrimers as potential delivery systems for bio-actives (New Delhi, CBS Publishers & Distributors).

Jevprasesphant R, Penny J, Attwood D, McKeown N.B, and D'Emanuele A. (2003). Engineering of dendrimer surfaces to enhance transepithelial transport and reduce cytotoxicity. *Pharmaceutical Research* **20:** 1543-1550.

Kawaguchi T, Walker K.L, Wilkins C.L, and Moore J.S (1995). Double exponential dendrimer growth. *Journal of the American Chemical Society* **117:** 2159-2165.

Khopade A.J, Caruso F, Tripathi P, Nagaich S, and Jain N.K (2002). Effect of dendrimer on entrapment and release of bioactive from liposomes. *International Journal of Pharmaceutics* **232:** 157-162.

Kojima C, Kono K, Maruyama K, and Takagishi T (2000). Synthesis of polyamidoamine dendrimers having poly(ethylene glycol) grafts and their ability to encapsulate anticancer drugs. *Bioconjugate Chemistry* **11:** 910-917.

Kukowska-Latallo J.F, Candido K.A, Cao Z, Nigavekar S.S, Majoros I.J, Thomas T.P, Balogh L.P, Khan M.K, and Baker J.R., Jr. (2005). Nanoparticle targeting of anticancer drug improves therapeutic response in animal model of human epithelial cancer. *Cancer Research* **65:** 5317-5324.

Kumar P.V, Asthana A, Dutta T, and Jain N.K (2006). Intracellular macrophage uptake of rifampicin loaded mannosylated dendrimers. *Journal of Drug Targeting* **14:** 546-556.

Kwon G, Naito M, Yokoyama M, Okano T, Sakurai Y, and Kataoka K (1997). Block copolymer micelles for drug delivery: loading and release of doxorubicin. *Journal of Controlled Release : Official Journal of the Controlled Release Society* **48:** 195-201.

Meijer E, Jansen J, and De Brabander-van den Berg E (1994). Encapsulation of guest molecules into a dendritic box. *Science* **266:** 1226-1229.

Milhem O.M, Myles C, McKeown N.B, Attwood D, and D'Emanuele A (2000). Polyamidoamine Starburst dendrimers as solubility enhancers. *International Journal of Pharmaceutics* **197:** 239-241.

Newkome G.R, Yao Z, Baker G.R, and Gupta V.K (1985). Micelles. Part 1. Cascade molecules: a new approach to micelles. A [27]-arborol. *The journal of Organic Chemistry* **50:** 2003-2004.

Nishiyama N, Stapert H.R, Zhang G.D, Takasu D, Jiang D.L, Nagano T, Aida T, and Kataoka K (2003). Light-harvesting ionic dendrimer porphyrins as new photosensitizers for photodynamic therapy. *Bioconjugate Chemistry* **14:** 58-66.

Ooya T, Lee J, and Park K (2003). Effects of ethylene glycol-based graft, star-shaped, and dendritic polymers on solubilization and controlled release of paclitaxel. *Journal of Controlled Release : Official Journal of the Controlled Release Society* **93:** 121-127.

Patri A.K, Kukowska-Latallo J.F, and Baker J.R, Jr (2005). Targeted drug delivery with dendrimers: comparison of the release kinetics of covalently conjugated drug and non-covalent drug inclusion complex. *Advanced Drug Delivery Reviews* **57:** 2203-2214.

Svenson S, and Tomalia D.A (2005). Dendrimers in biomedical applications--reflections on the field. *Advanced Drug Delivery Reviews* **57:** 2106-2129.

Tang M.X, Redemann C.T, and Szoka F.C, Jr (1996). *In vitro* gene delivery by degraded polyamidoamine dendrimers. *Bioconjugate Chemistry* **7:** 703-714.

Thiagarajan G, Greish K, and Ghandehari H (2013). Charge affects the oral toxicity of poly(amidoamine) dendrimers. *European Journal of Pharmaceutics and Biopharmaceutics : Official Journal of Arbeitsgemeinschaft fur Pharmazeutische Verfahrenstechnik* eV **84:** 330-334.

Thomas B.J, and Finnin B.C (2004). The transdermal revolution. *Drug Discovery Today* **9:** 697-703.

Tomalia D, Baker H, Dewald J, Hall M, Kallos G, Martin S, Roeck J, Ryder J, and Smith P (1985). A new class of polymers: starburst-dendritic macromolecules. *Polymer Journal* **17:** 117-132.

Turnbull W.B, and Stoddart J.F (2002). Design and synthesis of glycodendrimers. *Journal of Biotechnology* **90:** 231-255.

Vandamme T.F, and Brobeck L (2005). Poly(amidoamine) dendrimers as ophthalmic vehicles for ocular delivery of pilocarpine nitrate and tropicamide. *Journal of Controlled Release : Official Journal of the Controlled Release Society* **102:** 23-38.

Venuganti V.V, and Perumal O.P (2009). Poly(amidoamine) dendrimers as skin penetration enhancers: Influence of charge, generation, and concentration. *Journal of Pharmaceutical Sciences* **98:** 2345-2356.

Wang Z, Itoh Y, Hosaka Y, Kobayashi I, Nakano Y, Maeda I, Umeda F, Yamakawa J, Kawase M, and Yag K (2003). Novel transdermal drug delivery system with polyhydroxyalkanoate and starburst polyamidoamine dendrimer. *Journal of Bioscience and Bioengineering* **95:** 541-543.

Wiener E.C, Brechbiel M.W, Brothers H, Magin R.L, Gansow O.A, Tomalia D.A, and Lauterbur P.C (1994). Dendrimer-based metal chelates: a new class of magnetic resonance imaging contrast agents. *Magnetic Resonance in Medicine. Official Journal of the Society of Magnetic Resonance in Medicine / Society of Magnetic Resonance in Medicine* **31:** 1-8.

Wiwattanapatapee R, Carreno-Gomez B, Malik N, and Duncan R (2000). Anionic PAMAM dendrimers rapidly cross adult rat intestine *in vitro*: a potential oral delivery system? *Pharmaceutical Research* **17:** 991-998.

Wu G, Barth R.F, Yang W, Chatterjee M, Tjarks W, Ciesielski M.J, and Fenstermaker R.A (2004). Site-specific conjugation of boron-containing dendrimers to anti-EGF receptor monoclonal antibody cetuximab (IMC-C225) and its evaluation as a potential delivery agent for neutron capture therapy. *Bioconjugate Chemistry* **15:** 185-194.

Yiyun C, and Tongwen X (2005). Dendrimers as potential drug carriers. Part I. Solubilization of non-steroidal anti-inflammatory drugs in the presence of polyamidoamine dendrimers. *European Journal of Medicinal Chemistry* **40:** 1188-1192.

3

Liposomes: Manufacturing and Applications

Varsha Tilwani, Priyanka Jain, Darshana Jain, Nishi Mody and Aviral Jain

Pharmaceutics Research Laboratory, Department of Pharmaceutics,
Adina Institute of Pharmaceutical Sciences, Sagar (M.P.), India. 470002.

3.1 Introduction

With the advent of drug design, lipid based drug delivery system has gained immense impetus due to their ability to serve as efficient carriers for poorly water soluble drugs. They are competent in encapsulating the drug and providing important advantages of targeted delivery, long circulation, low toxicity, sustained-release, non-immunogenicity and protecting the encapsulated drugs from the destructive action of the external environment.

Liposomes are simply vesicles in which an aqueous volume is entirely enclosed by membrane composed of lipid molecules usually phospholipid (New, 1990). Liposomes were first discovered in 1960's by Bangham and Colleagues and were initially used as model for studying the biological membrane (Bangham *et al.,* 1965).

Liposomes are highly versatile structures for research, therapeutic, and analytical applications. They are basically composed of a lipid bilayer with the hydrophobic chains of the lipids forming the bilayer and the polar head groups of the lipids oriented towards the extravesicular solution and inner cavity (Edwards and Baeumner, 2006). Their structure is similar to that of cells, and thus can be used conviniently as a vessel for studying interactions between membrane lipids and biomolecules such as

DNA (Angelova and Tsoneva, 1999) and proteins (Fischer *et al.,* 2000) permeability of ions (Edwards and Baeumner, 2006; Toyran and Severcan, 2003) and drugs (Romanowski *et al.,* 1997), and elucidating the mechanism of action of pesticides (Braguini *et al.,* 2004) and antibiotics on target organisms (Grancelli *et al.,* 2002; Trombetta *et al.,* 2001).

3.1.1 Structure of Liposomes

Structurally, liposomes are defined as concentric bilayered vesicles in which an aqueous volume is enclosed by a membranous lipid bilayer. The vescicular size range can vary from few nanometers to tens of micron. The liposomes are so prepared that they can entrap quantities of material both within their aqueous compartment as well as in lipid membrane.

Liposomes are classified on the basis of size, number of bilayers present in the vescicle or the fabrication methods employed in development stage. When liposomes are described based on the number of bilayers they fall either under unilamellar vesicles (ULV) or multilamellar vesicles (MLV). When the description is based on their size, they are sectioned into large unilamellar vesicles (LUV) and small unilamellar vesicles (SUV).

3.1.2 Composition of Liposomes

The name liposome is derived from two Greek words: 'Lipos' meaning fat and 'Soma' meaning body. The lipid in the plasma membrane are chiefly phospholipids like phosphatidylethanolamine and phosphatidylcholine etc. along with the steroidal moiety mainly cholesterol.

3.1.2.1 Phospholipids

The general chemical structure of phospholipids has a glycerol backbone. Phosphatidic acid which might be the simplest phospholipid has a phosphoric acid moiety esterified to the hydroxl group present on carbon number 3 of glycerol molecule. The hydroxyl groups at positions 1 and 2 of the glycerol are then usually esterified with long chain fatty acids to build up more complicated phospholoipids. One of the remaining oxygen groups of phosphoric acid may further esterified to a variety of organic molecules including glycerol, choline, ethanolamine, serine and inositol. The phosphate moiety along with the attached alcohol represent the head group of phospholipid (Fig. 3.1). Various head groups and the name of phosphatidic acid with the head group are reported in Table 3.1. The most abundant phosphatide in plants and animals is phosphatidyl choline (also known as lecithin) and phosphatidyl ethanolamine. These two components constitute the major structural part of most biological membranes. In phosphatidyl serine the phosphoric acid moiety is esterified to the hydroxyl group of the amino acid L-serine and in phosphatidyl inositol to one of the hydroxyl groups of the cyclic sugar alcohol inositol. In the case of phosphatidyl glycerol the alcohol that is esterified to the phosphate moiety is glycerol. Phosphatidyl glycerol is found as a natural component of the lung surfactant of humans. The lipid nature of the phospholipid is due to the long chain fatty acids. Fatty acid chain length, saturation or branching of phospholipids molecule is important and differences in fatty acid part can change the characteristics of the phospholipids. Fatty acids differ in number of carbon atoms chain and degree of unsaturation (Florkin and Stotz, 1967). Fatty acid composition of phosphatidylcholines extracted from soybean oil and egg yolk are reported in Table 3.2.

There are a number of synthetic phospholipids available and utilized in the preparation of liposomes. The tissue distribution and clearance kinetics of drug containing liposomes are known to be affected by lipid composition and surface charge (Juliano and Stamp, 1975). Gangliosides are a class of sphingolipids, are sometimes included in liposome formulations to provide a layer of surface charged groups, to provide longer circulating liposomes in the blood stream (Vemuri and Rhodes, 1995).

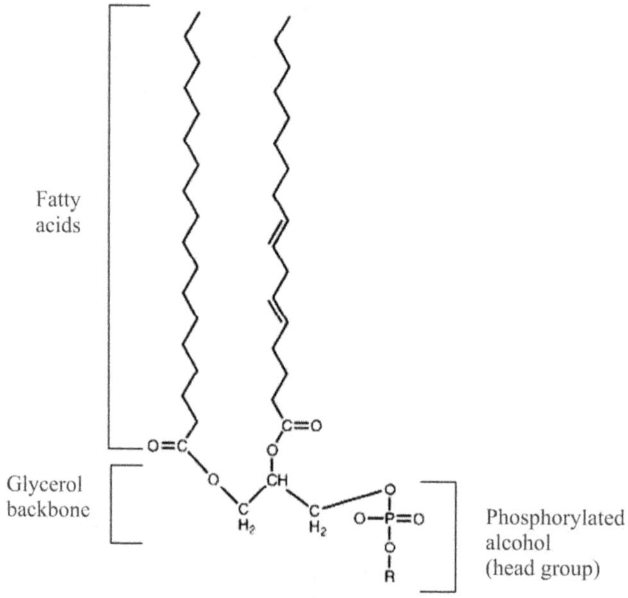

Fig. 3.1 Structure of phosphatidic acid (fatty acids, glycerol backbone & phosphorylated alcohol).

Table 3.1 Some common naturally occurring phosphatidyl phospholipids.

Common name	Abbreviation	Head group
Phosphatidyl ethanolamine	PE	$-CH_2-CH_2-NH_3^+$
Phosphatidyl glycerol	PG	$-CH_2-CHOH-CH_2OH$
Phosphatidyl choline	PC	$-CH_2-CH_2-N(CH_3)_3^+$
Phosphatidyl serine	PS	$-CH_2-CH-NH_2COOH$
Phosphatidyl inositol	PI	$-(CHOH)_6$
Phosphatidic acid	PA	O-H

Table 3.2 Fatty acid composition of phosphatidyl choline of egg yolk and soya bean oil origin

Fatty acid composition		Phosphatidylcholine	
		EGG	Soya bean
16:0	Palmitic	32	12
16:1	Palmitoleic	1.5	< 0.2
18:0	Stearic	16	2.3
18:1	Oleic	26	10
18:2	Linoleic	13	68
18:3	Linolenic	< 0.3	5
20:4	Arachidonic	4.8	< 0.1
22:5	Docosapentaenoic	4.0	< 0.1

3.1.2.2 Cholesterol

Cholesterol has a steroid backbone and its derivatives are included in liposome preparation. Cholesterol is found in animal membranes. It has been used in the preparation of liposomes to improve the bilayer characteristics of the liposomes. Cholesterol improves the fluidity of the bilayer membrane, reduces the permeability of water soluble molecules through the membrane, and improves the stability of bilayer membrane in the presence biological fluids such as blood/plasma. Liposomes without cholesterol tend to react with the blood proteins such as albumin, m-transferrin, and macroglobulin. These components tend to destabilize the liposomes and reduce the utility of liposomes as drug delivery systems. Cholesterol appears to reduce this type of interaction with blood proteins. Although the presence of a large quantity of cholesterol in a vesicle will effectively protect it against plasma-induced solute release, the loss of liposomal phospholipid cannot be entirely prevented (Damen *et al.,* 1981). Cholesterol molecule orients itself among the phospholipid molecules with its hydroxyl group facing towards the water phase, the tricyclic ring sandwiched between the first few carbons of the fatty acyl chains, into the hydrocarbon core of the bilayer (Vemuri and Rhodes, 1995).

3.1.3 Bilayer Properties of Liposomes

Liposomes in solution behave much like charged particles in colloid solutions. Two populations of liposomes bearing opposite charges tend to aggregate. The rate of aggregation is similar to that caused by the electrostatic attractive forces among the particles. The tendency of liposomes aggregation and fusion can be controlled by the addition of small amounts of acidic or basic lipids to the formulations. The magnitude of the electrostatic forces generated by the charged liposomes can be calculated and controlled by the 'double layer' theory of colloids.

Since liposomes are thermodynamically unstable, the method of their preparation will influence their physical structure. Surface chemistry of detergents offer information on monolayer films and perhaps that information can be used to learn about phospholipid bilayers. The surface chemistry of detergents, for example, suggest that the properties of liposomes made with phospholipids can be controlled by (a) increasing the hydrocarbon chain length of the fatty acid part of the phospholipid which in turn results in tighter film packing; (b) increasing the degree of unsaturation of the hydrocarbon chain of the phospholipid chain resulting in looser film packaging; (c) increasing the degree of branching of the hydrocarbon chain of the phospholipid which leads to slack film packing; (d) increasing the temperature of the system which results in looser film packing; and finally (e) by adding cholesterol to the phospholipid film which results in tighter film packing (Vemuri and Rhodes, 1995).

3.2 Method of Preparation of Liposomes

Numerous methods have been developed to prepare liposomes. Depending on the requirement in terms of type of drug loading or type/size of liposomal vesicles any of the following methods can be used.

3.2.1 Mechanical Dispersion

The mechanical dispersion method is simplest in concept in which lipids are dried down onto a solid dispersion and then dispersed by the addition of aqueous medium followed by shaking. Good entrapment of lipid soluble drugs can be achieved with this method. However, loading of water soluble drugs is compromised leading to low entrapment efficiencies. Hand shaking, sonication, freeze thawing and high pressure extrusion are covered under mechanical dispersion.

3.2.1.1 Hand Shaking Method

Hand shaken method is the simplest and most widely used method of mechanical dispersion for preparing liposomes. In this method, the lipids are dissolved in the organic solvents in a round bottom flask. The volatile organic solvent is evaporated using a rotary evaporator leading behind a thin film of lipid on the inner surface of round bottom flask. The flask is left on the rotary evaporator for 12-24 hr in order to remove traces of the organic solvent. Finally hydration of the lipid film is performed using aqueous medium leading to lipid swelling and peeling from the wall of the round bottom flask and formation of multi-lamellar vesicles (Bangham *et al.,* 1965).

For non-shaken method, the lipid film is exposed to a stream of water saturated nitrogen for 15 minutes which results in swelling of lipids without shaking. It is interesting to note that as compared to hand shaking method for preparing MLV, the vesicles produced by non-shaken method are LUV (Fig. 3.2).

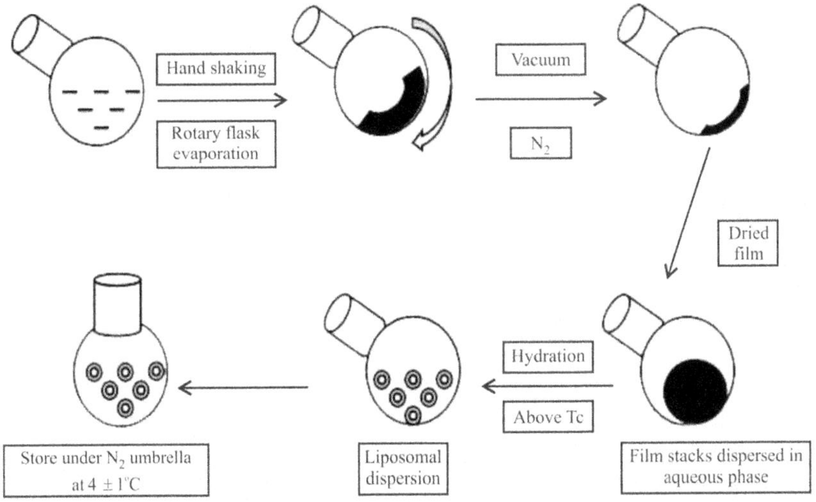

Fig. 3.2 Liposomes preparation using hand shaking method.

3.2.1.2 Non Shaking Method

This method is similar to the hand shaking method however it differs in terms of providing agitation. In the hand shaking method the agitation is provided by rotary evaporator whereas in non-shaking method a stream of nitrogen is used. The lipid is dissolved in a mixture of organic solvents in a conical flask and the organic solvent is evaporated at room temperature with the passage of nitrogen though the flask. After complete drying of the film, water saturated nitrogen is passed through the flask leading to hydration of the film and is continued until opacity of the dried film disappears. After hydrating the film, the liposomes are swelled by the addition of bulk of the swelling media. The content of the flask is flushed with nitrogen, sealed and allowed to stand for 2-4 hr at 35-40 °C for complete swelling and formation of stable liposomes (Reeves and Dowben, 1969).

3.2.1.3 Freeze Drying Method

The principle of formation of liposomal vesicles with mechanical dispersion method is to disperse the lipid in fine form. In the freeze drying method this particular objective is achieved by formation of solution of lipids in a suitable organic solvent followed by freeze drying in order to remove the solvent. Tertiary butanol is a suitable solvent to be used for preparation of liposomes by freeze drying method.

All the methods discussed above generally produce MLV with heterogeneous population. However as far as drug delivery is concerned SUV with homogenous population are preferred. Formulated MLV can be subjected to following techniques in order to produce liposomes with desired features.

3.2.1.4 Micro-Emulsification Method

Microfluidizer, a high pressure homogenizer manufactured by Microfludics, USA is now commonly used in order to reduce the size of various formulations including liposomes. The microfluidizer is a machine which pumps fluid at a very high pressure (10,000 psi, 600-700 bar), through a 5 μm filter flowed by movement through defined micro channels which direct the two streams of fluid to collide at right angles at a very high velocity, causing efficient transfer of energy. The lipids can be introduced into the fluidizer, either as a suspension of large MLV or as slurry of un-hydrated lipid in an aqueous medium. The fluid collected can be recycled through the pump and interaction chamber until vesicles of required dimensions are obtained (Mayhew *et al.,* 1984).

3.2.1.5 Sonicated Vesicles

Disruption of hydrated lipids using sonic energy (sonication) produces small unilamellar vesicles with diameter in the range of 20-200 nm. The most common instrument used for the preparation of sonicated particles is probe sonicator and bath sonicator to some extent. The probe sonicator is employed for suspension which requires high energy in small volume (e.g., high concentration of lipids or viscous aqueous phase), while the bath sonicator is more suitable for large volumes of dilute lipids. Probe sonication is very good method for reducing the size of large liposomes but it suffers from the drawback that it is impossible to completely eliminate the risk of lipid degradation when it comes in contact with hot probe and the contamination which occurs due to titanium that leaches from the probe. The rise in temperature can be controlled by placing the container having liposomal formulation in ice bath. The ice helps in dissipating the heat generated by ultrasonic waves. After sonication process the size of the vesicles is checked and the cycle can be repeated until desired size is achieved (Fig. 3.3).

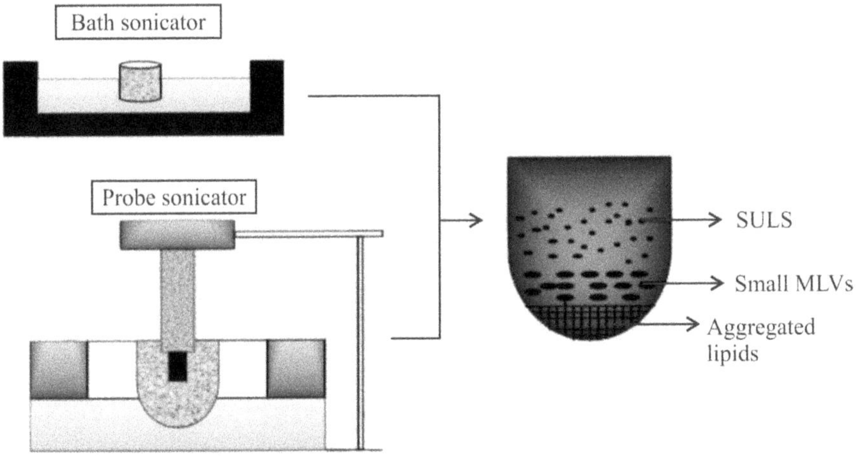

Fig. 3.3 Liposomes prepared by sonication method.

3.2.1.6 French Pressure Cell

In order to circumvent the degradation of lipids as well as macromolecules by ultrasonic radiation, other methods are developed which are able to cause fragmentation and restructuring of membrane under mild conditions. One of the first and very useful techniques developed is extrusion of preformed large vesicles in a French Press under generally high pressure. This technique yields rather homogenous uni-or-oligo lamellar liposomes preparation of intermediate size depending on pressure employed. The method is simple, rapid, and reproducible and involves gentle handling of unstable materials. Liposomes prepared by this technique are somewhat larger than vesicles prepared by sonication but are less likely to suffer from the structural defects and instabilities know to arise in sonciated vesicles. Leakage of the drug form liposomes prepared from French press has been found to be slower than sonicated liposomes. The French press has also been used to reduce the hetreogenicity of populations of proteoliposomes obtained by detergent analysis technique (Hamilton *et al.,* 1980) (Fig. 3.4).

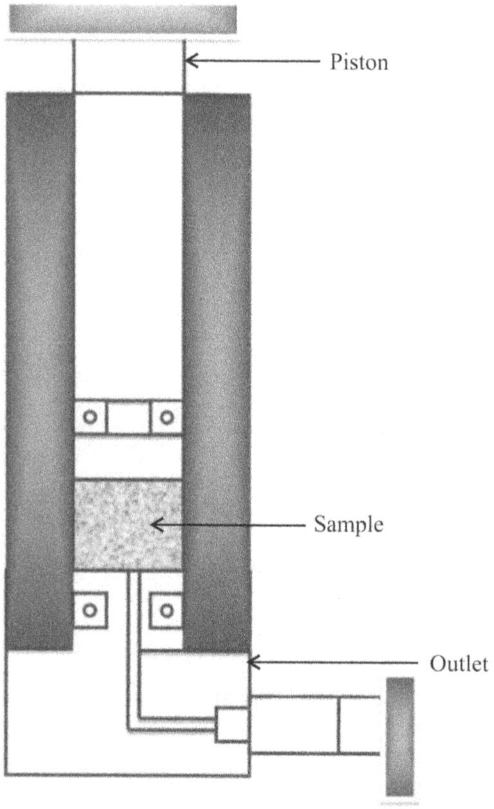

Fig. 3.4 Liposomes prepared by French pressure technique.

3.2.1.7 High Pressure Membrane Extrusion

It was demonstrated by several researchers that when MLV are repeatedly passed (5-10 passes) through very small pore polycarbonate membranes (0.2 to 1.0 μm) under high pressure the average diameter of the liposomes become progressively smaller reaching a minimum of 80-120 nm. As the average size is reduced the liposome vesicles tend to become unilamellar. Similar results were noted by other investigators when MLV were passed through a Microfluidizer that forces the feed material under high pressure through a narrow orifice (Vemuri *et al.,* 1990). When MLVs are forced, layers of bilayers are removed from the liposome structure. It was also suggested, that the mechanism of layer separation is only applicable to liposome vesicles made with positively charged phospholipids and the vesicles that are greater than 70 µm in size (Vemuri and Rhodes, 1995) (Fig. 3.5).

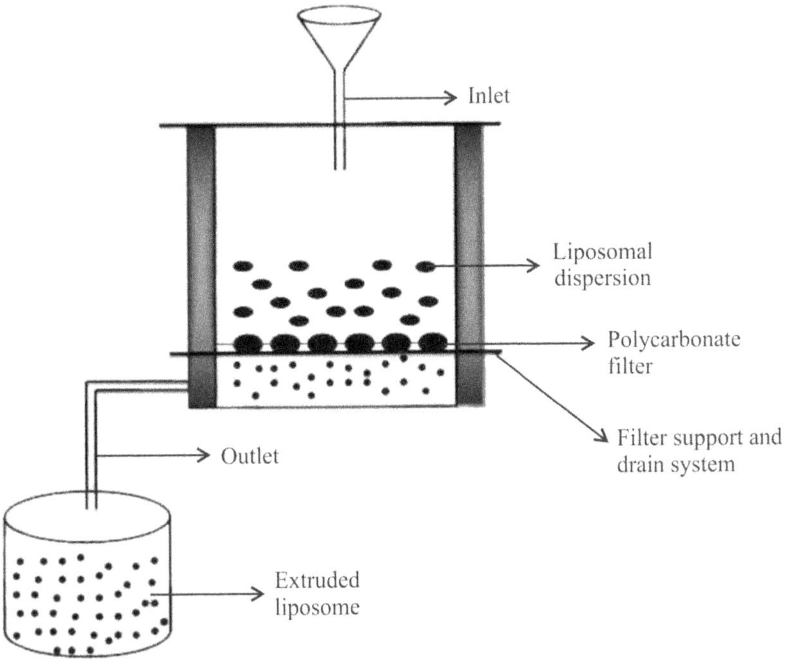

Fig. 3.5 Schematic representation of preparation of liposomes by high pressure membrane extrusion

3.2.2 Solvent Dispersion Methods

In these methods, the lipid(s) to be used for the preparation of liposomes are first dissolved in an organic solvent and the solution is brought in contact with aqueous phase containing drug or any other material to be entrapped within the liposomes. The phospholipids have the capability to self assemble and are therefore aligned at the interface comprising organic phase and aqueous phase into a monolayer leading to formation of lipid vesicles.

Methods employing solvent dispersion fall into one of the following categories.

(i) those in which the organic solvent is miscible with the aqueous phase

(ii) those in which the organic solvent is immiscible with the aqueous phase, the latter being in large excess

(iii) those in which the organic solvent is in large excess and is immiscible with the aqueous phase

3.2.2.1 Ethanol Injection Method

An alternative method for producing small liposomes that avoids both the sonication and exposure to high pressure is the ethanol injection technique. It was first described by Batzri and Korn in which the ethanol solution of lipids is injected rapidly into an excess of saline or other aqueous phase, through a fine needle (Batzri and Korn, 1973). The force of injection is usually sufficient to achieve complete mixing so that the ethanol is diluted almost instantaneously in water and phospholipid molecules are dispersed evenly through-out the medium. This procedure can yield a high proportion of SUV, although lipid aggregates and larger vesicles may form if the mixing is not thorough enough.

Ethanol injection method is simple, rapid and gentle to both lipids and the materials to be entrapped. Its major shortcoming is the limitation of the solubility of lipids in ethanol and the volume of ethanol that can be introduced into the medium which in turn limits the quantity of lipid dispersed so that the resulting liposomes suspension is usually dilute. Another drawback associated with this method is the difficult removal of ethanol from the phospholipid membranes and secondly the inactivation of some of the biologically active macromolecules in the presence of even low amounts of ethanol (Perrett *et al.,* 1991) (Fig. 3.6).

3.2.2.2 Ether Injection Method

This method was developed by Deamer and Bangham which provides a means of preparing the liposomes by slowly introducing a solution of lipids dissolved in diethyl ether into warm water (Deamer and Bangham, 1976). Typically it involves injecting the immiscible organic solution very slowly into an aqueous phase of the material to be encapsulated through a narrow size needle at such a temperature that the organic solvent is removed by vaporization during the process. The slow vaporization of solvent gives rise to an ether water gradient extending on both sides of the interfacial lipid monolayer resulting in the formation of bilayer sheet which folds itself to form a sealed vesicle. The diameter of the liposomes formed using this method is in range of 50-200 nm. The advantage of this method is that it is simple and can handle sensitive lipids very gently and possess very small risk of causing oxidative degradation. Since the solvent is removed at the same rate as it is introduced, there is no limit to the final concentration of lipid which can be achieved since the process can be run continuously for a long period of time, giving rise to a high percentage of the aqueous medium encapsulated within vesicles.

The primary shortcoming of the technique is that it takes long time for liposomal batch production. Another disadvantage is that the organic solvent used may be harmful for certain classes of solute and the method cannot be used to incorporate proteins into liposomes (Fig. 3.6).

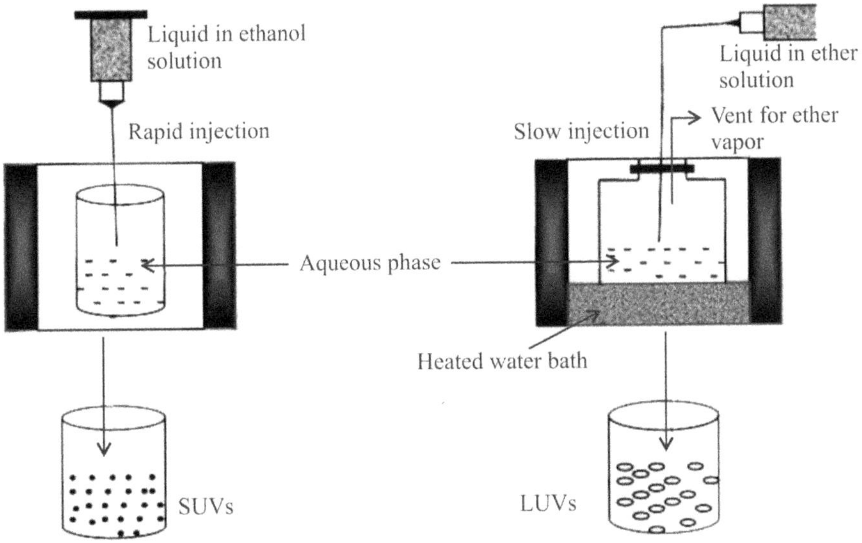

Fig. 3.6 Liposomes prepared by ethanol injection and ether injection method.

3.2.2.3 Double Emulsion Vesicles

In this method a double emulsion is formulated at room temperature (23 ± 2 °C) in two steps consisting of formulation of primary emulsion in first step followed by formulation of the double emulsion in second step. The double emulsion is usually water-in-oil-in-water ($W_1/O/W_2$) type of emulsion. In order to prepare the formulation, two phases, similar to conventional emulsion viz. oil phase and aqueous phase are used. Emulsifiers, co-emulsifiers, lyoprotectants, stabilizer, buffers and other pharmaceutical additives are also added to achieve stability. Water immiscible organic solvents viz. cyclohexane, ether, chloroform can be used as the oil phase. All oil soluble excipients including the phospholipids and drug are added to the oily phase and similarly the water soluble ingredients are dissolved in the aqueous phase. The aqueous phase is added to the oil phase slowly with constant stirring (speed is to be optimized) until a homogeneous emulsion (primary W_1/O

emulsion) is formed. The primary emulsion is very often sonicated (probe sonicator) to get a micro-emulsion. The primary micro-emulsion is observed for stability (phase separation) for at least 1-2 hr by visual observation. If emulsion is found to be stable, the second step is executed. The primary micro-emulsion (W_1/O) is slowly added to the specified quantity of aqueous phase and subjected to brisk homogenization. The double emulsion ($W_1/O/W_2$) is formed which can be sterilized by filtration. After formulation of the double emulsion, other techniques are adopted to get the liposomes such as solvent evaporation, lyophilization etc. In solvent evaporation method, the organic solvents of double emulsion are evaporated and the volume is adjusted with water. In the lyophilization technique the double emulsion is freeze dried and can be reconstituted with water whenever required. As a mechanistic view, the phospholipids dissolved in the organic solvent gets transported and spatially arranged at the interface between the organic and aqueous phase during continuous agitation. Due to high agitation the organic solvent is completely evaporated leaving a lipid film and hence a liposomal suspension is obtained (Fig. 3.7).

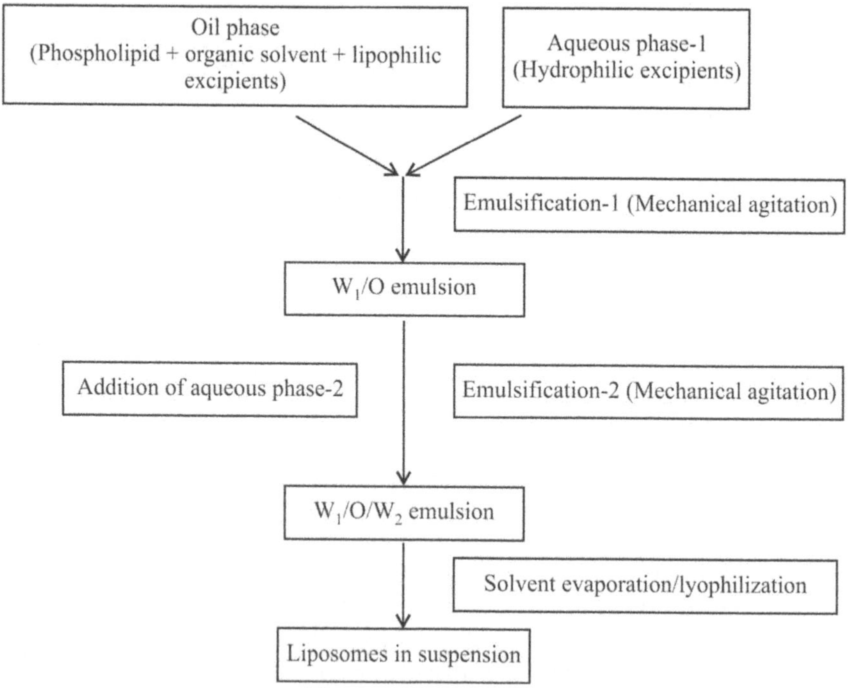

Fig. 3.7 Schematic representation of the steps of double emulsion method.

3.2.2.4 Multivesicular Liposomes

This technique is a variation of double emulsification method. The advantage of this method over double emulsion is that instead of just one single water droplet being entrapped in oil droplet of double emulsion several water droplets can be entrapped. Upon removal of the solvent by evaporation, these droplets remain intact and form multiple compartments within a single liposome. The authors of this technique have reported that a crucial ingredient of the lipid mixture is triolein a non-polar triglyceride which may accumulate at the junction where monolayers from three or more compartment interface and prevent rupture of these compartments during preparation. The multicompartment nature of the liposomes make them structurally more stable than single compartment liposomes of same size and have an entrapment yield of 50% or more (Kim *et al.,* 1983).

3.2.2.5 Reverse Phase Evaporation Method

Reverse phase evaporation (REV) method was developed by Szoka and Papahadjopoulos who were first to use 'water in oil' emulsion (Szoka and Papahadjopoulos, 1978). The droplets are formed by bath sonication of a mixture of two phases, followed by drying down of emulsion to a semi solid gel in a rotary evaporator under reduced pressure. At this stage the monolayers of phospholipid surrounding each compartment are closely opposed by each other and in the same case they already form part of a bilayer membrane separating adjacent compartments. The next step is to subject it to vigorous mechanical shaking using a vortex mixer in order to collapse a certain proportion of the water droplet. Under these circumstances, the lipid monolayer which enclosed the collapsed vesicles is contributed to adjacent intact vesicles to form the outer leaflet of the bilayer of large unilamellar liposomes. The aqueous content of the collapsed droplet provides the medium required for suspension of these newly formed liposomes. After the conversion of the gel into the homogenous free flowing fluid the dispersion is dialyzed to remove last traces of the solvent. The vesicles thus formed are unilamellar and have a diameter of 0.5μm with percentage entrapment of not more than 50% (Fig. 3.8).

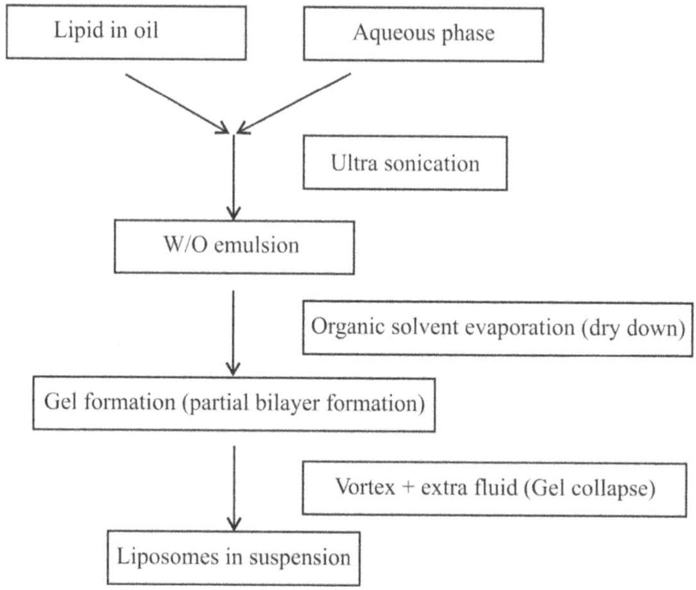

Fig. 3.8 Steps involved in the process of formulation of liposomes by reverse phase evaporation method.

3.2.2.6 Stable Plurilamellar Vesicles (SPLV)

In SPLV method, water in oil dispersion is prepared with lipid in excess, in which drying process is carried out using a stream of nitrogen accompanied by continuous bath sonication. The redistribution and equilibrium of aqueous solvent and solute occurs in between bilayer in each plurilamellar vesicle. Thus the internal structure of so formed plurilamellar differs from that of MLV-REV's as they are devoid of a large aqueous core. The majority of the entrapped aqueous medium being located in compartments is between the adjacent lamellae. Percentage entrapments are normally 30% (compared with $\geq$ 60% for MLV-REVs). The SPLV's have solute evenly distributed throughout the different compartments (Gruner *et al.,* 1985).

3.2.3 Detergent Removal (Depletion) Method

In this method, phospholipids are mixed together with the aqueous phase *via* detergent to form micellar mixtures. The detergent is then removed from the preparation and the micelles progressively become richer in phospholipid content and finally the lipids come together to form single bilayer vesicles.

Detergents that are commonly used for this purpose are those that have high critical micelle concentration (CMC). Materials such as sodium cholate, sodium deoxycholate, and octylglycoside and other detergents of high CMC (in the order of 10-20 mM) are suitable detergents for this work. The concentration of detergent in water at which micelles just start to form is known as "critical micelle concentration" (CMC). Below the CMC, the detergent molecules exist entirely in free solution. As the detergent is dissolved in water in higher concentration than the CMC, micelles form in more and more numbers, while the concentration of detergent in the free form remains essentially the same as it is at the CMC (Vemuri and Rhodes, 1994). A three stage model of the interaction for detergents with the lipid bilayers with increasing detergent/lipid radius has been proposed as discussed below:

- At low concentrations detergent equilibrates between vesicular lipid and water phase (stage-1). At this stage, mean vesicle size increases and functional properties of the bilayer changes.
- After reaching a critical detergent concentration (saturation of bilayers), membrane structure tends to be unstable and transforms gradually into micelles (stage-2). In this stage detergent saturated bilayers coexist with lipid saturated micelles.
- In stage-3, all the lipids exist in mixed micelle form.

This technique yields a homogeneous population of single layered vesicles. They are the best method for preparing liposomes with lipophilic proteins inserted into the membranes. Methods such as dialysis, column chromatography or adsorption onto biobeads can be used to remove the detergent from the preparation and transition of mixed micelles to concentric bilayered form. The main drawback of the method is the retention of traces of detergent(s) within the liposomes.

3.2.4 Active Loading

The methods described thus far have usually entrapped aqueous soluble entities, however certain modifications need to be adapted to ensure loading of ampiphillic entities. There are certain group of compounds which have both lipid as well as water solubility. Such compounds can be entrapped into liposomes only after the formation of an intact membrane which can control their movement. These compounds are often difficult to retain inside liposomes by normal means as they are able to pass in and out of the membrane readily because of their lipophilic behavior. Thus there exist an equilibrium between the interior and exterior of the liposomes (Mayer *et al.,* 1986).

The active loading method makes use of this behavior and creates such condition inside the vesicle that they remain in ionized form. Thus the solute after entering the liposomes membrane by diffusion in uncharged form is converted into charged form rendering it incapable to escape from liposomes as its lipophilicity is reduced. Therefore solutes accumulate inside the liposomes as long as pH difference is maintained between the interior and exterior of membrane. Such a difference can be brought about by entrappig a non-permeating buffer ion such as glutamate inside the liposomes at a low pH and replacing the extra liposomal buffer by one which is iso-osmolar at pH 7 (Fig. 3.9).

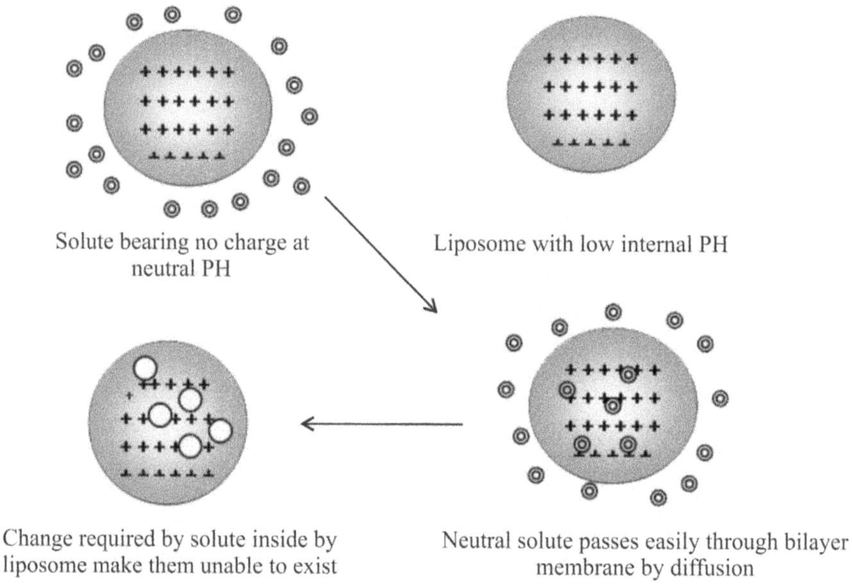
Solute bearing no charge at neutral PH
Liposome with low internal PH
Change required by solute inside by liposome make them unable to exist
Neutral solute passes easily through bilayer membrane by diffusion

Fig. 3.9 Principle of active loading.

Active loading methods have the following advantages over passive loading technique.

1. High encapsulation efficiency and capacity.
2. Reduced leakage of encapsulated compounds.
3. Encouraging Bed-side loading of drugs which restricts the loss of retention of drugs by diffusion or chemical degradation during storage.
4. It facilitates the development of transmembrane pH gradient using various methods depending upon the nature of the drug to be encapsulated.

3.2.5 pH Gradient Drug Loading

The use of transmembrane pH gradients to encapsulate drugs in liposomes is applicable to a wide variety of drug classes. A list of amine drugs (such as daunorubicin, doxorubicin, epirubicin, mitoxanthrone, vinblastine, chlorpromazine, dibucaine, lidocaine, quinidine, dopamine, serotonin, imipramine, diphenhydramine, quinine, and chloroquine) that respond to liposome preparations exhibit a pH-gradient effect (inside acidic) by accumulating protons inside the vesicle interior (Madden *et al.*, 1990). pH-gradient drug loading can be used to encapsulate a variety of antineoplastic, antianesthetics and antimalarials drugs.

Selection of buffer composition and pH during drug hydration and subsequent processing establishes the conditions of the vesicle size and interior composition of the vesicles. In order to create a pH gradient across the liposome membrane (inside acidic), the pH of the exterior aqueous compartment must be increased. This desired condition can be accomplished by more than one approach including addition of an alkaline buffer to increase the pH and exchanging the exterior media with the desired buffer by gel filtration technique or dialysis technique (Mayer *et al.*, 1993).

3.2.6 Lyophilization of Liposomes

Lyophilization yields high quality products with increased shelf-life. Lyophilized carrier is preferred when a drug is not stable in aqueous phase or it is not suitable for distribution in liquid state. If a drug molecule is not stable in aqueous media, it is very likely that it will be unstable when encapsulated in liposomes.

It has been reported that the liposomes containing drug molecules can be lyophilized and reconstituted with significant drug retention (measured as percent encapsulated drug) and without significant change in mean vesicle's size. Cryoprotection is needed during lyophilization and sugars such as sucrose, lactose and trehalose are used to protect the liposomes during freezing stage of lyophilization cycle. Upon rehydration water molecules quickly replace the sugars and liposomes appear to reseal before significant leakage occurs (Crowe *et al.*, 1985).

An important feature of phospholipid membrane is the existence of temperature-dependent reversible phase transition, where the hydrocarbon chains of the phospholipid undergo a transition from an ordered (gel) to a more disordered fluid (liquid crystalline) state. These changes have been documented by differential scanning calorimetry (DSC). The physical state of the bilayer affects the permeability, leakage and overall stability of the liposomes. Encapsulation of a drug in liposomes offers several advantages over conventional drug delivery systems. Sustained release and target delivery are good examples to name a few. However water soluble drugs tend to leak out during preparation as well as during shelf storage. The leakage problem is one of the limiting factors in commercial development of liposome products. Nevertheless, reasonable success has been attained to improve the long-term retention of encapsulated solutes by freeze-drying.

Freeze-dried phospholipid material and dry phospholipid films absorb water and swell. The degree of water absorption is a function of the hydrophilicity of the phospholipid's head group and the composition of the hydrocarbon chain.

3.3 Liposomes Scale up and Manufacturing Issues

3.3.1 Removal of Traces of Organic Solvents

Liposomal formulations contain a mixture of lipids, cholesterol and an anti-oxidant. In order to prevent oxidation of lipids during storage and to facilitate uniform and molecular dispersion, phospholipids are dissolved in organic solvents such as chloroform, ether, methylene chloride, methanol and their combinations. These organic solvents help in achieving a uniform distribution of lipids bilayer and the residual amounts of solvents left could pose health hazard to the user and the solvent residues must be kept below the toxic level of the solvents. But there are no set of higher acceptable limits for the organic solvents that can be ingested by a human being.

In the preparation of molecular mixtures of lipids, large volumes of solvents are used and then it is removed by solvent evaporation technique which tends to concentrate the lipids as well as the contaminants in the solvents. In order to avoid concentration of solvent impurities it is necessary to use highly pure solvents in the process. Ethanol can be used to improve the safety factor but it is not easy to remove it from the product as the product concentrates more and more into its final consistency. Residual solvents such as ethanol and hydrocarbons may lead to physical destabilization of liposomes by interfering with the cooperative hydrophobic interactions among the phospholipid methylene groups that hold the structure together (Vemuri and Rhodes, 1995).

Thus, it is important to set the specifications on the residual levels of solvent in the final product and establishing safety of the residual amounts. The permissible levels of residual solvent may vary depending upon the end use of the product. If possible, the best approach is to eliminate the use of solvents that are carcinogenic or teratogenic from the process even though the residuals can be removed as much as possible. Solvent residuals in the final product is an unavoidable troublesome situation to the liposome dosage form manufacturers, at this time.

3.3.2 Protection of Phospholipids from Oxidation

Most of the phospholipid dispersions contain unsaturated lipids (acyl chains) as part of the molecular chain. These unsaturated lipids undergo oxidative degradation or lipid peroxidation. These reactions can occur during preparation, storage or actual use. The oxidation peroxidation is a complex process involving generation of free radicals which result in the formation of cyclic peroxides and hydroperoxidase (New, 1990).

This oxidative degradation reaction takes place readily if the unsaturated lipids are not protected during manufacturing and storage. The various methods used for measuring the lipid peroxidation are non-specific based on either disappearance of unsaturated fatty acids or the appearance of conjugated dienes. The level of oxidation can be kept to a minimum by taking following precautions:

- Freshly purified lipid and freshly distilled solvents should be used
- High temperature procedures should be avoided
- Manufacturing should be done in absence of oxygen (using inert gases)
- Deoxygenation of aqueous solutions with nitrogen
- Liposomes suspension should be stored in an inert atmosphere
- Inclusion of antioxidant (alpha-Tocopherol or butylated hydroxytoluene) as a component of lipid membrane (Vemuri and Rhodes, 1995).

3.3.3 Removal of Endotoxins

Pyrogens are substances which cause a rise in temperature (fever) when injected. They are usually high molecular weight lipopolysaccharide (LPS) complexes associated with the cell walls of Gram negative bacteria and are often referred to by the generic term 'endotoxins'. The endotoxin isolated from Gramm negative bacteria contains three chemical regions. Lipid A, a central polysaccharide core and an O-antigenic side chain. It is reported that the lipid A is mostly responsible for the pyrogenic activity of endotoxin. This portion of the molecule also provides the basis for depyrogenation by membrane filters that can absorb endotoxin by the hydrophobic interaction of Lipid A with the uncharged membrane surface. Endotoxin molecules in solution may exhibit different states of aggregation. In the most aggregated form it can be as big as 0.1 μm in diameter. The addition of chelating agents breaks the aggregate into rod-shaped sub units, each 8-12 Å in diameter, and 200-700 Å in length, with an approximate molecular masses of 30000 to 1000000 dalton. Use of surface active agents such as sodium deoxycholate reduces the endotoxin to its smallest subunit, with a molecular mass of approximately 10000 dalton. Endotoxins in any state of aggregation can be removed by reverse-phase HPLC techniques and by ultrafiltration in aseptic pharmaceutical manufacturing (Martin, 1990). Since the endotoxin molecules are lipophilic and exhibit similar solubility behavior as phospholipids, liposomes may interfere with endotoxin assays, such as the Limulus amebocyte lysate tests (Pearson, 1985). The best way to control endotoxin levels in liposome preparations is by obtaining the raw materials of high quality and by carrying out the process under aseptic conditions with depyrogenated utensils.

3.3.4 Removal of Un-entrapped Drug

In order to use liposomes for controlled drug release, the complete removal of unentrapped drug is necessary. Various approaches have been explored to remove the unentrapped drug molecules in laboratory. Table 3.3 provides a brief account of various methods used for the separation of unentrapped drugs with their advantages and disadvantages.

Table 3.3 Various methods used to separate unentrapped drug from liposomes.

Method	Advantages	Disadvantages
Dialysis	Sample recovery	Inaccurate
Minicolumn centrifugation	Economical and sample recovery	Tedious only small sample volumes can be processed
Protamine aggregation	Economical and applicable to MLVs and LUVs	Slow with neutral and positively charged liposomes Causes contamination of liposomes
Gel chromatography	Sample recovery	Slow and tedious dilution of samples occur
Ultrafilration	Removal of water soluble drugs	Slow and tedious process

3.3.5 Sterilization of Liposomes

There are five different sterilization methods available including steam, dry heat, gas, ionizing radiation and filtration. Each of them differs in mechanisms of microbial removal, operation parameters and applicability to any given product. The selection of sterilization process is based on factors such as the impact of the method on product quality, the economics of the sterilization process and the logistics of sterilization.

Thermolabile liquids are typically sterilized by filtration technique. Liposome formulations are thermolabile and the lipids are likely to hydrolyze at the high temperature (121°C) of sterilization. It is reported that Gamma-Irradiation causes the hydrolysis as well as accelerates the peroxidation of unsaturated lipids. The only available sterilization technique for liposome formulations is filtration through 0.2 µm filter membrane. When filtering liposomes at a temperature above phase transition temperature, phospholipids larger than 2 µm can be filtered because of the increased flexibility of lipid membrane in its liquid crystalline membrane (Olson *et al.,* 1979). Alternatively, one can design an aseptic process from the beginning of lipids solubilization to the final filling of vials with product under aseptic conditions and in Class-100 environment. The best approach to scale-up the process to large scale production is by utilizing both the filtration technique as well as the aseptic process wherever applicable.

3.4 Characterizations of Liposomes

The behaviour of liposomes in both physical and biological system is determined to large extent by factors such as physical size, chemical composition, membrane permeability, quantity of entrapped solutes, as well as the quality and purity of the starting material. Therefore, it is important to have information regarding all these parameters.

3.4.1 Chemical Analysis

3.4.1.1 Quantitative Determination of Phospholipid

The accurate measurement of phoshpholipid concentration is quite difficult to estimate primarily because dried lipids can often contain considerable quantities of residual solvent and in case if derived from liposomes, contain high quantities of other contaminating lipids. Therefore the method most widely accepted for determination of phospholipid is an indirect one which involves the analysis of phosphorus using the Bartlett assay (Bartlett, 1959). In this method, phospholipid's phosphorus in the sample is first acid hydrolysed to inorganic phosphate. This is converted to phosphor-molybdic acid by the addition ammonium molybdate and the phospho-molybdic acid is quantitatively reduced to a blue-coloured compound by amino-naphthyl-sulphonic acid. The intensity of blue colour is measured spectrophotometrically and is compared with the calibration standard to yield phospholipid content.

3.4.1.2 Estimation of Phospholipid Oxidation

Oxidative deterioration is a complex process which involves the free radical generation resulting in the formation of cyclic peroxides and hydroxyperoxidase. Oxidation of the fatty acids of phospholipids in the absence of specific oxidants occurs *via* a free radical chain mechanism. In the initial step- abstraction of a hydrogen atom from the lipid chain can occur most commonly as a result of exposure to electromagnetic radiation or trace amounts of contamination with transition metal ions. Although any lipid can form radicals by this mechanism, the most susceptible to degradation are lipids containing double bonds i.e., polyunsaturated lipids and therefore these are more prone to oxidative degradation (New, 1990).

Oxygen is a stable diradical and its presence further adds to the process of degradation by generating initially hydroperoxides which finally get converted to the aldehydes with concomitant fission at the fatty acid chain on either side of the C-O bond and the overall process can be summarized into three steps viz., conjugation of isolated double bonds, formation of peroxides and aldehyde production which finally leads to chain scission.

Monitoring of the degradation process can be done either by UV spectroscopy, where the presence of conjugated dienes can be easily detected by the appearance of peak at 230 nm or by testing formation of peroxides (hydroperoxide and endoperoxides). The detection of hydroperoxides is based on their susceptibility to reduction by iodide as follows

$$2H^+ + ROOH + 3I^- \rightarrow H_2O + ROH + L_3$$

Under the condition used in this method, only lipid hydroperoxide react with iodide thus excluding the endoperoxide that form malondialdehyde from the assay. Endoperoxides are determined by reaction of their breakdown product at elevated temperature (malondialdehyde) with thiobarbituric acid giving a red chromophore which absorbs radiation at 532 nm.

3.4.1.3 Quantitation of α -Tocopherol

α-tocopherol (α-T) itself can be quantitated using specific tests for reducing power involving the formation of iron complexes as in the Emmeric-Engel reagent. However, the use of alternative antioxidant such as more stable hemisuccinate derivatives of tocopherol precludes the use of this type of test since the hemissucinate derivatives display little reducing activity until after it is hydrolysed to the free tocopherol. Quantitation using HPLC is the simplest alternative method for looking at both these compounds as well as their breakdown products (New, 1990).

3.4.2 Physical Characterization

3.4.2.1 Lamellarity Determination

The lamellarity of liposomes varies widely due to different lipids or preparation procedures. This is evident by reports showing that the fraction of phospholipid exposed to the external medium has ranged from 5% for large multilamellar vesicles (LMVs) to 70% for SUVs. Lamellarity of liposomes is often accomplished by ^{31}P NMR in which, the addition of Mn^{2+} quenches the ^{31}P NMR signal from phospholipids on the exterior face of the liposomes (Frohlich *et al.,* 2001). Mn^{2+} interacts with the negatively charged phosphate groups of phospholipids and causes a broadening and reduction of the quantifiable signal. The degree of lamellarity is determined from the signal ratio before and after Mn^{2+} addition. This technique has recently been found to be quite sensitive to the Mn^{2+} and buffer concentration and the types of liposomes under analysis. Other techniques for lamellarity determination include electron microscopy, small angle X-ray scattering (SAXS) and the methods that are based on the change in the visible or fluorescence signal of marker lipids upon the addition of reagents.

3.4.2.2 Size Determination

The average size and size distribution of liposomes are important parameters when the liposomes are intended for therapeutic use particularly if they are administered by inhalation or parenteral route. Several techniques are available for assessing submicrometer liposome size and size distribution. These include static and dynamic light scattering (Ruozi *et al.,* 2005) several types of microscopy techniques, size-exclusion chromatography, field-flow fractionation and analytical centrifugation. Several variations on electron microscopy (EM) such as transmission EM using negative staining, freeze-fracture TEM and cryo EM provide valuable information on liposome preparations since they yield a view of morphology and can resolve particles of varying sizes. Unfortunately, they require complicated sample preparation, remove the liposomes from their native environment, generate artifacts, can induce shrinkage and shape distortion and are time consuming to obtain a representative size distribution of the population thus are not amenable for being a routine measurement (Armengol and Estelrich, 1995; Egelhaaf *et al.,* 1996).

Another more recently developed microscopic technique known as atomic force microscopy has been utilized to study liposome morphology, size, and stability. This technique relies on the faster scanning of a nanometer sized sharp probe over a sample which has been immobilized onto a carefully selected surface, such as mica or glass, which is mounted onto a piezoelectric scanner. The end result is a high resolution three-dimensional profile of the surface under study. Zetasizer which works on the principle of dynamic light scattering is commonly used to determine the size and size distribution of the liposomal formulation. In order to measure the size, suitably diluted sample is transferred in the cuvette which is placed in the zetasizer and the sample is analyzed using software provided with the machine.

3.4.2.3 Determination of Residual Organic Phase in Phospholipid Mixtures

Chloroform is used as a solvent for egg phosphatidylglycerol and to protect the lipids from oxidation during storage as well as to facilitate the good molecular dispersion of various lipids during the process. Although chloroform is a good solvent to disperse the lipids, its complete removal from the lipid mixtures is imperative when the liposomes are intended for human use. The contaminant of chloroform is carbon tetrachloride and it is also a known carcinogenic material. A process that uses chloroform as a solvent in the preparation of liposomes should include a test method (Vemuri and Rhodes, 1995).

3.4.2.4 Surface Charge of Utilized Lipids

Lipids utilized to formulate liposomes are usually charge imparting and hence it is obvious to study the charge on the vesicle surface. In general two methods are used to access the charge namely free flow electrophoresis and zeta potential measurement. The surface charge of the vesicle can be calculated using Helmhoitz-Smoluchowski equation for which the mobility of the liposomal dispersion in a suitable buffer is required. The most reliable and simple method for determination of zeta potential is to use a zetasizer which gives quantitative value of zeta potential.

3.4.2.5 Percent Drug Encapsulation

The liposome preparations are a mixture of encapsulated and unencapsulated drug fractions. The unencapsulated drug fraction is also referred to as 'free' drug. In a majority of procedures the free and encapsulated drug fractions are separated to assess the free drug concentration as a first experimental step. Then the encapsulated fraction of the drug is treated with a detergent to lyse the liposomes and to completely discharge the drug from the liposomes into surrounding aqueous media. Thus exposed drug is assayed by a suitable technique. The free drug from the liposomal suspension is separated by either ultracentrifugation or mini column centrifugation method. For preparation of mini column, Sephadex G-25 is suspended in 100 ml saline and kept overnight. Subsequently supernatant is decanted and the swollen gel is poured in 1 ml syringe and centrifuged to get packed column free from saline. Formulation is placed on the top of Sephadex column and the formulation free from unentrapped drug is collected from the bottom (New, 1990).

3.5 Applications of Liposomes

3.5.1 Liposomes used in Antimicrobial Drug Delivery

Microbial infections can be broadly classified into bacterial, protozoal, fungal and viral. These intracellular pathogens harbor in the liver and spleen and thus therapeutic moieties can be targeted to these organs using liposomes as carrier system. Due to their intrinsic passive vectorization to RES predominant organs, liposomes offer enormous potential and opportunities for targeted drug delivery.

3.5.1.1 Viral

Viral infections are extremely difficult to treat and there are very few effective therapies. Antiviral therapy based on intracellular delivery of drugs may be enhanced through the use of liposomes. An ideal use of liposomes in the treatment of viral infection may be as carrier of topically administered antiviral agents. This is due to their ability to enhance local penetration while avoiding systemic absorption. Another potential advantage of liposomes is their ability to transport extremely lipophilic drugs. Targeted or regular liposomes bearing idoxuridine or acyclovir applied to corneal cell infected with *Herpes simplex* inhibited viral replication more effectively than the application of free drug. In the treatment of recurrent genital HSV-2 infection in guinea pigs, interlukin-2 encapsulated liposomes in combination with HSV recombinant glycoprotein greatly reduced the disease. The therapy was much more successful than the use of free interlukin-2 (Ho *et al.,* 1992).

3.5.1.2 Protozoal

A parasitic disease leishmaniasis is a major cause of morbidity and mortality world-wide. In this disease, the organism grows and multiply within the macrophages of the RES (Reed, 1988). Leishmaniasis infection in humans are manifested in three forms: visceral (kala-azar caused by *L. donovani*), mucocutaneous (caused by *L. mexivane*) and cutaneous (caused by *L. tropica*).

The gold standard drug for the treatment of visceral leishmaniasis is Amphotericin B. However its application is restricted due to its wide spread toxicity to normal body cells. To avoid such toxicities, liposomes are used to direct such drugs to their site of action. Evidence suggests that after the liposomes are taken up by the macrophages, it enters the parasite itself through endocytosis. The passive targeting approach is based on the behaviour of macrophages to engulf foreign particles as soon they appear in the systemic circulation. The engulfment of the carrier system bearing drug by the macrophages ultimately leads to delivery of the drug to the parasites residing in the macrophages. Similarly incorporating Amphotericin B in liposomes shows promising result in visceral leishmaniasis which was unresponsive to conventional therapy. Another advantage of using liposomes as carrier is the prolongation of the therapeutic effect (Rathore *et al.,* 2011).

3.5.1.3 Bacterial

The resistance posed by intracellular bacterial infection to antibiotics therapy is due to poor intracellular uptake of these drugs. Liposomal encapsulation of these drugs may improve their uptake and increases the duration of action of antibiotics by providing the drug reservoir and decreasing their toxicity by reducing their accumulation in sensitive tissues. Native gentamycin causes toxicity to kidney nephron and auditory cells. Encapsulation of gentamicin in liposomes decreases the amount of free drug and less amount is distributed to kidney nephron and auditory cells leading to reduced toxicity to these organs.

Liposomes may widen the therapeutic margin of currently available antibiotics. Some of the strains of bacteria (especially *Pseudomonas aeruginosa*) can produce phospholipase that may actually facilitate the release of therapeutic agent from liposomes in area of high bacterial density. There are several studies which shows that liposomes effectively increases the antibiotic therapy.

3.5.1.4 Fungal

Another very promising use of liposomes is as carrier for antifungal drugs, especially Amphotericin B. Systemic fungal infections are associated with increasing frequency in the immune-compromised patients. Candida and Aspergillus are the most common causative organism for the systemic infections. Amphotericin B is effective against these organisms but has limited utility due to acute reactions such as fever and chills and severe toxicity such as nephrotoxicity which occurs on chronic administration. Therefore, this drug should be targeted to the macrophages in such a way that the interaction of free drug with the non-targeted tissues could be minimized. Treatment of disseminated fungal infection by liposomal Amphotericin B results in lower toxicity and significant increase in the concentration of drug in macrophages through passive uptake which therefore increases the therapeutic index.

3.5.2 Use of Liposomes in Cancer Therapy

Most of the medical applications of liposomes that have reached the pre-clinical and clinical stages are in cancer treatments. There are three general approaches for increasing the effectiveness of chemotherapy of malignant diseases (Schwendener, 1992).

(a) To implement new therapy combinations with different dosing and treatment regimens for existing drugs.

(b) To develop new drugs with different pharmacological properties.

(c) To improve the effectiveness of existing drugs by altering drug dispersion pharmacokinetics and toxicity to maximize their therapeutic activity.

In the treatment of cancer even small alteration in the therapeutic index of the drug can be of great benefit. Encapsulation of chemotoxic agent is very much beneficial as it protect sensitive tissue from toxicity. For example, the chemotherapeutic agent doxorubicin (adriamycin) is extremely effective but when used as free drug it causes severe cardiotoxicity. Liposomes do not concentrate in the myocardium after IV administration and offer a promising method in enhancing doxorubicin utility. Not only does encapsulation of drug in liposomes dramatically decrease the doxorubicin induced cardiotoxicity, it also enhances the drug activity against liver metastases.

Liposomes can be targeted to the cancer cells either by passive or by active targeting. Passive targeting utilizes the leaky vasculature property of cancer cells by which the liposomes can get entry into the target area. This phenomenon is known as enhanced permeability and retention effect (EPR). In the active targeting process, a ligand, having affinity to the receptors over-expressed in the cancer cells is attached to the surface of liposomes. Upon entry into systemic circulation, the carrier system i.e., liposomes is moves towards cancer cells due to affinity of the ligand to the over-expressed receptors. The entrapped drug along with carrier system is available in the vicinity of the target area. The presence of liposomes or other carrier systems activate defense system of the body and macrophages which are the main component of the body's defense system engulf and try to remove the carrier system from body. This process of opsonization can be overcome by surrounding the liposomes with some hydrophilic molecules like polyethylene glycol. Macrophages cannot recognize these molecules and the liposomes can remain in circulation for longer period of time. Such stealth or long circulating liposomes are one of the most explored particulate drug carriers which can reach to the tumor site by both active as well as passive means thereby releasing the entrapped drugs in the tumor vicinity. The range of diameters of drug-containing liposomes is approximately 100-200 nm which is large enough to allow the extravasation of most liposomes from the vessel into the tumor interstitial space. Passively targeted liposomal systems can be used to treat cancer, but the selectivity can be enhanced by active targeting incorporating ligand to the surface of liposomes (Lee *et al.,* 2004). Targeting moieties can include; monoclonal antibodies or antibody fragments such as scFv, peptides, growth factors, carbohydrates, glycoproteins, or receptor ligands which get overexpressed or selectively expressed on cancer cells (Sapra and Allen, 2004). Ligand-mediated targeting of liposomal anti-cancer drugs such as doxorubicin or vincristine has resulted in improved survival times in a variety of disease models relative to non-targeted liposomal therapeutics (Sapra *et al.,* 2004).

Another use of liposomes in the treatment of cancer is the slow or sustain release of the drug from the membrane. This property can increase the potency of cell-cycle-dependent drugs such as methotrexate and cytarabine without increasing drug toxicity. Liposomes could also be used as carriers for unstable drugs such as alkylating agents and cisplatin.

Liposomes have also displayed its potential when used as carrier for immunosuppressant such as macrophages activating factor which render normal macrophage tumoricidal in anticancer therapy. Encapsulating immunomodulators in liposomes is much more effective than administration of free agents. Liposomes encapsulating interlukin-2 administered with T-activated killer cell was effective in treating the MCA-38 murine colon adenocarcinoma cell line (Loeffler *et al.,* 1991).

3.5.3 Liposomes in Oxygen Transport

Liposomes exhibit vast similarity between its membrane structure and that of RBC and hence they can be used as a carrier for hemoglobin (hemosomes) to be used as erythrocytes substitutes. Protoheme moieties of haemoglobin and myoglobin are completely surrounded by hydrophobic residue of the globin chains and this hydrophobic environment effectively prevents the irreversible oxidation of iron to ferric state and promotes the reversible formation of oxygen adducts. In haemoglobin vesicles, this hydrophobic environment is provided by lipid bilayer and thus they mimic the red cells. Tsuchida reported that the aggregation and fusion of haemoglobin vesicles and the leakage on long term storage can be prevented using either polymerized phospholipids or polyphospholipids or by introduction of oligosaccharides type of glycolipid in the bilayer membrane (Tsuchida, 1995).

3.5.4 Liposomes in Enzyme Replacement Therapy

Many of the genetic diseases surface due to the deficiency of lysosomal enzymes in the patient. For example, patient with Pompe's disease lack α-glucosidase enzyme and the patient with Gaucher's disease lack specific lysosomal β-glucosidase enzyme. Such enzymes when injected in patient in the free form get degraded. Therefore, the liposomal form of these enzymes for their transport to the specific site seems more feasible as the liposomes are carried to the lysosomes after endocytosis by the cell.

3.5.5 Liposomes in Metal Poisoning

The chelating agent such as EDTA and DTPA use to chelate metals often has difficulty in crossing the cell membrane. Such membrane often gets degraded in plasma and are toxic due to their lack of specificity. Liposomal entrapment of such chelating agents allows these agents to cross cell membrane and allows the natural targeting to the RES cells of the liver, which are primary site of metal disposition in poisonings such as iron and plutonium overdose (Rahman, 1988).

3.5.6 Liposomes in Diagnostic Applications

The radiolabelled liposomes can be used to detect tumors if the liposomes are selectively taken up by the tumors. The most successful use of liposomes are diagnostic tool was Tc-labelled small neutral liposomes for lymph node imaging in patients with breast cancer. In computer tomography, multilamellar liposomes were successful as carrier for ^{125}I labelled X ray contrast agent for imaging liver and spleen.

Immunoassay such as Enzyme Linked Immunosorbent Assay (ELISA), Radioimmuno Assay (RIA) and Liposome Immune Lysis Assay (LILA) are based on the selective interaction of an analyte antigen with corresponding antibodies. The concentration of antigens and antibodies is normally determined by competition of analyte with known concentration of radio or fluorescent labelled receptor in the binding to the immobilized antibody. Liposomes can be useful analytical reagent as they can encapsulate upto a million markers and can therefore serve as signal amplifier. Liposome is well recognized as a model membrane and its lytic ability inculcated through various lytic agents such as complement led to the development of the efficient assay system known as LILA. The technique is based upon specifically engineered liposomes constructed with a marker inside and either antigen/antibody appended to the liposomal surface. Addition of either antibody/antigen along with a lytic substance such as complement (an opsonin) will lyse liposome with a release of marker which can be monitored.

3.5.7 Liposomes to Inhibit Immune Reactions

After undergoing organ transplant procedure, patients normally are dosed with cyclosporine to prevent rejection of the transplant. Cyclosporine is one of the most effective immunosuppressive agents available but has severe toxicities. These toxicities include nephro, neuro and hepato toxicities. Incorporation of cyclosporine into MLVs not only decreased the toxicity but also increased the effectiveness (Gorecki *et al.,* 1991).

3.5.8 Liposomes as Vaccine Carriers

Liposomes may also be used as a vaccine carrier. This concept of liposomes has been examined since 1974 by various researchers but there has not been a direct medical application of liposomes in a practical vaccine for humans or animals. The use liposomes as carrier offer the theoretical advantage of presenting the antigen in its natural membrane configuration. Insertion of purified cell membrane molecule into liposome can induce an *in vivo* antibody response (Gregoriadis, 1990).

Liposomal enhancement of the response to an antigen may be due to the attachment of the antigen to the liposome, rendering the antigen particulate and readily captured by the RES.

Some antigens used in vaccines are not capable of eliciting an antibody response when administered alone. For such antigens, it is necessary to include an adjuvant which increases the immune response. Liposome can function as adjuvants and unlike some presently used adjuvants, are non-toxic.

In general, liposomes used as vaccine carrier have produced functional results. The frequency of serum antibody response and the level of antibody titers obtained with protein antigen entrapped in liposomes are superior to the use of use of aqueous antigen solution. The immune response can be enhanced by using unilamellar rather than multilamellar vesicles.

3.6 Stability of Liposomes

The stability of liposomes is a major consideration in all steps of their production and administration i.e., from processing step to storage and delivery. Stability of lyophilized powders and its controlled release at the time of usage is a serious issue. When a pharmaceutical dosage form is altered the stability of the drug may be changed. A stable dosage form maintains its physical integrity and does not adversely influence the chemical property of the active ingredient during its life on the shelf. Researchers are attempting to deliver low and high molecular weight drugs in a variety of polymer matrices and liposome delivery systems. The successful introduction of new dosage form in the market depends upon a well-defined stability study that can establish product's integrity, without ambiguity at the end of the study. In designing a stability study one must consider to evaluate physical, chemical, and microbial parameters.

A stability study program must include a section for product characterization and another section to study the product stability during storage. As a first step of product stability program one must identify various parameters of the product that characterize the drug as well as the dosage form. Develop and validate each of the product parameters of interest prior to their use in the stability study. Liposomes are vesicles formed from amphiphilic substances like phospholipids dispersed in aqueous medium. All liposome preparations reported in the literature are heterogeneous in size with potential physical and chemical stability problems. Average size distribution of liposomes determined at the time of preparation which changes upon storage. Liposomes tend to fuse and grow into bigger vesicles, which is a thermodynamically more favorable state. Fusion and breakage of liposomes on storage also poses a more important problem of drug leakage form the vesicles. Interactions of drug with the phospholipid also creates the chemical stability problems. Chemically, phospholipids are susceptible to oxidation and hydrolysis reactions. Majority of therapeutic liposomal formulations are parenteral products (either injectable or inhalation dosage forms) and thus they must be sterilized to remove the microbial contamination from the product.

Other factors to be taken into consideration prior to starting a stability study are the formulation factors and environmental conditions which may influence the stability of liposomes. Influence of formulation factors such as pH, buffer species, ionic strength, and solvent system and their influence on the liposomes play a major role in stabilizing a liposome formulation. For example, the liposomes prepared with distearoyl-phosphatidylcholine (DSPC) showed an optimal stability at pH 6.5 in aqueous solutions at 70 °C (Frokjaer *et al.,* 1982). Influence of environmental factors such as temperature, light, oxygen and heavy metal ions may initiate chemical or physical reactions. These reactions may include changes in size distribution of vesicles and oxidation and hydrolysis of lipids.

3.6.1 Chemical Stability

The major ingredient in the liposomal formulation is the lipid. The lipid portion of liposomes is derived from natural and/or synthetic phospholipid sources. Phospholipids containing unsaturated fatty acids are known to undergo oxidative reactions. The reaction products can cause permeability changes in the liposome bilayers. Furthermore, the reaction products can also alter the shelf-life of liposomes. It has been identified that the lipid peroxidation and the lipid hydrolysis are the two major routes of lipid degradation. Firstly, oxidative degradation of the lipids in general can be minimized by protecting the lipid preparations from light; by adding antioxidants such as alpha-tocopherol or BHT; by adding EDTA to lipid formulations to remove heavy metals and by producing the product under nitrogen or argon environment. Secondly, hydrolysis of lipids leads to the formation lysophosphatidylcholine. The presence of lysophosphatidylcholine enhances the permeability of liposomes and thus it is essential to keep its level to a minimum in a given preparation which makes it extremely important to keep lyso-PC levels to a minimum during storage also. Finally, the chemical stability profile of a drug molecule may entirely be different from the stability profile after entrapment inside lipid vesicles. Thus, it is essential to develop stability protocols to study the chemical integrity of the active drug molecule over a period of time.

3.6.2 Physical Stability

The visual appearance, average size and size distribution are important parameters to examine. There are a number of methods to follow the physical stability of liposomes. For instance, the size distribution of MLVs is much wider as compared to the ULV. The liposomal vesicles have tendency to aggregate in long term storage until unless the formulation is completely optimized. The arrangement of bilayers can be disturbed upon storage and the same can be investigated using electron microscopy. The shape and surface morphology of formulation after storage can be compared with the freshly prepared formulation. The changes in size and size distribution after storage can be assessed by measurement of vesicle size with the help of DLS using a zetasizer (Szoka and Papahadjopoulos, 1980).

3.7 Conclusion

The development of 'pharmaceutical' liposomes is now an explored area in drug delivery therapeutics. Clinical efficacy of liposomal formulations will be judged ultimately by its ability to deliver the drug to the desired site of action which may be in the liver, the lung, the reticuloendothelial system, or some other remote tissue of the body, over a prolonged period of time. Pharmacokinetics of the liposomal formulation depends upon the drug lipid ratio, drug concentration in the formulation and route of administration. The increasing variety of suggested applications and encouraging results from early clinical applications and clinical trials of different liposomal drugs, need to be augmented by simple production processes and a variety of quality control assays for liposomal formulations. With these requirements met, we are surely likely to see more liposomal pharmaceuticals on the market in the foreseeable future. Also the stability of liposomes in blood stream dictates the pharmacokinetics of the drug in liposome dosage form. The entrapped drugs are expected to remain encapsulated by the phospholipid bilayers and slowly diffuse out of bilayers. Contrary to the desired expectations, the lipoproteins of the blood destabilize the liposomes when they are administered systemically. The pharmaceutical scientists must overcome this barrier to successfully deliver bioactives *via* liposome dosage forms.

References

Angelova M.I, and Tsoneva I (1999). Interactions of DNA with giant liposomes. *Chemistry and Physics of Lipids* **101:** 123-137.

Armengol X, and Estelrich J (1995). Physical stability of different liposome compositions obtained by extrusion method. *Journal of Microencapsulation* **12:** 525-535.

Bangham A.D, Standish M.M, and Watkins J.C (1965). Diffusion of univalent ions across the lamellae of swollen phospholipids. *Journal of Molecular Biology* **13:** 238-252.

Bartlett G.R (1959). Phosphorus assay in column chromatography. *J biol Chem* **234:** 466-468.

Batzri S, and Korn E.D (1973). Single bilayer liposomes prepared without sonication. *Biochimica et Biophysica Acta* **298:** 1015-1019.

Braguini W.L, Cadena S.M, Carnieri E.G, Rocha M.E, and de Oliveira M.B (2004). Effects of deltamethrin on functions of rat liver mitochondria and on native and synthetic model membranes. *Toxicology Letters* **152:** 191-202.

Crowe L.M, Crowe J.H, Rudolph A, Womersley C, and Appel L (1985). Preservation of freeze-dried liposomes by trehalose. *Archives of Biochemistry and Biophysics* **242:** 240-247.

Damen J, Regts J, and Scherphof G (1981). Transfer and exchange of phospholipid between small unilamellar liposomes and rat plasma high density lipoproteins. Dependence on cholesterol content and phospholipid composition. *Biochimica et Biophysica Acta* **665:** 538-545.

Deamer D, and Bangham A.D (1976). Large volume liposomes by an ether vaporization method. *Biochimica et Biophysica Acta* **443:** 629-634.

Edwards K.A, and Baeumner A.J (2006). Analysis of liposomes. *Talanta* **68:** 1432-1441.

Egelhaaf S.U, Wehrli E, Mu¨ller M, Adrian M, and Schurtenberger P (1996). Determination of the size distribution of lecithin liposomes: a comparative study using freeze fracture, cryoelectron microscopy and dynamic light scattering. *Journal of Microscopy* **184:** 214-228.

Fischer A, Oberholzer T, and Luisi P.L (2000). Giant vesicles as models to study the interactions between membranes and proteins. *Biochimica et Biophysica Acta* **1467:** 177-188.

Florkin M, and Stotz E.H (1967). Comprehensive Biochemistry (Elsevier Publishing Company).

Frohlich M, Brecht V, and Peschka-Suss R (2001). Parameters influencing the determination of liposome lamellarity by 31P-NMR. *Chemistry and Physics of Lipids* **109:** 103-112.

Frokjaer S, Hjorth E.L, and Worts O (1982). Stability and storage of liposomes. In Optimization of Drug Delivery, H. Bundgaard, A. Bagger Hansen, and H. Kofod, eds. (Munksgaard, Copenhagen: Alfred Benzon Symp), p. 384.

Gorecki D.C, Jakobisiak M, Kruszewski A, and Lasek W (1991). Evidence that liposome incorporation of cyclosporine reduces its toxicity and potentiates its ability to prolong survival of cardiac allografts in mice. *Transplantation* **52:** 766-769.

Grancelli A, Morros A, Cabañas M.E, Domènech Ò, Merino S, Vázquez J.L, Montero M.T, Viñas M, and Hernández-Borrell J (2002). Interaction of 6-fluoroquinolones with dipalmitoylphosphatidylcholine monolayers and liposomes. *Langmuir* **18:** 9177-9182.

Gregoriadis G (1990). Immunological adjuvants: a role for liposomes. *Immunology Today* **11:** 89-97.

Gruner S.M, Lenk R.P, Janoff A.S, and Ostro M.J (1985). Novel multilayered lipid vesicles: comparison of physical characteristics of multilamellar liposomes and stable plurilamellar vesicles. *Biochemistry* **24:** 2833-2842.

Hamilton R.L, Jr, Goerke J, Guo L.S, Williams M.C, and Havel R.J (1980). Unilamellar liposomes made with the French pressure cell: a simple preparative and semiquantitative technique. *Journal of Lipid Research* **21:** 981-992.

Ho R.J, Burke R.L, and Merigan T.C (1992). Liposome-formulated interleukin-2 as an adjuvant of recombinant HSV glycoprotein (gD) for the treatment of recurrent genital HSV-2 in guinea-pigs. *Vaccine* **10:** 209-213.

Juliano R.L, and Stamp D (1975). The effect of particle size and charge on the clearance rates of liposomes and liposome encapsulated drugs. *Biochemical and Biophysical Research Communications* **63:** 651-658.

Kim S, Turker M.S, Chi E.Y, Sela S, and Martin G.M (1983). Preparation of multivesicular liposomes. *Biochimica et Biophysica Acta* **728:** 339-348.

Lee T.Y, Wu H.C, Tseng Y.L, and Lin C.T (2004). A novel peptide specifically binding to nasopharyngeal carcinoma for targeted drug delivery. *Cancer Research* **64:** 8002-8008.

Loeffler C.M, Platt J.L, Anderson P.M, Katsanis E, Ochoa J.B, Urba W.J, Longo D.L, Leonard A.S, and Ochoa A.C (1991). Antitumor effects of interleukin 2 liposomes and anti-CD3-stimulated T-cells against murine MCA-38 hepatic metastasis. *Cancer Research* **51:** 2127-2132.

Madden T.D, Harrigan P.R, Tai L.C, Bally M.B, Mayer L.D, Redelmeier T.E, Loughrey H.C, Tilcock C.P, Reinish L.W, and Cullis P.R (1990). The accumulation of drugs within large unilamellar vesicles exhibiting a proton gradient: a survey. *Chemistry and Physics of Lipids* **53:** 37-46.

Martin F.J (1990). Pharmaceutical manufacturing of liposomes. In Specialized drug delivery systems: manufacturing and production technology, F.J. Martin, ed. (New York: Marcel Dekker Inc.), pp. 267-316.

Mayer L.D, Bally M.B, and Cullis P.R (1986). Uptake of adriamycin into large unilamellar vesicles in response to a pH gradient. *Biochimica et Biophysica Acta* **857:** 123-126.

Mayer L.D, Madden T.D, Bally M.B, and Cullis P.R (1993). pH gradient-mediated drug entrapment in liposomes. In liposome technology: Entrapment of drugs and other materials (Boca Raton, FL: CRC Press), pp. 27-44.

Mayhew E, Lazo R, Vail W.J, King J, and Green A.M (1984). Characterization of liposomes prepared using a microemulsifier. *Biochimica et Biophysica Acta* **775:** 169-174.

New R.R.C (1990). Characterization of Liposomes. In Liposomes: A Practical Approach, R.R.C. New, ed. (New York: Oxford University Press), pp. 105-161.

Olson F, Hunt C.A, Szoka F.C, Vail W.J, and Papahadjopoulos D (1979). Preparation of liposomes of defined size distribution by extrusion through polycarbonate membranes. *Biochimica et Biophysica Acta* **557:** 9-23.

Pearson F.C (1985). Pyrogens: Endotoxins, LAL Testing and Depyrogenation (New York: Marcel Dekker).

Perrett S, Golding M, and Williams W.P (1991). A simple method for the preparation of liposomes for pharmaceutical applications:

characterization of the liposomes. *The Journal of Pharmacy and Pharmacology* **43:** 154-161.

Rahman Y.E (1988). Use of liposome in metal poisoning and metal storage diseases. In Liposomes as drug carrier, G. Gregoriadis, ed. (New York: John Wiley and Sons Ltd.), pp. 485-495.

Rathore A, Jain A, Gulbake A, Shilpi S, Khare P, Jain A, and Jain S.K (2011). Mannosylated liposomes bearing Amphotericin B for effective management of visceral Leishmaniasis. *Journal of Liposome Research* **21:** 333-340.

Reed R.G (1988). Liposome encapsulated lymphokine for treatment of experimental visceral leishmaniasis. In Liposomes as drug carrier, G. Gregoriadis, ed. (New York: John Wiley and Sons Ltd.), pp. 337-344.

Reeves J.P, and Dowben R.M (1969). Formation and properties of thin-walled phospholipid vesicles. *Journal of Cellular Physiology* **73:** 49-60.

Romanowski M, Zhu X, Ramaswami V, Misicka A, Lipkowski A.W, Hruby V.J, and O'Brien D.F (1997). Interaction of a highly potent sdimeric enkephalin analog, biphalin, with model membranes. *Biochimica et Biophysica Acta* **1329:** 245-258.

Ruozi B, Tosi G, Forni F, Fresta M, and Vandelli M.A (2005). Atomic force microscopy and photon correlation spectroscopy: two techniques for rapid characterization of liposomes. *European Journal of Pharmaceutical Sciences : Official Journal of the European Federation for Pharmaceutical Sciences* **25:** 81-89.

Sapra P, and Allen T.M (2004). Improved outcome when B-cell lymphoma is treated with combinations of immunoliposomal anticancer drugs targeted to both the CD19 and CD20 epitopes. *Clinical Cancer Research : An Official Journal of the American Association for Cancer Research* **10:** 2530-2537.

Sapra P, Moase E.H, Ma J, and Allen T.M (2004). Improved therapeutic responses in a xenograft model of human B lymphoma (Namalwa) for liposomal vincristine versus liposomal doxorubicin targeted via anti-CD19 IgG2a or Fab' fragments. *Clinical Cancer Research : An Official Journal of the American Association for Cancer Research* **10:** 1100-1111.

Schwendener R.A (1992). Liposomes and Immunoliposomes as carriers for cytostatic drugs, magnetic resonance contrast agents, and fluorescent chelates. *CHIMIA International Journal for Chemistry* **46:** 69-77.

Szoka F, Jr, and Papahadjopoulos D (1978). Procedure for preparation of liposomes with large internal aqueous space and high capture by reverse-phase evaporation. *Proceedings of the National Academy of Sciences of the United States of America* **75:** 4194-4198.

Szoka F, Jr, and Papahadjopoulos D (1980). Comparative properties and methods of preparation of lipid vesicles (liposomes). *Annual Review of Biophysics and Bioengineering* **9:** 467-508.

Toyran N, and Severcan F (2003). Competitive effect of vitamin D2 and Ca^{2+} on phospholipid model membranes: an FTIR study. *Chemistry and Physics of Lipids* **123:** 165-176.

Trombetta D, Arena S, Tomaino A, Tita B, Bisignano G, De Pasquale A, and Saija A (2001). Effect of the exposure to gentamicin and diltiazem on the permeability of model membranes. *Farmaco* (Societa chimica italiana : 1989) **56:** 447-449.

Tsuchida E.E., UK, (1995). Liposomes in biochemical application (UK: Harwood Academic Publisher).

Vemuri S, and Rhodes C (1994). Separation of liposomes by a gel filtration chromatographic technique: a preliminary evaluation. *Pharmaceutica Acta Helvetiae* **69:** 107-113.

Vemuri S, and Rhodes C (1995). Preparation and characterization of liposomes as therapeutic delivery systems: a review. *Pharmaceutica Acta Helvetiae* **70:** 95-111.

Vemuri S, Yu C.D, Wangsatorntanakun V, and Roosdorp N (1990). Large-scale production of liposomes by a microfluidizer. *Drug Development and Industrial Pharmacy* **16:** 2243-2256.

4

Carbon Nanotubes and their Applications in Drug Delivery

J.G. Meher[1], Nitin K. Jain[2] and Manish K. Chourasia[1]

[1]Pharmaceutics Division, CSIR-Central Drug Research Institute, Lucknow-226031, India.

[2]Department of Biotechnology, Ministry of Science & Technology, New Delhi-400003, India.

4.1 Introduction

Conventional drug delivery systems of many drug molecules in some specific diseases/disorders (cancer, infectious/metabolic diseases etc.) are reported to be either ineffective or to cause serious adverse reactions in human beings. The reasons might be the action of these drugs at the non-target sites along with the desired sites of action (Bertrand *et al.,*; Ruenraroengsak *et al.,* 2010). Search for better alternatives in facilitating the availability of these drugs at required site of action (receptor sites) has led to the advent of a new facet called as "*targeted drug delivery* or *drug targeting*". Now, targeted drug delivery has become a very broad topic for research/trade and vesicular as well as particulate delivery systems of drugs have come up as the major pillars in this field. In these categories, nanotechnology (various polymeric/metallic nanoparticles) shares a major segment because of many advantages over other systems. Passive targeting (only because of size of nanoparticles) as well as active targeting (because of any specific ligand attached to nanoparticles) are employed successfully *via* nanoparticle drug delivery. Nanotechnology has evolved into many drug delivery systems viz. nanoemulsions, nanosuspensions, nanocrystals, nanoballons, nanospheres, nanocapsules, nanorods, nanocore shells, nonodots, nano cells, nanohorns, nano devices as well as nanotubes (Alkilany *et al.,* 2012; Asthana *et al.,* 2013; Gao *et al.,* 2012; Guo *et al.,* 2013).

Carbon nanoparticles have attracted the attention of researchers as a promising drug delivery tool owing to their specific features viz. high aspect ratio, biocompatibility, flexibility in functionalization, capability of carrying drugs of wide categories as well as drug release modification capability. Among the various carbon nanoparticles, carbon nanotubes (CNTs) have emerged as a novel system in drug delivery and their special architecture (hollow interior and cage structure) as well as physicochemical properties (discussed later in this chapter) have made them eligible to be used as potential drug carriers. With this background information readers may be interested in knowing what exactly CNTs are, how these look, what characteristics theses possess and how these are useful for drug delivery?

CNTs belong to Fullerenes (molecules composed of carbon atom and exist in the form of a hollow sphere, ellipsoid, or tube) families, which are cylindrical in shape and composed of a hexagonal arrangement of sp^2-hybridized carbon atoms. CNTs are formed by rolling single or multiple layers of graphene sheets into seamless cylinders (Foldvari and Bagonluri, 2008a, b). Graphene is a basic structural arrangement as a 2 dimensional crystalline allotrope (different structural modifications of an element) of carbon, or in a simpler term it may be called as one-atom thick layer of graphite, where carbon atoms are bonded together in sheets of a hexagonal lattice. In the CNTs carbon atoms are connected evenly to three carbon atoms in the x-y plane, and a weak π bond is present in the z-axis (this free electron is responsible for electrical conductivity of CNTs). These sp^2 hybridized bonds are strong bonds and are responsible for exceptional strength and features of CNTs. Readers are encouraged to brush up their memories of quantum chemistry, specifically, orbital hybridization that would be helpful in understanding the chemical bonding in nanotubes. Figs. 4.1a to 4.1f represent the software generated graphical orientation of various Fullerenes including nanotubes (both 2-D and 3-D views). The graphene sheets of CNTs are rolled at definite and distinct ("chiral") angles, consequently the combination of these rolling angle and radius adopt various physico-chemical/-mechanical properties of CNTs.

The CNTs, which are around $1/50{,}000^{th}$ the thickness of a human hair, have wide applications in healthcare sector staring from pharmaceutical companies in developing target oriented drug delivery medicines, biotech companies in developing many novel vaccine and blood products as well as biomedical industries in designing nano-sensors (glucose sensors, blood pressure/temperature sensor), nano-diagnostic tools, nano-probes and nano-robots.

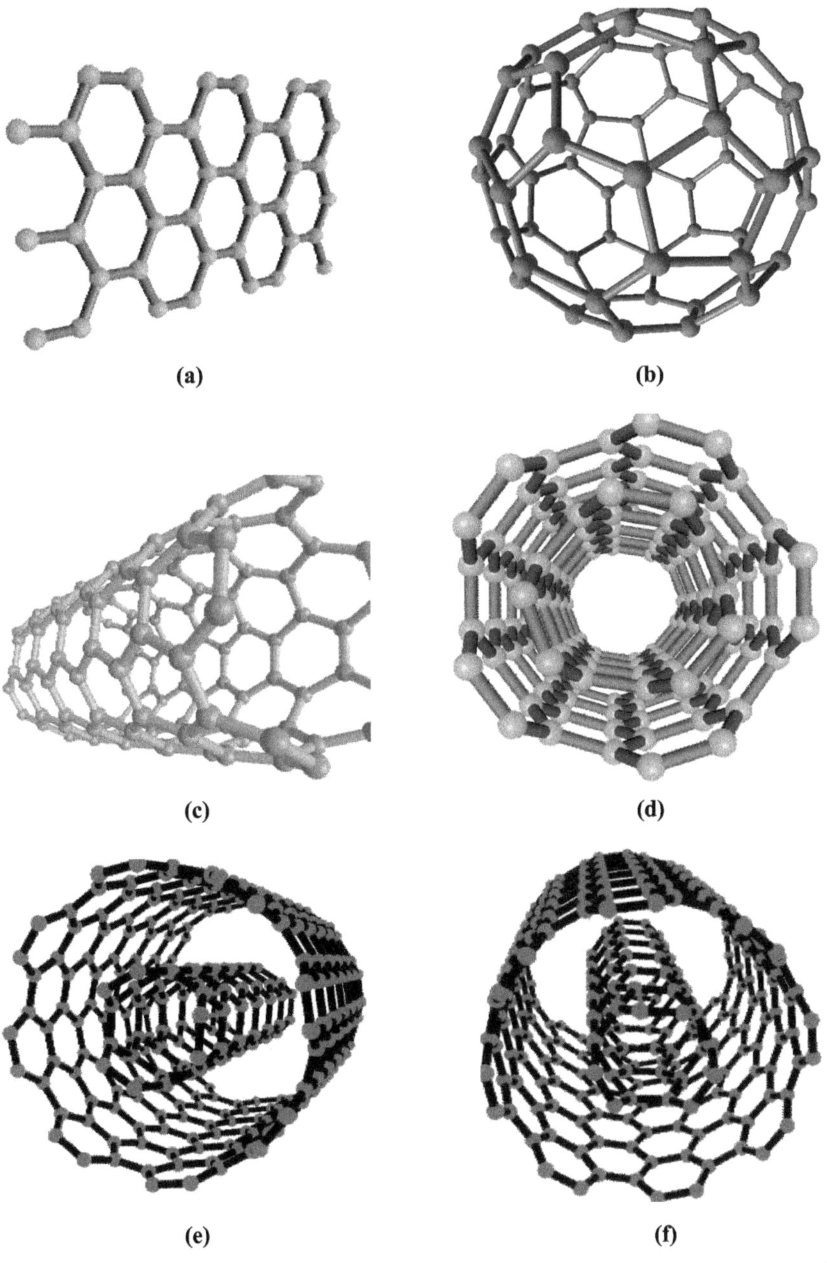

Fig. 4.1 Computer software generated representative graphics of (a) graphene sheets, (b) spherical Fullerene (60 carbon atoms in a series of interlocking hexagons and pentagons), (c) 3-D view of single walled CNTs, composed of a single cylindrical graphene layer, (d), (e), and (f) 3-D view of multi walled CNTs, composed of concentric cylinders of graphitic shell.

4.2 Brief History of CNTs

Carbon, the sole constituent of CNTs was believed to exists in two physical forms (allotropes) viz. diamond and graphite. The basic difference in these two forms is the arrangement of carbon atoms, which is also responsible for dissimilarity in their properties. Diamond is the metastable allotrope, and here the carbon atoms are arranged in cubic crystal structure, whereas graphite is composed of sheets of carbon atoms arranged in a hexagonal fashion. These differences make diamond the strongest, beautiful and non-conductive, on the contrary graphite is soft, conductive and lubricating in nature. Up to early 1980s this conception was continued but in 1985, Richard Smalley and Robert Curl (Rice University, Houston) and Harry Kroto (University of Sussex, England) reported a different allotrope of carbon composed of 60 carbon atoms, C60. The newly reported C60 was spherical in shape and formed a ball with 32 faces among which 12 were pentagons and 20 were hexagons exactly like a soccer ball (Fig. 4.1b). This was considered as a major discovery, which opened avenues for the development of other allotropes of carbon. These molecules were named after an architect, Buckminster Fuller, and became known as "buckminsterfullerene" or "buckyball". Later the same were also developed with C36, C70, C76 and C84 and known as "fullerenes". Further these fullerenes are developed in various other structures such as nanohorns, nanobuds, nanotubes etc. The history of CNTs is bit controversial as there are many claims on the discovery of CNTs. The information we are presenting may contradict with other existing literature but to the best of our knowledge and belief as well as published papers, this is the correct story behind discovery of CNTs. It has been mentioned in literature that in 1991 Sumio Iijima (Japanese physicist) had reported using carbon nanotubes in his work "Helical microtubules of graphitic carbon" published in Nature (Iijima, 1991). These were multi walled CNTs (MWCNTs) and later single walled CNTs (SWCNTs) were reported in the 17th issue of Nature in June 1993 by two papers submitted independently, one by Iijima and Ichihashi, at the time affiliated to NEC (Japanese multinational provider of information technology), the other by Bethune *et al.,* from IBM, California (Bethune *et al.,* 1993; Iijima and Ichihashi, 1993). Later many researchers reported synthesis and development of CNTs and many reviews came to limelight in this field.

4.3 Classification

CNTs can be classified in various ways but the standard classification is based on (1) structure and arrangement of atoms and (2) functionalization of CNTs. As per the first classification, CNTs are basically of two types viz. SWCNTs and MWCNTs. Further the SWCNTs are classified based on the arrangement of atoms as armchair (n = m), zigzag (n, 0) and chiral (n, m) nanotubes. Similarly MWCNTs are also classified as Russian-doll and parchment model. Based on functionalization the CNTs may be classified as target oriented CNTs, ligand attached CNTs, solvent dispersed CNTs, and surfactant grafted CNTs etc. Table 4.1 gives a brief classification of various CNTs.

Now it's very much crucial to understand what "n" and "m" are? These are best described by the chiral vector (n, m), where "n" and "m" are integers of the vector equation "$R = na_1 + ma_2$". To understand this concept we have to imagine the CNTs in 2-D planner dimension. Fig. 4.2 depicts the planner view of the CNTs that we are going to understand. The lines X1-X2 and X3-X4 are two parallel lines along the axis of CNT. Point "A" is a carbon atom on the X1-X2 line. An armchair line is drawn from point "A" to the line X3-X4 which travels across each hexagon, separating them into two equal halves. Another point "B" is spotted out on line X3-X4 which is a carbon atom nearer to the armchair line. Both the points "A" and "B" are joined with chiral vector "R". Now the angle between chiral vector R and armchair line decides the type of CNTs. If the angle is 0°, it's an armchair CNT, while with angle 30°, it's a zigzag CNT and lastly it is a chiral CNTs if the angle is between 0° and 30° (Wilder *et al.,* 1998). Fig. 4.3 depicts the 2-D and 3-D views of types of SWCNTs based on configuration of graphene.

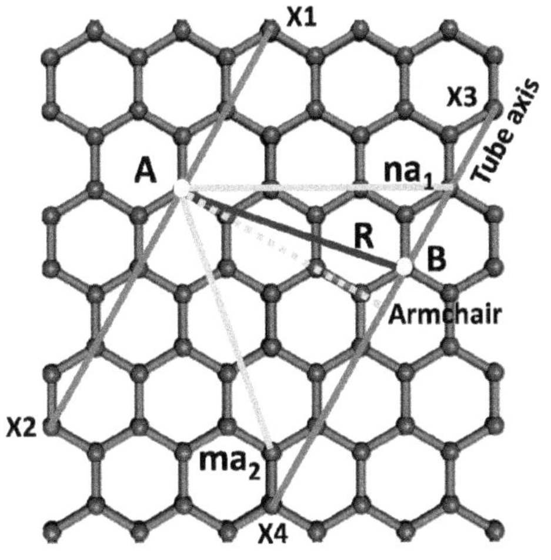

Fig. 4.2 Planner view of the CNTs depicting the various types of SWCNT viz. armchair, zigzag and chiral CNTs.

The "n" and "m" are not only important in depicting the types of CNT but also suggest the physicochemical properties (chirality/twist which decides the conductivity, lattice structure, density etc.) of the same. These values can also be used in determining the diameter of CNTs by the following formula.

$$d = \sqrt{(n^2 + m^2 + nm)} \times 0.0783 \text{ nm}$$

Table 4.1 A brief classification of CNTs.

<table>
<tr><th colspan="6">Based on structure (layers of CNTs)</th></tr>
<tr><th colspan="3">SWCNTs</th><th colspan="3">MWCNTs</th></tr>
<tr><td colspan="3">Single layer of graphene capped at both ends in a hemispherical arrangement of carbon linkages</td><td colspan="3">Multiple layer of graphene arranged in concentric cylinders of graphitic shells</td></tr>
<tr><td colspan="3">Dimension: diameter 0.6-2.4 nm, defined nanostructure, length up to few micrometers</td><td colspan="3">Dimension: diameter 2.5-100 nm, interlayer separation between SWCNTs: ~ 0.34 nm, nanostructure is not properly defined, length up to few micrometers</td></tr>
<tr><th colspan="6">Types of SWCNTs based on configuration of graphene</th></tr>
<tr><th colspan="2">Armchair</th><th colspan="2">Zigzag</th><th colspan="2">Chiral</th></tr>
<tr><td colspan="2">n = m</td><td colspan="2">n, 0</td><td colspan="2">n, m</td></tr>
<tr><td colspan="2">Angle* = 0°</td><td colspan="2">Angle* = 30°</td><td colspan="2">Angle* is between 0° and 30°</td></tr>
<tr><td colspan="2">Shown in Fig. 4.3a</td><td colspan="2">Shown in Fig. 4.3b</td><td colspan="2">Shown in Fig. 4.3c</td></tr>
<tr><th colspan="6">Types of MWCNTs based on configuration of graphene</th></tr>
<tr><th colspan="3">Russian-doll model MWCNTs</th><th colspan="3">Parchment model MWCNTs</th></tr>
<tr><td colspan="3">In this type, sheets of graphite are arranged in concentric cylinders. For example a smaller SWCNT is placed within a larger SWCNT. The graphical representation is shown in Fig. 1e and 1f</td><td colspan="3">In this type, single sheet of graphite is rolled around itself, resembling a scroll of parchment or a rolled newspaper</td></tr>
<tr><th colspan="6">Based on functionalization of CNTs</th></tr>
<tr><td colspan="6">Target oriented CNTs: To enhance the therapeutic efficacy of CNTs. pH responsive or temperature sensitive CNTs are prepared for this purpose. Magnetic CNTs are special types of CNTs in this category.</td></tr>
<tr><td colspan="6">Ligand attached CNTs: Various ligands like antibody, mannose, transferrin etc., are used for this purpose which increase the targeting efficiency of CNTs.</td></tr>
<tr><td colspan="6">Solvent dispersed CNTs: To increase the dispersibility of the CNTs, various solvents such as dimethyl sulfoxide, dimethylformamide, methylpyrrolidone, chloroform etc., are used.</td></tr>
<tr><td colspan="6">Surfactant grafted CNTs: To increase the dispersibility of the CNTs, various surfactants are employed. Pluronic, spans and tweens have been employed for this purpose.</td></tr>
</table>

*Angle between chiral vector R and armchair line (Fig. 4.2)

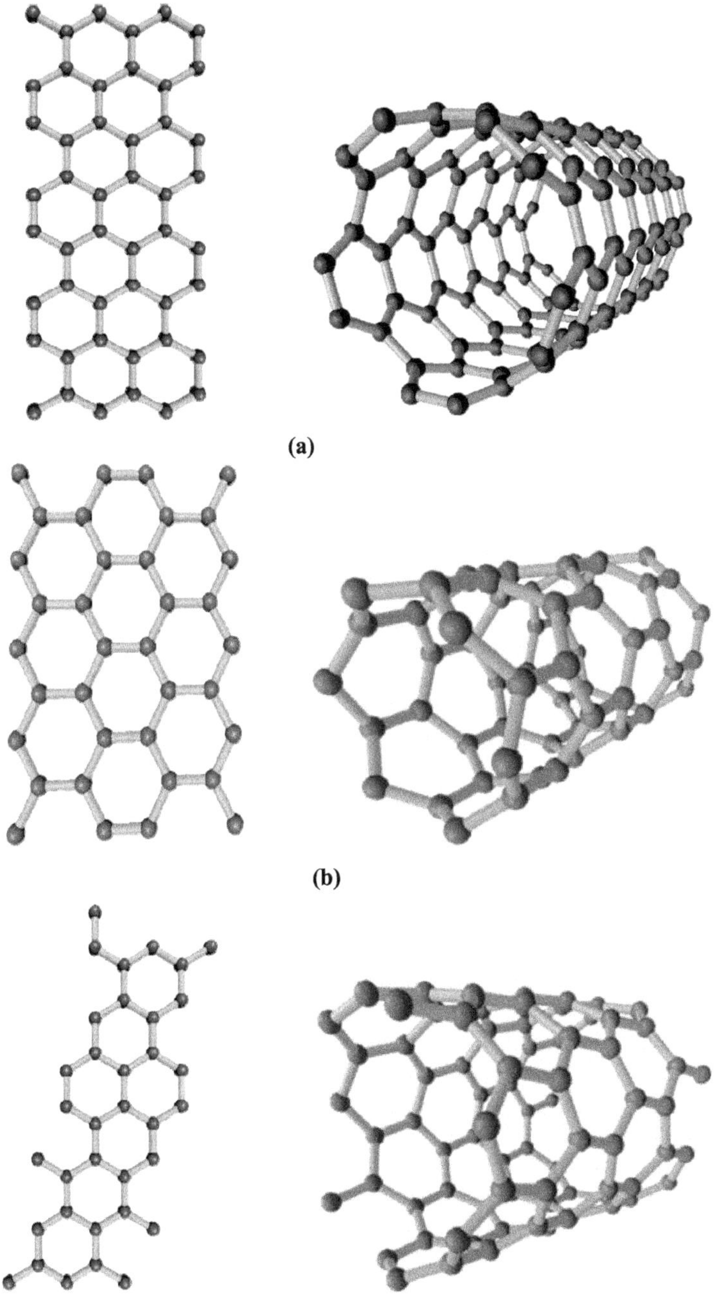

(c)

Fig. 4.3 2-D and 3-D views of SWCNTs based on configuration of graphene, (a) armchair (n = m), (b) zig-zag (n, 0) and (c) chiral (n, m) SWCNTs.

4.4 Physicochemical Properties of CNTs

The physicochemical properties of CNTs are governed by diameter, degree of chirality, and types of CNTs. As discussed in classification section, the orientation of the graphene sheets with respect to axis of CNTs, may have different chirality which leads to formation of armchair or zigzag, or chiral CNTs. It has been observed that the armchair CNTs are metallic, while CNTs with either zigzag or chiral conformations are semiconducting or metallic. Arrangement of different diameters along with chirality leads to the development of a variety of nanotubes exhibiting distinct mechanical, electrical, and optical properties. In general CNTs have got many advantageous physicochemical properties. Their tensile strength is extremely larger than high-strength steel alloys (45 billion pascals versus ~2 billion pascals). The current carrying capacity is estimated to be 1 billion amps per square centimeter which is quite more than copper wires (copper wires burn out at about 1 million amps per square centimeter). The heat transmission efficiency and temperature stability are substantially larger than other materials.

In SWCNTs there are two distinct regions viz. sidewalls and the end regions (end caps).

There is major variation in reactivity between the sidewalls and end regions/caps due to the fact that the difference in the surface curvature influences the chemical reactivity of CNTs. Similarly the differences in chirality of atoms which ultimately cause alteration in molecular structures (band structure and band gap), lead to variation in the electrical properties of CNTs. SWCNTs are metallic (armchair) and semi-conducting (zigzag) in nature, whereas the MWCNTs are the mixture of both conducting and semi-conducting CNTs. As far as the organoleptic properties are concerned both the SWCNTs and MWCNTs are granular or fluffy black powder. The optical activity of CNTs is supposed to decrease with increase in diameter of tubes, which influences other physical parameters. CNTs show a very high Young's modulus in the axial direction but remain flexible, in part due to their length. The physicochemical properties are affected by defects in the CNTs and also due to the interference of impurities (Chowdhury, 2011; Foldvari and Bagonluri, 2008a).

Aqueous solubility of CNTs is a major concern as it is well known that these are strongly hydrophobic in nature due to the graphene sheets. The strong p-p interactions between the individual tubes also cause assembly of CNTs as bundles. In drug delivery, aqueous solubility is essentially needed for formulation development as well as therapeutic effect and such behavior of CNTs is undesirable. Aqueous solubility can be increased by increasing the wettability and decreasing the inter bond attraction (by modifying the surface of CNTs) which avoid aggregation of the CNTs. In this regard many approaches have been worked out which are of pharmaceutical significance. The foremost approach in increasing the solubility of CNTs is the employment of surfactants. While it is risky to use the ionic surfactants owing to their reactivity, the non-ionic surfactants are found to be suitable for this purpose. These surfactants act *via* their well-known traditional mechanism to increase solubility whereas they tend to decrease the aggregation of the tubes by interfering with the inter-bond forces. Surfactants with high molecular weight are found to be more effective in managing the solubility of the CNTs. Other approaches in manipulating solubility of CNTs are modification of the surface by introduction of the polar functional groups such as carboxylic group, hydroxyl group etc. The presence of these polar groups reduces the hydrophobic interactions of the CNTs and increase solubility as well as minimize the aggregation. PEGylation of the CNTs is another approach which can be utilized for solubility enhancement. There are certain other approaches, such as employment of biomolecules but are not much efficient in fulfilling the purpose. Fig. 4.4 illustrates the approaches for improving solubility and dispersibility of CNTs.

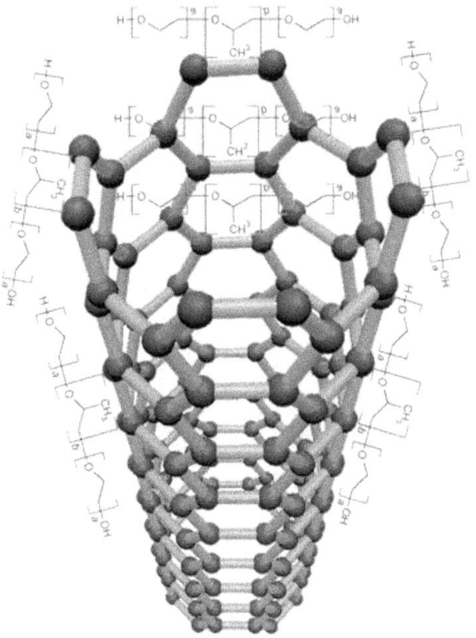

(a)

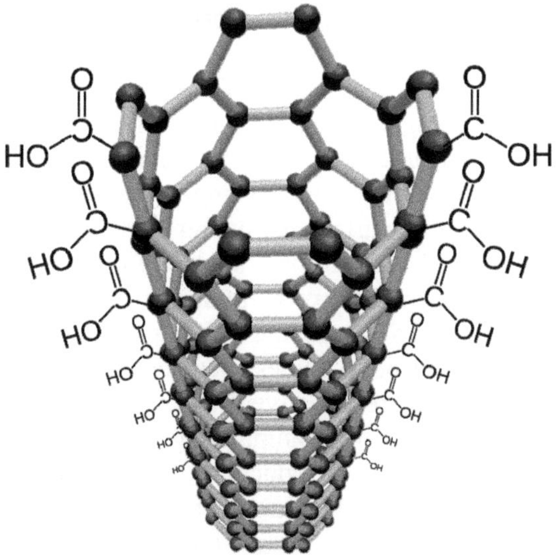

(b)

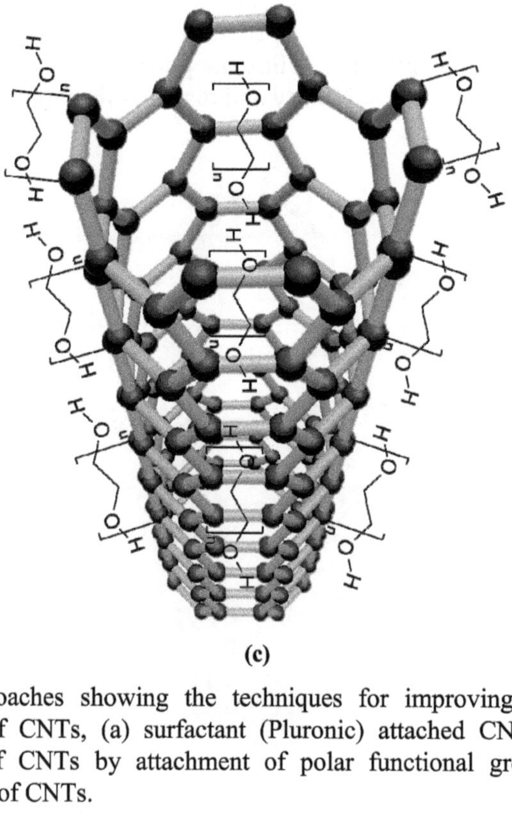

(c)

Fig. 4.4 Approaches showing the techniques for improving solubility and dispersibility of CNTs, (a) surfactant (Pluronic) attached CNTs, (b) surface modification of CNTs by attachment of polar functional groups (-COOH), (c) PEGylation of CNTs.

4.5 Manufacturing Methods

CNTs are manufactured by various methods (synthetic methods) and most popular among these are electric-arc discharge, catalytic chemical vapor deposition, and laser ablation methods. Purification is the subsequent process in the manufacturing of CNTs which facilitates in removing the undesired impurities and improves the quality of the CNTs. The purification techniques include high-temperature annealing, chromatography, microfiltration, microwave-assisted purification as well as oxidative purification. Depending upon the manufacturing techniques the characteristics of the CNTs vary, hence it is very much crucial to select suitable methods in synthesizing CNTs for specific purposes. There have been many advancements in the synthesis/manufacturing as well as purification techniques (Baddour and Briens, 2005).

4.5.1 Production Methods

4.5.1.1 Electric-arc Discharge

Electric-arc discharge method is the first and most widely used method for manufacturing of CNTs. This is based on the concept that at very high-discharge temperatures, carbon starts sublimating from the negative electrode leading to development of CNTs. Both SWCNTs and MWCNTs are synthesized by this method and the production yield is upto 30% by weight, however there is difference in opinion regarding the yield by this method. CNTs of various lengths and diameters can be produced by this technique and comparatively a few structural defects are found in CNTs prepared by this technique. The instrumental set up for electric-arc discharge method is shown in Fig. 4.5. There are two graphite electrodes separated by a distance of 1 mm. These electrodes are placed in a chamber filled with inert gas (helium/argon) and maintained at a pressure of 50-800 mbar. A current flow of 50-100 amps is supplied through this electrode which causes a high temperature discharge leading to evaporation of anode. This phenomena is responsible for deposition of carbon tubes on the cathode. These are further collected and subjected to purification. This method is very efficient in production of both MWCNTs and SWCNTs in laboratory as well as bulk scale.

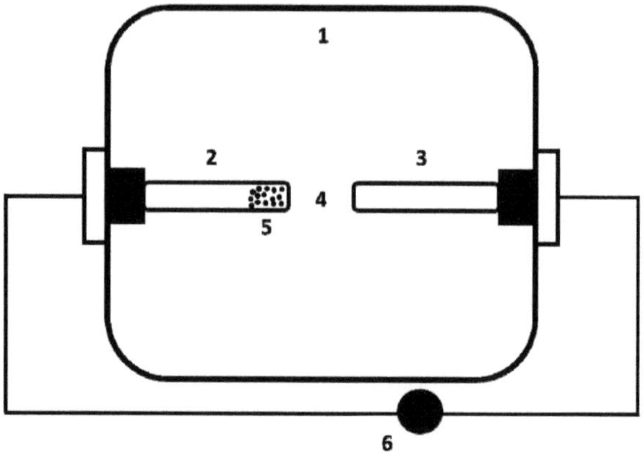

Fig. 4.5 Diagrammatic representation of electric-arc discharge method for synthesis of CNTs. (1) the reaction chamber filled with inert gas (Ar, He etc.) and maintained at 50-800 mbar pressure, (2) cathode (graphite), (3) anode (graphite), (4) space between anode and cathode i.e., 1 mm, (5) CNTs deposited on the cathode, (6) DC current supply for application of 50 to 100 amps driven by 20V.

4.5.1.2 Catalytic Chemical Vapor Deposition

Catalytic chemical vapor deposition is not that much popular as the previously discussed electric-arc discharge method. The reasons might be the use of various catalysts and lengthy process in comparison to the electric-arc discharge technique. In the chemical vapor deposition method, first of all a catalyst (Fe, Co, Ni etc.) is activated by some multi-step process and is deposited on the surface of substrate where nucleation of catalyst occurs. This activated catalyst is used further in the development of CNTs. As like in electric-arc discharge method, a reaction chamber is filled with inert gas. The carbon source (carbon monoxide, acetylene, methane, etc.) is then put inside the reaction chamber and high temperature of around 600-850 °C is supplied. The carbon source is allowed to diffuse in atomic level to the catalyst coated substrate. Progressively carbon tubes get deposited on the surface of substrate which can be collected and subjected to purification. In this method the yield is comparatively low (there is no specific Figure) than electric-arc discharge method of CNTs synthesis.

4.5.1.3 Laser Ablation

Laser ablation technique is quite similar to the electric-arc discharge method. In this technique a laser source is employed for the vaporization of carbon source which leads to the production of CNTs. Fig. 4.6 shows a diagrammatic arrangement of laser ablation technique. As shown in the

Figure there is a reaction chamber filled with inert gas, and inside the chamber the carbon source (graphite) is placed. There are laser sources which could supply laser either continuously or in a pulsatile manner as per requirement. CNTs collectors are also integrated inside the chamber which are made up of copper materials. After making all set up, the reaction is started and the carbon source is exposed to laser which produces a temperature around 1000-1200 °C. To facilitate the reaction a pressure of 400-500 torr is maintained throughout the experiment.

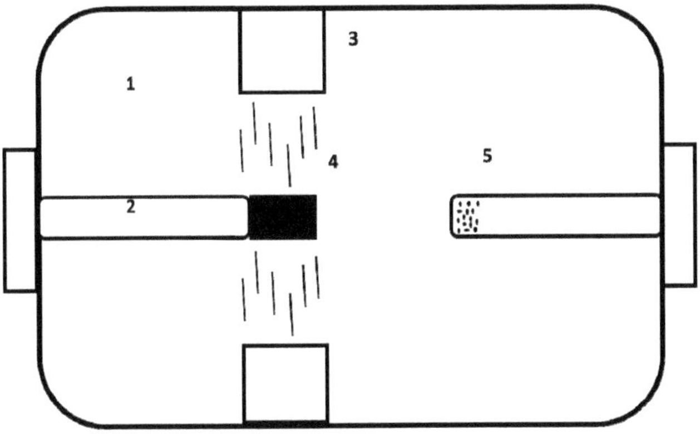

Fig. 4.6 Diagrammatic representation of laser ablation technique. (1) Container filled with inert gas (He/Ar etc.), (2) rod holding the graphite source, (3) laser source, (4) laser light falling on the graphite target, (5) CNTs collector.

In comparison to the two previously mentioned methods viz. electric-arc discharge and catalytic chemical vapor deposition, this technique is expensive. It is usually employed for the production of the SWCNTs as the vaporization caused by laser application is capable of producing ultra-small size CNTs with uniform size and shape. There is no common agreement on the yield of CNTs by this process, but it is usually expected that ~30 yield is achieved by this process. The developed CNTs are further subjected to purification to get good quality products.

4.5.2 Purification Techniques

As discussed in earlier sections, the yield of CNTs is not more than 30% irrespective of types of manufacturing techniques and there is presence of many impurities in the synthesized CNTs. It is obligatory to remove these impurities to get good quality CNTs products. Functionalization of the CNTs is done after the purification process is over so that efficacy and safety can be ensured. Many techniques are adopted for this purpose and most widely used among these are sonication, oxidation as well as acid refluxing methods. However several other purification techniques are also reported based on special type of manufacturing of CNTs and the number of such processes is so vast that all of them cannot be narrated. The commonly used technique in purification is the oxidation method. In this method, the raw CNTs produced after synthesis is subjected to air oxidation to remove the undesired impurities. The oxidized products are removed carefully by various means of separation. Application of some surfactants along with organic solvents followed by sonication also causes solubilization of impurities, which could be removed later. Some researchers have employed the acid refluxing method to remove the undesired impurities like amorphous carbon, metal catalyst or any other materials used in the synthesis process.

4.6 Functionalization of CNTs

There are two basic reasons for functionalization of CNTs viz. changing physicochemical properties, and to attach drug molecules/ligands for therapeutic action. Changing the physicochemical properties especially increasing solubility and dispersibility are intended to make these suitable for formulation development. At the same time, it is also desirable to make these CNTs biodegradable which is possible by rational functionalization with biomolecules as well as various functional groups. Attachment of any drug molecules to the CNTs is done by this functionalization approach.

As far functionalization of CNTs is concerned, there are two distinct parts in the CNTs to which any drug, ligand or bio-molecule can be attached. These two parts are the tip (end part) and side walls of the CNTs. It has been observed that the side walls are less reactive than the tip part, therefore maximum reactions usually occur in that area. Many research reports demonstrate that the more efficient the functionalization is, the more safe (non-toxic) and effective the CNTs will be. Functionalization of CNTs with various chemical or biological moieties are found to endow the ability to penetrate the cell membrane in an energy dependent way, however the extent of such activity is yet to be analyzed and quantified. There are three basic approaches for functionalization of the CNTs viz. (i) covalent functionalization (direct attachment), (ii) non-covalent functionalization (adsorption of molecules on the side walls) and (iii) entrapment of molecules in the internal cavity of CNTs. The non-covalent functionalization is based on the π-π interactions and are comparatively less robust/perfect than the covalent functionalization. One of the main drawbacks of non-covalent functionalization is its possibility of dissociation in the biological fluid environment. However, in some cases such non-covalent functionalized CNTs are required for specific purposes in employing targeted drug delivery.

In the covalent functionalization process, the CNTs are subjected to oxidation reaction or 1,3-dipolar cycloaddition of azomethine ylides (nitrogen-based 1,3-dipoles, consisting of an iminium ion next to a carbanion). In the oxidation reaction -COOH functional groups are generated which are employed for attachment of drug/bio-active molecules whereas the cycloaddition reaction leads to the development of biocompatible CNTs. In the oxidation reactions the CNTs are treated with acids like HNO_3, H_2SO_4/HNO_3, $KMnO_4/H_2SO_4$ and the functional groups such as -COOH are introduced in to the CNTs. These functionalized CNTs are observed to be non-toxic and biocompatible than the pristine CNTs. In order to investigate the *in vivo* bio-distribution, CNTs are labeled with the radio isotopes. The radioactivity can be measured by the suitable techniques such as gamma scintigraphy. The biocompatibility as well as therapeutic activity of CNTs are also enhanced by PEGylation techniques. PEGylation of CNTs (Fig. 4.4c) leads to delay in the opsonization and further engulfment by phagocytes. Proteins-peptides, DNA, carbohydrates, enzymes, as well as polymers have successfully been attached to the CNTs *via* covalent linkages. Gonadotropin releasing hormone which is overexpressed in the plasma membrane of some cancer cells, has been covalently grafted to the surface of oxidized MWCNTs. This functionalized MWCNTs efficiently penetrates the prostate cancer cells and exhibits better therapeutic effect. Other examples of covalent functionalization include conjugation of anti-HER2 IgY antibody to the surface of SWCNTs by amidation reaction which is facilitated via formation of NHS-esters on oxidized CNTs. Apart from these, many drug molecules are also attached to the surface of CNTs. Dapsone, an anti-microbial drug is successfully conjugated to MWCNTs by amidation. This is found to exhibit higher activity than the drug alone. In the covalent functionalization of CNTs the carbon lattice is usually disrupted leading to change in the characteristics of the CNTs. The sp^2 hybridization of the carbon atom in the CNTs are sometimes converted to the sp^3 hybrids and thus may compromise some of the physicochemical characteristics.

In the non-covalent functionalization of CNTs, adsorption of the functional groups/bio-molecules or polymers takes place. Here the reaction is based on the hydrophobic interactions and *via* π-stacking. The biggest advantage of non-covalent functionalization is that it does not affect the carbon lattice and hence the electrical properties remain same.

This method is very much useful to achieve good dispersibility and effective debundling of CNTs. Supramolecular complexes have been formed between CNTs and DNA where the nucleo-bases directly interact with the carbon scaffold, whereas the sugar-phosphate backbone is oriented towards the solvent. This non-covalent interaction leads to functionalized CNTs with more efficiency in terms of attachment of DNA. Similarly, dispersions of CNTs are achieved by physisorption of a series of surfactants viz. gum arabic, amylose, polyvinyl pyrrolidone, and dispersions were found to be stable for several weeks, without any precipitation of CNTs. Apart from these, the non-covalent functionalization of CNTs is also employed in cell targeting. Functionalization of CNTs with carbohydrates viz. α-N-acetyl-glucosamine, glucose, or mannose have been implemented for cell recognition by adsorbing mucinmimics adsorbed onto the CNTs surface. Such functionalization increases the interaction of CNTs with the living cells and support their adhesion to the surface. Various other events such as adsorption of drugs, polymers, bio-molecules, ligands are also worked out and found to be effectively done *via* this non-covalent approach.

The advantage of CNTs in drug delivery is to utilize both the surface and internal cavity for functionalization as well as encapsulation of drugs. The hollow cage like structures are well recognized and employed by researchers to entrap various drug molecules especially the chemotherapeutic drugs. The hydrophobic drug molecules are efficiently encapsulated in the hollow cavity and get adhered by the van der Wall forces. In some instances such encapsulation protects the drug from degradation, aggregation, enzymatic/pH dependent cleavage etc. Many drugs are reported to perform better after encapsulation in the CNTs. Carboplatin, an anticancer drug was encapsulated inside the MWCNTs after treatment of the CNTs with nitric acid at 90 °C which helps in opening of the tips of CNTs. The cytotoxic effect of functionalized CNTs to various cancer cell lines was higher than free drug which might be attributed to a protective action of CNTs. Other anticancer drugs such as oxaliplatin, cisplatin, and taxols are encapsulated in the similar manner to CNTs and their pharmacological activity is observed to be superior in comparison to free drug. The encapsulation approach is utilized not only for filling the cavities of CNTs with drugs, but it has also been employed for filling of polymers, genetic materials, and magnets for drug targeting. One such approach was reported by Li and co-worker (Li *et al.,* 2011) where they covalently derivatized doxorubicin on the side walls of MWCNTs with folate, as targeting agent of cancer cells. In the inner cavity of CNTs they incorporated iron nanoparticles. This was a very novel approach in drug targeting to cancer cells by bimodal approach employing folate and magnetic field. A 6-fold higher delivery efficiency of doxorubicin compared to free drug into cancer cells was observed by this approach. CNTs conjugated covalently to transferrin were employed for delivery of doxorubicin and these CNTs were encapsulated with Fe_3O_4 nanoparticles. The synergistic effects of transferrin and magnetic properties of CNTs significantly increased the cytotoxic effects of the developed target oriented CNTs. As such functionalization can be done in a variety of ways but it is expected to ensure biocompatibility and increased therapeutic efficacy. Fig. 4.7 illustrates the diagrammatic representation of functionalization of CNTs.

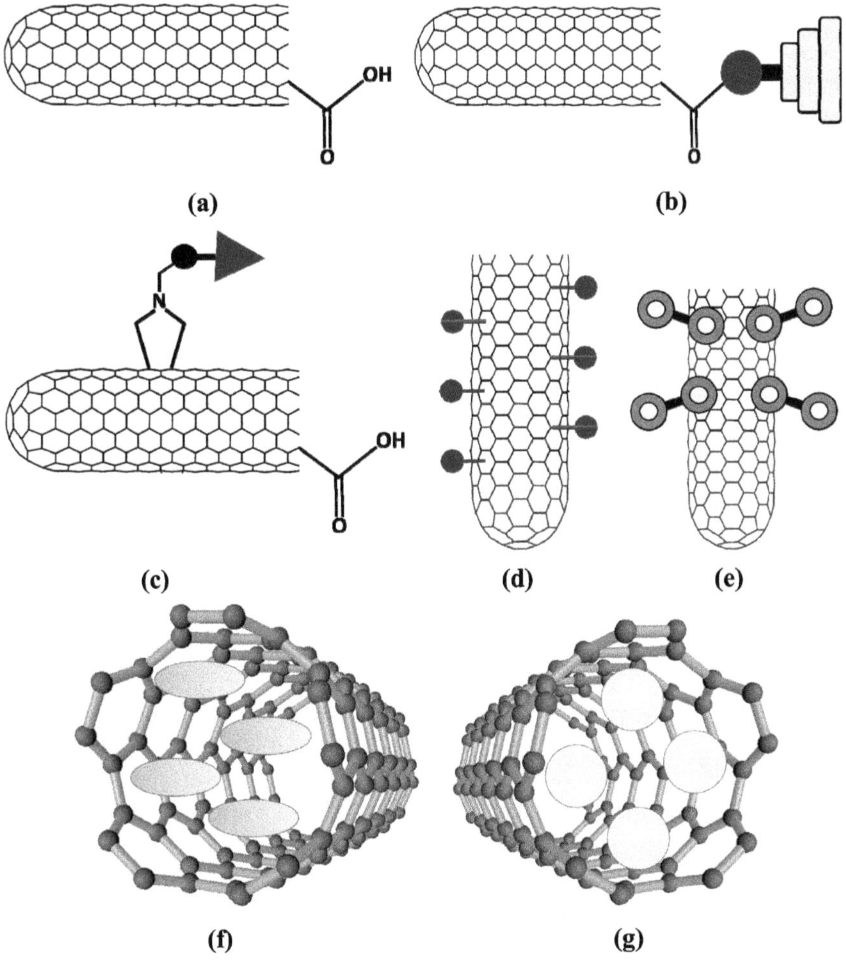

Fig. 4.7 Functionalization of CNTs by various approaches (a) oxidized CNTs with covalently attached -COOH group, (b) oxidized CNTs with covalently

conjugated drug/polymer/ligand *via* -COOH group, (c) covalent functionalization of CNTs by 1,3-dipolar cycloaddition of azomethine yields, (d) non-covalent functionalized CNTs with surfactant molecules, (e) non-covalent functionalized CNTs with bio-active molecules, (f) biomolecules encapsulated inside the hollow cavity of functionalized CNTs, (g) polymer conjugated drug encapsulated inside the empty cavity of CNTs.

4.7 Characterization Parameters

In a broad sense CNTs should be characterized for both physicochemical and functional parameters. Being nanomaterial, CNTs must be characterized for size, charge, morphology, purity, yield, and toxicity. However, the functionalized and drug bearing CNTs are to be characterized for several other parameters including drug content, entrapment efficiency, drug release, *in vivo* efficacy and toxicity in animals. Apart from these parameters, CNTs must be checked for surface defects, electronic characteristics, mechanical strength, and thermal conductivity.

4.7.1 Size, Charge and Size Distribution

CNTs are intended to be in nanometer range. The size and size distribution is evaluated by laser diffraction technology. The sample is suitably diluted and placed in the cuvette for analysis in the instrument. The polydispersity index which is a measure of size distribution is the output which is generated for the subjected sample in laser diffraction technology. The charge of the CNTs in dispersion is examined by micro-electrophoretic technique where the movement of oil CNTs is measured under the influence of a known electric field. The other techniques include electrophoretic light scattering technique which is employed for the same purpose.

4.7.2 Morphology

The internal as well as surface morphology of the CNTs can be investigated by any of the electron or atomic microscopic techniques. Scanning electron microscopy (SEM) is used to study surface properties. It also shows the presence of other impurities and routinely employed for quality control purpose in CNTs production. The process of analysis by SEM is simple and solely depends on the preparation of the samples. The sample is fixed on stubs and coated with gold palladium with the help of a gold sputter module in a high vacuum evaporator which is further analyzed using secondary electron imaging. Similarly, TEM is employed to determine the size, shape and internal features of CNTs. An appropriately diluted sample is adsorbed onto a grid. Excess sample is blotted off and the grid is covered with a small drop of staining solution. It is kept on the grid for few minutes and excess solution is drained off. The grid is put aside to dry thoroughly followed by examination in TEM.

4.7.3 Spectroscopic Evaluation

Various spectroscopic evaluations such as NMR, FTIR and Raman spectroscopy are employed for the characterization of CNTs. The Raman spectroscopy is widely used for the evaluation of synthesis and purification of CNTs. The ratio of intensities of the D-band (ID) to G-band (IG) is used for determination of impurity content as well as defects of CNTs. However, the impurities of amorphous carbon and metallic catalysts sometimes cause interference in the Raman spectra and make it complicated for interpretation. NMR and FTIR are very often employed for the characterization of functionalization of CNTs. FTIR is successfully employed for the identification of attached/grafted functional groups in the CNTs.

4.7.4 Miscellaneous Characterization

Apart from the parameters we have discussed, some other attributes are also evaluated in order to characterize the CNTs. The first among these is thermo gravimetric analysis, which is used for quantitative determination of the amount of carbon and non-carbon materials in the bulk samples of CNTs. This is also helpful in evaluation of the homogeneity and thermal integrity of the CNTs. One of the disadvantages of this method is that it is unable to identify the metallic impurities present in CNTs. The UV-VIS spectroscopy can be employed for the determination of dispersity of the CNTs, however it is always preferable to use diffraction techniques discussed earlier for this purpose.

4.8 Release of Drug from CNTs

As per the requirement, CNTs can be functionalized by covalent, non-covalent interactions or even adsorption on the surface can be employed for this purpose. In any of the cases the drug is attached/conjugated or grafted on the surface or even encapsulated inside the hollow cavity of the CNTs. These drug molecules are required to be released in a desired manner at the site of action. The functionalized CNTs work by successfully transporting the drug to the target site but the next crucial question is the release of drug from the CNTs to elicit therapeutic effects.

In order to facilitate the release of drug from the CNTs, some researchers suggest the use of an external force either in the form of magnetic field or NIR irradiation (Boncel *et al.,* 2013). An example in this regard is the development of CNTs encapsulating taxol. The drug molecule "taxol" is incorporated in gelatin and this temperature sensitive hydrogel is encapsulated in the MWCNTs. An external magnetic field is applied to facilitate the drug release from CNTs in the *in vivo* environment. A significant cytotoxic effect was observed after 48 hr, with these CNTs, whereas in the absence of magnetic stimulation a less cytotoxic effect was observed. Similarly, indole was encapsulated inside the CNTs and employed for cancer targeting by the application of NIR light. The indole molecule is efficiently transported to the target site and it caused disruption of the cell membrane leading to inhibition of cell growth. The NIR irradiation (10-s pulsed) facilitated the release of indole from the functionalized CNTs. Experimentally it was observed that incubation with the HeLa cells these functionalized CNTs caused significant cell death, however the same CNTs did not perform well in absence of NIR irradiation. The mechanism behind the effect of NIR in drug release from CNTs has been investigated and it was found that heat generated by NIR is responsible for drug release either by breaking bonds or enhancing permeability of the drugs. It has also been realized that the living systems are highly transparent in the NIR region whereas, the CNTs (ideal black body) strongly absorb the NIR radiation. Exposure of NIR light to CNTs causes significant rise in temperature of these materials which if accumulated in the cancer cells may cause overheating and explosion of the cells.

The wide variations in the pH of living systems viz. buccal, gastric, intestinal, lacrimal and intracellular pHs have been successfully employed in drug targeting by various approaches like pH responsive nanoparticles, microparticles, micells, liposomes etc. In recent years, the CNTs are also employed for drug targeting utilizing this pH variation especially to cancer cells. Usually the pH of cytoplasm is neutral but the disease conditions like cancer causes lowering of pH (~ 6.5) making it different from the other cells. MWCNTs are functionalized with pH responsive polymers like poly (N-isopropylacrylamide) and poly-L-lysine with simultaneous grafting to the chemotherapeutic drug. The polymer in the CNTs is subjected to meet up favorable pH conditions in the biological medium leading to release of the drug from CNTs. Molecular structure of drug, surface characteristics of CNTs and drug grafting/ conjugating methods play important role in the development of targeted CNTs delivery systems.

Some of the delivery systems like hydrogel, microparticles, tablets, and microcapsules have been reported as carrier of CNTs. Here in these cases, the functionalized CNTs carrying the drug molecules are incorporated in any of the mentioned delivery system which acts as carrier vehicle for CNTs. Release of the drug from the CNTs is also influenced by the type of carrier which is used to incorporate CNTs. The release of the drug from the polymeric carriers including hydrogels, microparticles and microcapsules is based on diffusion controlled, dissolution controlled and environmental responsive or chemical controlled mechanism. Release of the entrapped CNTs within these carriers will adopt one or combination of the mentioned mechanisms depending on the type of polymers used to fabricate the delivery carrier.

4.9 Fate of CNTs *In vivo*

Anything that enters the living system must be eliminated either intact or in degraded form and CNTs are not any exception. However, there is a long debate on the biodegradation of CNTs due to their unique physicochemical properties including aggregation, charge, lack of solubility and optical properties. There is no specific mechanism reported till date for biodegradation of CNTs, rather a series of postulations exist for the same. When CNTs are administered in the living system, they follow the bio-distribution as well as clearance mechanism of body, but the route of administration decides many issues like the time of clearance, toxicity and the therapeutic activity as well. CNTs may be cleared through lymphatic, biliary, or renal pathways depending on the route through which theses are administered into body (Kotchey *et al.,* 2013). As CNTs (any other nanomaterial and pathogens) enter the systemic circulation they are treated as intruders by immune system and as the first step towards immune response, a group of proteins (mannose-binding protein, ficolins etc.) cover these CNTs. After being recognized as foreign particles, a complement cascade is initiated. This cascade results into clearance of CNTs, either directly through the formation of the "membrane attack complex", or indirectly through opsonization leading to engulfment by macrophages or other phagocytes (Dumortier, 2013). Fig. 4.8 exhibits the diagrammatic representation of fate of CNTs *in vivo* after being administered *via* intravenous route. Being a foreign material to the biological system, CNTs after intravenous administration are opsonized and captured by the reticulo enthelial system (RES) in an attempt to flush it out of body. On the contrary, CNTs administered *via* intratracheal or peritoneal routes do not follow the above said path and cause severe inflammatory reactions. Physicochemical properties and the surface functionalization of CNTs also have influence on the biodistribution and clearance. CNTs functionalized with functional groups like -COOH, -OH etc. and having short length are subjected to quicker elimination from the body in comparison to the longer and non-functionalized CNTs. Functionalization with DNA, protein, or polymers have shown to improve the dispersion and biocompatibility of CNTs. PEGylation of CNTs is also found to significantly influence the clearance by interfering with their uptake by RES (Kotchey *et al.,* 2013; Liu *et al.,* 2009).

It has also been demonstrated that CNTs after being administered *in vivo* cause inflammatory events leading to increased production of macrophages and neutrophils. The macrophages play a vital role by either engulfing the CNTs or by imparting oxidative stress to cause biodegradation. On the other hand the neutrophils produce high, local concentration of hypochlorous acid (HClO), which causes biodegradation of the CNTs. Some studies have reported that after being engulfed, the macrophages undergo apoptosis and cause degradation of the CNTs. Dendritic cells and eosinophils are also reported to participate in biodegradation of some CNTs. Theses CNTs, especially MWCNTs are observed to be degraded into smaller CNTs after being exposed to macrophages and neutrophils which can be confirmed by TEM and AFM analysis. However, over activation of the immune cells may lead to undesired or even serious allergic reactions leading to anaphylaxis.

The enzymes, plant peroxidase, horseradish peroxidase, animal peroxidases, myeloperoxidase and eosinophil peroxidase are found to catalyze the biodegradation of the CNTs. Many *in vitro* studies are reported showing the action of these enzymes in degradation of functionalized CNTs. These enzymes are released by neutrophils and eosinophils, during the inflammatory response and cause formation of reactive enzymatic intermediates and oxidants like hydroxyl radicals and HClO which actively participate in CNTs degradation (Kotchey *et al.,* 2013; Rothen-Rutishauser *et al.,* 2010).

Deng and co-workers (Deng *et al.,* 2007) have demonstrated the biological behavior and consequences of CNTs *in vivo*. By using [^{14}C-taurine]-MWCNTs as tracer, they have shown the bio-distribution and translocation pathways of MWCNTs in mice by different routes. They concluded that after intravenous injection, MWCNTs predominately accumulated in the liver and retained there for long a time. Yang and team researchers (Yang *et al.,* 2007) examined bio-distribution of pristine SWCNTs and ^{13}C-enriched SWCNTs in mice by using isotope ratio mass spectroscopy. They also found that CNTs were majorly accumulated in the liver, lungs, and spleen over an extended period of time. They also agreed that biological consequence of pristine SWCNTs is obviously very different from that of their chemically modified or functionalized counterparts.

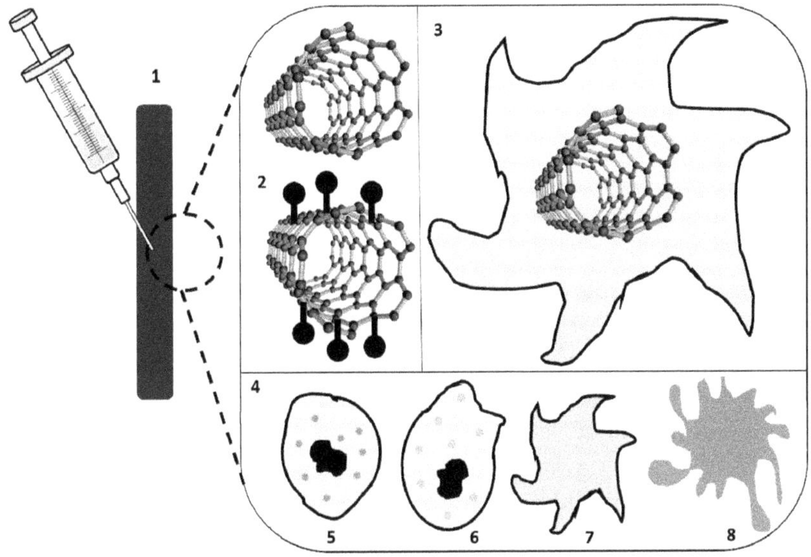

Fig. 4.8 Pictorial representation of fate of CNTs *in vivo*. (1) CNTs injected through intravenous route, (2) CNTs degradation by membrane attack complex, (3) engulfment and biodegradation of CNTs by macrophages, (4) immune cells participating in biodegradation of CNTs (5) neutrophil, (6) eosinophil, (7) macrophage, (8) dendritic cell.

4.10 Applications

Owing to their unique characteristics of being smaller in size, high strength, higher surface area, electrical conductivity, optical activity, hydrophobicity and ability to undergo functionalization, CNTs have gained a wide space for application in pharmaceutical, biomedical as well as biotech fields. Their smaller size and ability to get targeted even to nuclei of cells make them an attractive option for targeted delivery in many diseases like cancers, infectious as well as metabolic diseases. Electrical conductivity and optical activity make them eligible for easy detection and hence create scope for application in development of diagnostic tools, sensors and imaging tools. CNTs are also reported to act as a carrier for genetic materials, proteins and other biomolecules which can be accommodated on the walls (side walls in SWCNTs or even internal walls in MWCNTs) either by covalent or non-covalent linkages. The following section put emphasis on some of the important applications of CNTs in drug delivery and related areas.

4.10.1 Role of CNTs in Drug Delivery

Some drug molecules are notorious in nature. The term "Notorious drug molecules" is used for those molecules which are difficult to handle for formulation development owing to their inherent characteristics like poor aqueous solubility leading to poor and erratic absorption, poor permeability, higher cytotoxicity, enhanced biodegradability in physiological pH, un-predictable thermal and pH sensitivity, photosensitivity etc. Such molecules need special attention during the development of stable and effective pharmaceutical products. In spite of many efforts these physicochemical hitches as well as cytotoxicity of chemotherapeutic agents could not be controlled due to the failure in targeting the drugs to the desired site of action. Nanoparticles, especially CNTs bring new hopes in this area of research and reported to be useful in handling these drugs to get desired therapeutic effects. Amphotericin B (AmB) is one of such drugs which shows poor aqueous solubility and erratic absorption from the GI tract. Although very much effective in leishmaniasis, its aggregated form is reported to harm host cells and cause serious adverse effects. In liposomal form it is comparatively less toxic but its stability always remains a question. CNTs functionalized with specific functional groups carrying AmB are reported to be less toxic than the free form. The free AmB was found to be toxic (40% cell mortality) at 10 μg/mL, whereas the functionalized CNTs carrying AmB was found to be non-toxic up to 40 μg/mL. There are other reports also in agreement with this fact that, AmB is effective and better tolerated with functionalized CNTs (Wong *et al.,* 2013).

The anticancer drug 10-hydroxycamptothecin was covalently conjugated to MWCNTs *via* a cleavable ester bond, and exhibited a better release rate after coming in contact with esterase enzyme. A successful internalization of the active drug conjugates with CNTs has been seen with human gastric carcinoma MKN-28 cells. Other anticancer molecules viz. methotrexate, camtothecin, irinotecan, doxorubicin, daunorubicin, and epirubicin have been incorporated in the CNTs by either covalent or non-covalent functionalization. These are found to exhibit better therapeutic efficacy by successfully getting targeted to cancer cells. The higher accumulation of the CNTs at the cancer tissues as well as internalization into cancer cells due to the surface decoration by some special ligands or because of EPR effect mediated small size lead to high efficacy and better tolerability.

CNTs delivery is not confined to the anticancer drugs alone, rather it has been explored for other drug molecules such as anti-inflammatory, anti-hypersensitive, antimicrobials drugs as well as for antioxidants. The antimicrobials viz. AmB, pazufloxacin mesylate, gentamicin are attempted to be developed in form of CNTs delivery system and found to be very much effective against specific microorganisms. Similarly the glucocorticoid and non-steroidal anti-inflammatory drugs (NSAIDs) have been functionalized into CNTs and examined for therapeutic efficacy. These oxidized and functionalized CNTs have shown strong anti-inflammatory action in *in vitro* conditions. In this category, CNTs have been used as an additive in electro-responsive gel systems to control and improve the release of several NSAIDs at a moderately low voltage that is non-irritating to skin. Diclofenac sodium has been incorporated into spherical gelatin/MWCNTs hybrid microgels to form an electro-responsive systems and was demonstrated to be appreciably effective (Wong *et al.,* 2013).

Antihypertensive drug molecules have also been grafted to the CNTs. In this case a transdermal composite membrane made up of polyvinyl alcohol and oxidized MWCNTs was prepared. The antihypertensive drug diltiazem hydrochloride was loaded in the CNTs and therapeutic efficacy was investigated. The results were encouraging and it has been found that the CNTs grafted with drug exhibited higher anti-hypertensive action than free drug alone. A sustained release of diltiazem hydrochloride was seen in this experiment and apart from that incorporation of CNTs increased the tensile modulus/strength, percent elongation and viscosity of the composite membrane, resulting in low bursting tendency. Carvedilol, a β blocker was conjugated to MWCNTs and its drug loading mechanism was investigated. Carvedilol was distributed both on the surface and inside of CNTs using the fusion method, with higher drug content. The *in vitro* dissolution and drug loading was found to be satisfactory with this approach. Tocopheryl PEG succinate, a water soluble precursor of the α-tocopherol was found to disperse MWCNTs/ SWCNTs higher than the conventional surfactant triton X-100. This molecule formed amorphous coating on the CNT surface after drying, and predicted to be a potential delivery system for α-tocopherol.

4.10.2 Boosting up Immunity and Vaccination

T lymphocytes are the major components of immune system as they actively participate in the initiation and maintenance of immune responses. These are employed as targets in vaccination and anti-tumor immunotherapy. Specific antibodies are entrapped with CNTs which mimic the physiological activation of T cells by antigen-presenting cells. In comparison to the free antibody, those attached with functionalized CNTs are found to be more efficient in initiating immune response. The spatial configuration achieved by the stimulatory antibody attached to CNTs in *in vivo* condition is the key element in boosting up the immune response. Vaccination can be achieved *via* CNTs as it is reported in many research publications/reports. A stronger immune response was observed when CNTs functionalized with a peptide derived from the foot-and-mouth disease virus were injected to mice in comparison to free peptide. Peptide conjugated CNTs have also been tried in antitumor immunotherapy where tumor lysate proteins were conjugated to CNTs and a significant increase in efficacy was observed (Dumortier, 2013). The ability of CNTs to get inside the nuclei of cells is employed in boosting immune response. Cationic CNTs functionalized with oligodeoxynucleotides containing CpG motifs were found to exhibit higher immune-stimulatory action and this might be due to the enhanced delivery of therapeutic agents at intracellular targets. Gene knockdown could also be efficiently done by the use of PEGylated CNTs. Recent studies also have witnessed employment of siRNA attached CNTs in silencing genes in some specific diseases. Although these studies are to be recurrently validated in different animal models as well as human and positive results in this may lead to major breakthrough in drug delivery (Delogu *et al.,* 2009; Liu *et al.,* 2007).

4.10.3 Gene Delivery

CNTs functionalized with some specific functional groups such as polyethyleneimine, polyallylamine, chitosan and poly (L-lysine), are cationic in the physiological environment. These cationic CNTs are successfully employed as carrier for gene delivery owing to ability of forming complex with genetic materials as well as to translocate inside the cells. Prato and co-workers have successfully employed cationic functionalized CNTs for delivery of plasmid DNA for expression of β-galactosidase marker gene. They observed that expression of the marker gene was around 5-10 times higher levels than the plasmid DNA delivered alone (Prato *et al.,* 2007). Similarly Behnam and team have worked out on the non-covalent functionalization of SWCNTs with modified polyethyleneimines for efficient gene delivery (Behnam *et al.*, 2013). In their research they found functionalized CNTs exhibited increased transfection efficiency up to 19-fold in comparison to non-functionalized CNTs. Gene silencing is also explored by the application of CNTs. SWCNTs are functionalized with poly(ethylene glycol) and phospholipid (PL-PEG) molecules which bind together by van der Waals and hydrophobic interactions between two phospholipid alkyl chains and the SWCNTs sidewall. The amine or maleimide terminal of PL-PEG on SWCNTs surface is employed to conjugate a wide range of biological molecules such as siRNA, DNA, and antibodies. It has been found that these functionalized CNTs are quite efficient in penetrating the cells and exerting the desired therapeutic action. In an interesting research carried out by Varkouhi and fellow researchers, it was seen that functionalized CNTs complexed siRNA showed 10-30% gene silencing activity. The same research also reported that a cytotoxicity of 10-60% was seen with these functionalized CNTs. These researchers apart from approving gene silencing by CNTs, advocated for the development of comparatively more biodegradable CNTs which could show less cytotoxicity (Varkouhi *et al.*, 2011). Dendron-functionalized MWCNTs with numerous positively charged tetraalkyl ammonium salts at the periphery of the dendron, have been reported for siRNA delivery to cells. The researchers demonstrated an increased penetration and availability of the developed CNTs in cell because of surface functionalization. This is reported to be a very efficient carrier for siRNA to cells as the internalization of MWCNTs bearing siRNA was found to be increased which was confirmed by TEM, AFM and fluorescence microscopy (Herrero *et al.*, 2009).

4.10.4 Imaging Tools

A considerable work has been reported in the field of imaging science with CNTs. These CNTs have been found to be a suitable tool for imaging owing to their inherent characteristics. CNTs functionalized with fluorescent compounds have been investigated for use as radio-opaque substances. This technique is employed for *in vivo* imaging of the organs and tissues. Many anticancer drug molecules are grafted with fluorescein probe functionalized CNTs and it has been observed that these could exhibit better visibility *in vivo* because of fluorescence produced by the probe on CNTs. Raman scattering of SWNTs has been explored for *in vitro* and *in vivo* imaging of biological samples. The strong absorbance of CNTs in the NIR region is also used for photoacoustic imaging. A further advancement in this field is imaging of several body parts with administration of CNTs encapsulating miniaturized video systems as a pill. This novel system can be swallowed, and helps in visualizing the disease area of a particular tissue or organ. CNTs labeled with radioactive isotopes have also been employed for nuclear imaging applications. CNTs are becoming unique imaging probes with tremendous prospects in biomedical imaging (Gong *et al.,* 2013).

4.10.5 Biomedical Applications

In the sections above we have been informed regarding the various applications of CNTs starting from delivering drug molecules to *in vivo* imaging. Apart from these applications CNTs also share a major application in the biomedical segments. CNTs are reported to be employed as nano-sensors where the device is designed in such a way that the change in temperature is correlated to sensing pressure. A novel device viz. "piezoelectric pressure sensor" is developed by employing pressure sensing capacity of CNTs (Liu and Dai, 2002). Recent advancements in biomedical sciences have employed CNT-based nano-biosensors in detection of DNA sequences, especially those related to cancer, and human autoimmune diseases. Nano-robots, nano-probes, nano-tweezers and actuators have been developed for biomedical applications employing CNTs. Actuators usually work by converting electrical energy to mechanical energy and after the energy conversion, actuator utilizes mechanical energy in performing useful work. CNTs perform like artificial muscle which generates higher mechanical stress after the energy conversion (Beg *et al.,* 2011). The CNTs are found to be best materials for actuators owing to capacity in withstanding higher stress-strain forces, electromechanical properties and higher electrochemical coefficients. Nanoprobes use CNTs as raw materials and such probes are very much successful in diagnostic applications.

4.11 Toxicity Aspects

CNTs have been appeared as a key player in various disciplines of science and technology, especially for "theranostics" i.e., combined diagnostic and therapeutic uses. Their usefulness in drug delivery and biomedical applications have been established at pre-clinical measure and continuous efforts are put in order to develop them as successful delivery systems in nanotechnology at clinical level. However, because of their ability to interact with biological nano-machinery (membranes, intracellular organelles and macromolecules) in an uncontrolled manner, these nano-carriers sometimes behave as potential toxic substances. The toxicity of CNTs might be attributed to their length/diameter, incompatibility with biological components, surface characteristics, agglomerated architecture and presence of harmful residue on surface.

The biological components of cells viz. mitochondria, ribosomes, nuclear pore, receptors, channels and structural proteins have size in nanometer range. The engineered CNTs have similar size and when get into the body, start navigating through bio-fluids, tissues or targeted cells, and interact with a wide variety of biological nano-objects of cells. The length of the CNTs is found to be one of the major factors of toxicity. Larger and aggregated CNTs are not efficiently engulfed by macrophages leading to long stay of CNTs in the vicinity of biological components and this prompts to the release of IL-1ß, TNF-α, IL-6 and IL-8. This pro-inflammatory response results in allergic reactions and toxicity (Lanone *et al.,* 2013). Some reports related to diameter of CNTs and toxicity are also available in literature. For instance fullerenes and SWCNTs with a diameter of around 0.7-1 nm efficiently interact with the ligand binding sites of the enzyme. Such interaction was found to interfere with the active site of enzyme in binding with polypeptides leading to blockage of enzyme activity. CNTs are predicted to affect the channels or pores (0.3-1.2 nm) formed by membrane proteins involved in transporting molecules as well as various ions. Based on some molecular docking studies, it has been anticipated that SWCNTs interact with potassium channel and block the entrance for K^+ ions (Yanamala *et al.,* 2013). Cells are equipped with multi-protein intracellular assemblies including exosomes and proteasomes which are responsible for degradation of obsolete RNA and proteins. These assemblies have interior hydrophobic hollow cavity (1.2-5 nm) surrounded by catalytic site residues that are capable of degradation of biomolecules. CNTs effectively bind to these sites and interfere with the normal functioning of multi-protein intracellular assemblies. Other cellular components like voltage dependent ion channels of mitochondria, DNA and RNA interact with CNTs leading to conformational changes and altered function of these components. Van der Waal's forces and hydrophobic interactions are the major driving forces involved in the infraction of CNTs with DNA and RNA whereas the surface modified CNTs may interact *via* electrostatic forces. These genotoxicity accounts for carcinogenesis and inflammation caused by CNTs. Durability of the CNTs in the body is another determinant of toxicity. It has been observed that pristine CNTs have a much higher time of stay inside the body in comparison to the functionalized CNTs. Such conditions increase the chances of augmented exposure of CNTs to the biological components of body and consequently cause higher toxicity. On the contrary the functionalized

CNTs are comparatively more biodegradable and expected to cause less toxicity to host cells, however the complete eradication of toxicity in either cases cannot be assured.

Apart from the cellular toxicity, there are possibilities of skin, lung as well as eye toxicity of the CNTs. Because of the ultra-small size the CNTs are expected to get deposited in the lung and these are very slowly eliminated by macrophage phagocytosis. The retention of these CNTs further causes inflammatory response and may lead to chronic lung infection. Similar to that of lung toxicity, the entry of CNTs into skin *via* stratum corneum leads to deposition in the epidermis causing various skin infections due to inflammatory response. Deposition of CNTs in the ocular tissues may cause eye infection, glaucoma as well as alteration in the properties of aqueous humor. So deposition of the CNTs in any region of living system and slow removal process may lead to severe toxicity.

4.12 Future Prospects

The future progress of CNTs in drug delivery is beyond our imagination. We cannot exactly predict the fate of this novel nano-drug delivery system in the field of drug delivery sciences. Although a handsome numbers of publications, reports and parents are available in literature but their practical applicability and feasibility to reach pharmaceutical pipelines for mass production is questionable. The major hindrance in CNTs is to tame their tremendous ability to interact with nano-architecture of living cells. The so called toxicity (uncontrolled/ aggravated immune response causing allergic reactions) of CNTs in living system has got close proximity to their therapeutic action. Induction of immune response is desired but beyond a certain limit it may be fatal and the boundary of this has to be setup. However, development of safe, effective and stable CNTs will be the future need/scope in this field of research. Design and development of short, functionalized, highly dispersible in the physiological environment, biocompatible and biodegradable CNTs is challenging but needful task for scientists, healthcare professionals as well as engineers in realizing theses nano-carriers in service to human being.

References

Alkilany A.M, Thompson L.B, Boulos S.P, Sisco P.N, and Murphy C.J (2012). Gold nanorods: Their potential for photothermal therapeutics and drug delivery, tempered by the complexity of their biological interactions. *Advanced Drug Delivery Reviews* **64:** 190-199.

Asthana S, Jaiswal A.K, Gupta P.K, Pawar V.K, Dube A, and Chourasia M.K (2013). Immunoadjuvant chemotherapy of visceral leishmaniasis in hamsters using amphotericin B-encapsulated nanoemulsion template-based chitosan nanocapsules. *Antimicrobial Agents and Chemotherapy* **57:** 1714-1722.

Baddour C.E, and Briens C (2005). Carbon nanotube synthesis: a review. *International Journal of Chemical Reactor Engineering* **3**.

Beg S, Rizwan M, Sheikh A.M, Hasnain M.S, Anwer K, and Kohli K (2011). Advancement in carbon nanotubes: basics, biomedical applications and toxicity. *Journal of Pharmacy and Pharmacology* **63:** 141-163.

Behnam B, Shier W.T, Nia A.H, Abnous K, and Ramezani M (2013). Non-covalent functionalization of single-walled carbon nanotubes with modified polyethyleneimines for efficient gene delivery. *Int J Pharm* **454:** 204-215.

Bertrand N, Wu J, Xu X, Kamaly N, and Farokhzad O.C (2013). Cancer nanotechnology: The impact of passive and active targeting in the era of modern cancer biology. *Advanced Drug Delivery Reviews* **66:** 2-25.

Bethune D, Klang C, De Vries M, Gorman G, Savoy R, Vazquez J, and Beyers R (1993). Cobalt-catalysed growth of carbon nanotubes with single-atomic-layer walls. *Nature* **363:** 605-607.

Boncel S, Zajac P, and Koziol K.K (2013). Liberation of drugs from multi-wall carbon nanotube carriers. *Journal of Controlled Release : Official Journal of the Controlled Release Society* **169:** 126-140.

Chowdhury D.F (2011). Carbon Nanotube for Drug Delivery and Controlled Release. In Comprehensive Biotechnology pp. 643-655.

Delogu L.G, Magrini A, Bergamaschi A, Rosato N, Dawson M.I, Bottini N, and Bottini M (2009). Conjugation of Antisense Oligonucleotides to PEGylated Carbon Nanotubes Enables Efficient Knockdown of PTPN22 in T Lymphocytes. *Bioconjugate Chemistry* **20:** 427-431.

Deng X, Jia G, Wang H, Sun H, Wang X, Yang S, Wang T, and Liu Y (2007). Translocation and fate of multi-walled carbon nanotubes *in vivo*. *Carbon* **45:** 1419-1424.

Dumortier H (2013). When carbon nanotubes encounter the immune system: desirable and undesirable effects. *Adv Drug Deliv Rev* **65:** 2120-2126.

Foldvari M, and Bagonluri M (2008a). Carbon nanotubes as functional excipients for nanomedicines: I. Pharmaceutical properties. *Nanomedicine* **4:** 173-182.

Foldvari M, and Bagonluri M (2008b). Carbon nanotubes as functional excipients for nanomedicines: II. Drug delivery and biocompatibility issues. *Nanomedicine* **4:** 183-200.

Gao L, Liu G, Ma J, Wang X, Zhou L, and Li X (2012). Drug nanocrystals: In vivo performances. *Journal of Controlled Release* **160:** 418-430.

Gong H, Peng R, and Liu Z (2013). Carbon nanotubes for biomedical imaging: the recent advances. *Adv Drug Deliv Rev* **65:** 1951-1963.

Guo J.J, Yue P.F, Lv J.L, Han J, Fu S.S, Jin S.X, Jin S.Y, and Yuan H.L (2013). Development and *in vivo/in vitro* evaluation of novel herpetrione nanosuspension. *International Journal of Pharmaceutics* **441:** 227-233.

Herrero M.A, Toma F.M, Al-Jamal K.T, Kostarelos K, Bianco A, Da Ros T, Bano F, Casalis L, Scoles G, and Prato M (2009). Synthesis and characterization of a carbon nanotube-dendron series for efficient siRNA delivery. *Journal of the American Chemical Society* **131:** 9843-9848.

Iijima S (1991). Helical microtubules of graphitic carbon. *Nature* **354:** 56-58.

Iijima S, and Ichihashi T (1993). Single-shell carbon nanotubes of 1-nm diameter. *Nature* **363:** 603-605.

Kotchey G.P, Zhao Y, Kagan V.E, and Star A (2013). Peroxidase-mediated biodegradation of carbon nanotubes *in vitro* and *in vivo. Advanced Drug Delivery Reviews* **65:** 1921-1932.

Lanone S, Andujar P, Kermanizadeh A, and Boczkowski J (2013). Determinants of carbon nanotube toxicity. *Advanced Drug Delivery Reviews* **65:** 2063-2069.

Li R, Wu R.a, Zhao L, Hu Z, Guo S, Pan X, and Zou H (2011). Folate and iron difunctionalized multiwall carbon nanotubes as dual-targeted drug nanocarrier to cancer cells. *Carbon* **49:** 1797-1805.

Liu J, and Dai H (2002). Design, fabrication, and testing of piezoresistive pressure sensors using carbon nanotubes (Stanford Nanofabrication Facility).

Liu Z, Tabakman S, Welsher K, and Dai H (2009). Carbon nanotubes in biology and medicine: *In vitro* and *in vivo* detection, imaging and drug delivery. *Nano Res* **2:** 85-120.

Liu Z, Winters M, Holodniy M, and Dai H (2007). siRNA Delivery into Human T Cells and Primary Cells with Carbon-Nanotube Transporters. *Angewandte Chemie International Edition* **46:** 2023-2027.

Prato M, Kostarelos K, and Bianco A (2007). Functionalized carbon nanotubes in drug design and discovery. *Accounts of Chemical Research* **41:** 60-68.

Rothen-Rutishauser B, Brown D.M, Piallier-Boyles M, Kinloch I.A, Windle A.H, Gehr P, and Stone V (2010). Relating the physicochemical characteristics and dispersion of multiwalled carbon nanotubes in different suspension media to their oxidative reactivity *in vitro* and inflammation *in vivo*. *Nanotoxicology* **4:** 331-342.

Ruenraroengsak P, Cook J.M, and Florence A.T (2010). Nanosystem drug targeting: Facing up to complex realities. *Journal of Controlled Release* **141:** 265-276.

Varkouhi A.K, Foillard S, Lammers T, Schiffelers R.M, Doris E, Hennink W.E, and Storm G (2011). SiRNA delivery with functionalized carbon nanotubes. *Int J Pharm* **416:** 419-425.

Wilder J.W, Venema L.C, Rinzler A.G, Smalley R.E, and Dekker C (1998). Electronic structure of atomically resolved carbon nanotubes. *Nature* **391:** 59-62.

Wong B.S, Yoong S.L, Jagusiak A, Panczyk T, Ho H.K, Ang W.H, and Pastorin G (2013). Carbon nanotubes for delivery of small molecule drugs. *Adv Drug Deliv Rev* **65:** 1964-2015.

Yanamala N, Kagan V.E, and Shvedova A.A (2013). Molecular modeling in structural nano-toxicology: Interactions of nano-particles with nano-machinery of cells. *Advanced Drug Delivery Reviews* **65:** 2070-2077.

Yang S.T, Guo W, Lin Y, Deng X.Y, Wang H.F, Sun H.F, Liu Y.F, Wang X, Wang W, Chen M, *et al.,* (2007). Biodistribution of Pristine Single-Walled Carbon Nanotubes *In vivo*. *The Journal of Physical Chemistry* **C 111:** 17761-17764.

5

Target Oriented Nano-Carrier based Drug Delivery Systems

P. Khare[1], V.K. Pawar[2] and M. Chaurasia[3]

[1]Truba Institute of Pharmacy, Karond - Gandhi Nagar By Pass Road, Bhopal-462038, India.

[2]Pharmaceutics Division, CSIR-Central Drug Research Institute, Lucknow-226031, India.

[3]Amity Institute of Pharmacy, Amity University, Lucknow-226028, India.

5.1 Introduction

Targeted drug delivery is a method of delivering medicine to a patient in a manner that increases the concentration of the drug in specific parts of the body relative to others. In other words, to optimize a drug's therapeutic index by strictly localizing its pharmacological activity to the site or organ of action. A targeted drug delivery system offers various advantages like reduction in the frequency of the dosages taken by the patient, having a more uniform effect of the drug, minimising drug adverse effects, reduced fluctuation in circulating drug levels and increased safety. The drug which have narrow therapeutic window like anti-cancer, anti-tubercular and antileishmanial drugs need to be localized to particular site of body in adequate quantity and targeted delivery systems are beneficial in terms of achieving this goal. There are different types of drug delivery vehicles, such as, polymeric micelles, liposomes, lipoprotein-based drug carriers, nanoparticle drug carriers and dendrimers that can be used to achieve controlled and targeted drug delivery. An ideal drug delivery vehicle must be non-toxic, biocompatible, non-immunogenic, and biodegradable and should be able to avoid recognition by the host's defence mechanisms. The chapter focuses on the various nano-carriers based targeted drug delivery systems, biological processes involved in drug targeting and their pharmacokinetic/pharmacodynamic considerations.

Nanotechnology offers a solution to allow for safe, effective dose, site-specific drug delivery of pharmaceuticals to the target tissue. Nano-carriers composed of biodegradable polymers can be designed and engineered with various layers of complexity to achieve drug targeting. They offer aid by providing multiple mechanisms to encapsulate and strategically deliver drugs, proteins, nucleic acids, or vaccines while improving their therapeutic index. Targeting of nanoparticles to diseased tissue and cells assumes two strategies: physical and chemical targeting. Physical targeting is achieved through nanoparticle fabrication techniques. It includes using size, shape, charge, and stiffness among other parameters to influence tissue accumulation, adhesion, and cell uptake. Physical targeting can be more economically viable when certain fabrication techniques are used. Chemical targeting can employ molecular recognition units to decorate the surface of particles or molecular units responsive to diseased environments or remote stimuli.

5.2 Rationale for Nanocarrier based Targeted Drug Delivery

Conventional therapies have been administered *via* an oral route (tablets, pills and oral liquids) or via injections. These traditional drug delivery systems have certain disadvantages. The drugs are delivered to the entire body *via* the blood circulation and only a small proportion of the total dose reaches the site where it is required. Secondly, the high doses often required to achieve the requisite therapeutic effect at the site of action has the potential to cause toxic side effects.

Targeted drug delivery can overcome these shortcomings by delivering the drugs right where it is needed, with minimal side effects. The aim is to maximize the therapeutic effect in the patient whilst minimizing the potential side effects of the intervention and increase patient compliance and satisfaction with the therapy. Nanotechnology has witnessed development in the therapeutic field and possesses potential to improve the drug development as well as modify the scenario of the pharmaceutical field. Nanoparticles possess such physicochemical properties which allow them to be targeted to specific part/sites of the body and carry different molecules. Such aspects of the nanoparticles are advantageous in improving of the therapeutic efficacy through enhanced bioavailability and higher drug carrying capacity. To add to this nanoparticles can also be helpful in the protection of the therapeutic molecules from the physiological barriers as well as delivery of the novel macromolecules including DNA and siRNA (Lee *et al.,* 2013). Nowadays, drug-delivery systems with nanoparticles show a clear potential for cancer treatments (Aslan *et al.,* 2013; Chen *et al.,* 2013) in view of advantages such as,

(i) the ability of targeting specific locations in the body,
(ii) the ability of reducing the quantity of drug that needs to be delivered to attain a particular concentration level in the vicinity of the target, and
(iii) the ability of decreasing the concentration of the drug at non-target sites.

Drug carriers include micro and nanoparticles, micro and nanocapsules, lipoproteins, liposomes, and micelles, which can be engineered to degrade slowly, react to stimuli and be site-specific. Targeting mechanisms can also be either passive or active (Fig. 5.1). An example of passive targeting is the preferential accumulation of chemotherapeutic agents in solid tumors due to the differences in the vascularization of the tumor tissue compared with healthy tissue. Active targeting involves the chemical linking of the surface of drug carriers with molecules specifically known as ligands which enable the carriers to be recognized by the receptors and get selectively attached to diseased cells.

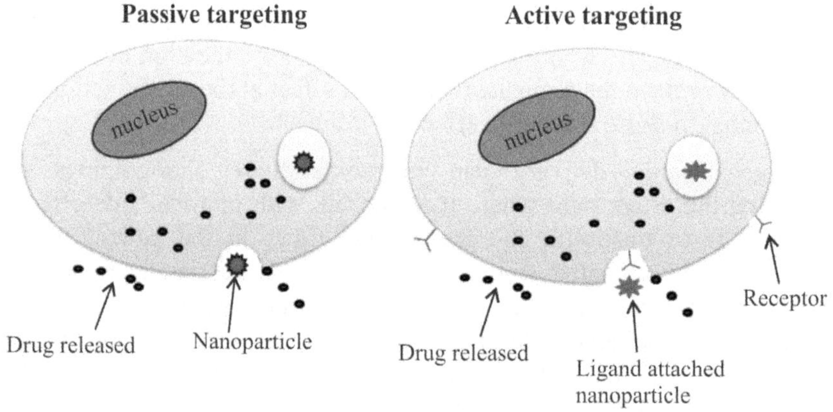

Fig. 5.1 Types of nanocarrier targeting.

5.2.1 Passive Targeting

Passive targeting as the name implies uses carrier systems for drug targeting without any external impetus. Drug targeting to macrophages for the treatment of leishmaniasis is an excellent example of passive targeting which utilizes the inherent defence capability of the body. As soon as the carrier system appears in systemic circulation, it is phagocytosed leading to accumulation of drug bearing carrier in macrophages which is the target site for leishmania parasites. In order to be effective the carrier systems may have to be specially formulated for sustained delivery of the drug or to enhance their permeability. Methods of delivery include: nasal sprays, inhalation systems such as nebulizers, dry powder inhalers and metered dose inhalers, and vesicular and particulate carrier systems. Nanomedical technologies are witnessing increased use of these systems as nanoparticles engineering can help to maximize drug bioavailability at the site of action. Passive targeting thus employs and utilises normal mechanism and pathophysiology of the organs for effective localization. In case of tumor the vasculature has wide fenestrations due to which the nanocarriers preferentially accumulate inside the tumor rather than the normal tissues. This leads to passive targeting of the carrier bearing drug to the target site. However these nano carriers are considered as foreign particles by the body and are quickly eliminated by the macrophages. In order to achieve efficient targeting, the carrier has to remain in circulation for longer period of time by avoiding the defence system of body i.e., macrophages. This particular property can be endowed by attaching or coating the carrier with some hydrophilic polymers like polyethylene glycols (PEGs). Attachment of such polymers inhibits the process of opsonisation which means the macrophages can not recognize the carrier and consequently the carrier can remain in circulation for longer period of time. There are some delivery systems which have demonstrated considerable level of drug targeting based on the passive targeting concept. Doxorubicin loaded PEG coated long circulatory liposomes displayed excellent effects in tumor therapy (Gabizon, 1992). Gupta and Vyas in 2007 developed amphotericin B emulsomes for passive targeting of the drug to be concentrated in infected macrophages of liver and spleen for better systemic anti-fungal activity (Gupta and Vyas, 2007).

5.2.2 Active Targeting

Active targeting is mediated by utilizing some ligands having specificity to the receptors which get over-expressed on the surface of target cells. Such ligands are attached with the carrier and the carrier bearing drug is carried to the specific biological sites due to the affinity of the ligand with the receptors on target cells. The carriers are designed to be highly specific for the intended target, minimizing side effects. Monoclonal antibodies and RNA interference therapies are examples of this category. This type of the targeting is highly sought after since this is very specific for the tissue. As already mentioned that the targeting is brought by the interaction of the ligand with that of the receptor and hence it is necessary to mention some of the ligands which have been utilised by the researchers for the active targeting of the biomolecules. Literature holds a number of such targeting moieties or ligands which are specific for a particular receptor present over a specific cell or organ viz. transferrin, specific antibodies, lectins, glycoconjugates, amino acids etc. Some of the targeted delivery systems along with the ligand utilised are being mentioned here. Tomasina *et al.,* in 2013 developed folate-functionalized nanoparticles in order to deliver a poorly water soluble cytotoxic agent, tripentone against the ovarian carcinoma *via* targeting of the nanoparticles bearing folate which is specific for the folate receptors present over the surface of the carcinoma cells. It was observed that the nanoparticles displayed potential in the targeting of the drug to the carcinoma cells where a rapid delivery of the drug tripentone was achieved which was confirmed by the *in vitro* real time cellular activity assay. A number of the studies have been performed for the targeting of the biomolecules by the active deployment of the folate as a targeting ligand. Folate receptors have also been reviewed for their utilization in the active targeting of cancer cells and in cancer nanotherapeutics (Zwicke *et al.,* 2012). In another study related to the targeting of the drugs block copolymer micelles were developed for the transport of the drugs to the solid tumors. Trastuzumab Fab fragments were linked or grafted over the surface of the micelles which provided internalization of the micelles into the breast cancer cells (Hoang *et al.,* 2013). Human serum albumin has been utilised for use as ligand. PLGA nanoparticles loaded with docetaxel were developed and the surface was conjugated by the human serum albumin. Results displayed a lower toxicity of the human serum albumin conjugated nanoparticles as compared to the unconjugated nanoparticles and free drug showing human serum albumin a promising ligand for targeting of the bioactives (Manoocheheri *et al.,* 2013). Hydrolyzed galactomannan (GalM-h), which is a polysaccharide of mannose and galactose are recognized by lectin-like receptors and so was utilised as ligand for the modification of the flower-like polymeric micelles coated with chitosan or GalM-h/chitosan directed toward the macropahges for the delivery of the rifampicin against tuberculosis. It was found that the surface engineered systems were taken up by the macrophages (Moretton *et al.,* 2013). Antibodies also find use as targeting ligands. Employment of the target oriented nano-devices or nano-systems for the diagnostic purpose have played a crucial role. Humanized monoclonal antibody trastuzumab has been utilized for the similar purpose. Multifunctional nanoparticles linked with different variants of the antibody or antibody fragment have been used for the breast cancer detection. Enzyme directed nanoparticle targeting has also been explored which displayed that the retention of the particles in the tumor cells was enhanced (Chien *et al.,* 2013). Pullulan has been conjugated with that of the doxorubicin and the conjugate was developed in the nanoparticles with the pullulan on the surface. These nanoparticles were utilized for the delivery of the drug to the hepatic cells. The pullulan has specific interaction with the asialoglycoprotein receptors present on the membrane of the hepatic cells and this leads to the targeting of the drug to the liver for antitumor chemotherapy (Li *et al.,* 2013). It is a known fact that the ligands play a vital role for the targeting of the drugs. Use of double ligands has also been used to modify the surface of the nanosystem for targeting of the therapeutics. In a study transferrin and mannan were linked to polyethylene glycol-phosphatidylethanolamine and phospahtidylethanolamine respectively. Solid lipid nanoparticles were formulated with these dual ligands. The efficiency of these nanoparticles was assessed in the tumor bearing mice. It was shown that the engineered nanosystem with dual ligands displayed higher transfection efficiency and that the ligands functioned as promising targeting moieties (Jing *et al.,* 2013). Antibody functionalized nanoparticles have proven to possess potential in delivery of anti-neoplastic agents. Chitosan nanoparticles conjugated with cetuximab has been utilized for the delivery of paclitaxel in the neoplastic cells with over-expressed epidermal growth factor receptors. Results indicated that nanosystems resulted in enhanced cell death which was due to higher cell uptake in case of the cetuximab linked chitosan nanoparticles (Maya *et al.,* 2013). Cancer specific phage fusion proteins have been recently evaluated as targeting ligands. The work focussed on the development of complexes of siRNA and phage protein which were formulated into nanoparticles/nanophages. It was found that the protein as targeting ligand specifically introduced the siRNA into the cancer cells. Lectin mediated drug targeting has been achieved for the delivery of the bioactives to colon. Wheat germ agglutinin was used and conjugated with doxorubicin which was targeted to the colon carcinoma cells. The conjugate demonstrated significantly higher cytostatic activity as compared to that of the free drug (Wirth *et al.,* 1998).

5.3 Biological Processes Involved in Drug Targeting by Nanocarriers

Drug targeting by nanocarriers can be of following three types:

5.3.1 Organ and Tissue Targeting

Organ or tissue targeting is meant to target the organ as a whole to deliver the bioactive specifically to the organ wherein the disease or infection may involve or effect the total organ as a whole. The organ targeting can be brought about through the deployment of different strategies in general. These can be included under the following head groups:

(i) Direct application of the drugs or introduction of the bioactives into the organ.

(ii) Therapeutics introduced into the organ through infiltration of the carrier system which accumulates into the leaky areas of the tissue. This is also known as passive targeting involving enhanced permeability and retention effect (EPR) i.e., accumulation through mechanical process.

(iii) Targeting can also be done utilising the change in the pH or temperature of the tissue environment by the use of the pH/temperature sensitive drug carrier system.

(iv) An altogether different strategy involves the use of the specific ligand attached to the carrier or the drug or through the surface modification of the carrier which may preferentially be directed to the organ. This type of the targeting involves drug delivery to specific tissue or organ in the body which can be exemplified through the examples such as pulmonary delivery of nanocarriers loaded with drug to lungs in case of tuberculosis, asthma, and brain specific drug delivery for treatment of Alzheimer disease. Another example in this category is targeting of vascular endothelium in inflamed tissue for site selective delivery of drugs for rheumatoid arthritis and osteoporosis, and colon-specific delivery systems for peptide and protein drugs. There are numerous reports related to the targeting of the drugs/drug loaded delivery systems to a specific tissue or organ for one or other cause. Colon specific delivery of the 5-Aminosalicylic acid has been achieved by the utilization of the dextran wherein the dextran was conjugated to the drug by the p-aminobenzoic acid and benzoic acid as linkers. Drug release and other results indicated towards the specificity of the conjugate in targeting of the drug to the colon (Shrivastava *et al.*, 2013). Targeted delivery of methotrexate has been achieved through the fabrication of drug loaded calcium pectinate cross linked microspheres intended to release the drug in colonic environment (Chaurasia *et al.*, 2008). Eudragit coated cross linked chitosan microspheres have been developed for combining pH-sensitive property and specific biodegradability for colon-targeted delivery of metronidazole (Chourasia and Jain, 2004). Delivery of the therapeutics to the pulmonary part has also been explored widely apart from the approach that utilizes aerosols. Lactose conjugated PLGA nanoparticles have been formulated for the lung specific delivery of rifampicin. The linking of the lactose as ligand on the surface of the PLGA nanoparticles significantly enhanced the lung uptake of drug, which is indicated by the fact that the recovery of dose from the lungs was higher as compared to the dose recovered in the case of uncoupled drug-loaded NPs and plain drug solution (Jain *et al.*, 2010). In a similar way brain delivery of anti antiparkinson drug dopamine HCl has been performed through the active deployment of the amino acid coupled liposomes. The results demonstrate that the highly hydrophilic drug dopamine can be effectively targeted to the brain. Coupled liposomes displayed superiority over the uncoupled formulation and plain drug (Khare *et al.*, 2009b). A wide number of the conjugates with effective targeting to different organs have been reviewed in the literature (Khare *et al.*, 2009a).

5.3.2 Cellular Targeting

There are infections occurring in the body which affect only a specific part of the organ or specific cells of a particular organ. The causative organism or infection can be localized in a particular cell of the organ or the tissue. Therefore it is wise to target that particular cell(s) so as to spare the normal cells of the tissue from the effect of the drug. Since each cell type possesses different characteristics and hence can be targeted through the use of such biomaterials which have specificity to particular cell(s). The most common type of the targeting strategy is through the use of cell specific targeting moieties attached to the drug or drug carrier. In general this refers to targeting of drug using nanocarriers to specific cells in the tissues or organs e.g., receptor mediated macrophage cell targeting using ligand coated nanocarriers in tuberculosis and leishmaniasis, drug targeting specifically to cancerous cells, hepatic endothelial and kupffer cells for the treatment of inflammatory liver diseases. Targeting of kupffer cells has been done through the effective use of fucosylated carbon nanotubes for the management of liver damage induced by cytokine. Deployment of modified carbon nanotubes resulted in the higher inhibition of the cytokines and indicated that these could be promising delivery systems for targeting of kupffer cells (Gupta *et al.,* 2013). Targeting of antitubercular drug isoniazid was brought about by the mannosylated gelatin microspheres. It has been suggested that these delivery systems could be a potential tool for drug targeting to alveolar macrophages (Tiwari *et al.,* 2011).

5.3.3 Intracellular Targeting

This type of targeting is known as the cell organelle targeting also regarded as the third order of targeting. It implies delivery of drug into specific organelles of the cell like nucleus, mitochondria, phagosomes etc. Nanocarrier can gain access to and get inside the cytoplasm of a target cell in order to release the drug at the optimum rate for pharmacological effectiveness. This type of delivery can be of intracellular receptor specific, enzyme specific or pH dependent. Subcellular delivery is gaining impetus and recently has become a potential tool for the delivery of genes in case of gene therapy which is advancement of the therapeutic regimen. Much of the research is being conducted for the targeting of the organelles for a specific cause. Although the targeting to the organelle is brought about by the targeting ligands it involves some processes which are instrumental in such type of targeting. The drug should reach to a specific cell and thereafter it should get into the cell to reach the specific cell organelle. Majority of such targeting are based on the endocytosis of the drug or drug/biomolecule loaded carrier system wherein the carrier is absorbed into the cell through engulfment. The molecule is invaginated to form an endosome which after fusion with the lysosome gradually releases the bioactive into the cell. The endocytosis can take place in three different ways i.e., phagocytosis, pinocytosis and receptor mediated endocytosis (Neekhra and Padh, 2004). The delivery of the bioactive through the endocytic pathway involves the formation of the endolysosome and the engulfed substances are lysed through the enzymes present inside the lysosome and therefore limited delivery of the therapeutics may occur. Hence attempts have been made to deliver the bioactives or target them to the cell such that they escape the endosomal pathway i.e., following a nonendosomal route. In relation to the above context cell penetrating peptides which are also known as protein transduction domains with the ability to cross the biological cell membrane have attracted the interest of the research workers. The cell penetrating peptides cross the biological membranes in an energy independent non-toxic way and possess capacity for the internalization of the biomolecules attached to them (Lindgren *et al.,* 2000). A study has shown that an engineered chimeric protein was efficiently taken up by the cardiac cells *in vivo* for the purpose of control of stress (Bian *et al.,* 2007). Targeting of nucleus is often practised for delivery of the drugs that act on DNA and prevent its replication. Also this is helpful in the inhibition of the transcription of the some of the genes to block the production of some of the proteins. Since most of the drugs do not gain entry into the nucleus and in many cases the drug resistance is also acquired due to genetic changes and hence there is need for such targeting which allows the bioactives to be delivered in the nucleus. In this context the nuclear localization sequence has been of immense importance which is recognised by the nuclear localization signal receptor and is allowed to enter into the nucleus. Some of the peptides which display nuclear localization include KKKRKV peptide from SV40 large T antigen used for nuclear localization and delivery (Sakhrani and Padh, 2013). On the other hand cationic lipids conjugated with DNA (lipoplex) and cationic polymers complexed with DNA (polyplex) have been utilised for the delivery of DNA into the nucleus (Li and Huang, 2000). These have also been used in clinical trials for treatment of melanoma. Another nuclear localisation sequence i.e., nucleoplasmin has been used for the delivery of the DNA, oligonucleotide and peptide. The other organelle which has been explored for targeting is mitochondria. Mitochondria is involved in production of ATP and also plays vital or key roles in different processes and malfunctioning of mitochondria has been found in different diseases viz. obesity, cardiomyopathy, migraine, parkinsonism etc. This has been attributed to the mutation in the genome of the mitochondria which could be brought about by the targeted delivery of such drugs to mitochondria which could prevent the effect of the mutant genes. The mitochondrial targeting has been achieved through the covalent coupling of the Vitamin E to triphenylphosphonium cation (Smith *et al.,* 1999). Targeting to mitochondria can also be achieved by using the mitochondria targeting sequence which directs the moiety attached to it specifically to the mitochondria. This concept was utilised for targeting restriction endonuclease sma1 to the mitochondria by fusing it to the MTS (mitochondrial targeting sequence) for the elimination of the mutant DNA (Tanaka *et al.,* 2002). Targeting of the cellular components/ organelles is being explored widely for the betterment of the therapy and other cellular parts are also being subjected to targeting for one or the other reason.

5.3.4 Cellular Uptake and Processing

Several membrane layers provide an obstacle for therapeutic agents attempting to target intracellular structures. Generally low molecular weight drugs can easily penetrate cell membrane *via* diffusion. During this process, compound is lost due to ineffective partitioning across biological membranes. Nanocarriers present opportunity for eliminating much of this 'waste' due to masking of the therapeutic agent from its biological environment; this effectively limits the influence of a drug's physical properties on intracellular drug concentrations. Instead, the properties and surface characteristics of the nanoparticles play a greater role in compound delivery and resulting intracellular drug concentrations. Since nanocarriers are formed of molecular assemblies, hence cannot enter the cells *via* simple diffusion process. It requires a complex procedure of endocytosis which includes both membrane manipulation to envelope the entering nanocarrier and its internalizations. It includes three subtypes: phagocytosis, pinocytosis, and receptor-mediated endocytosis. Different mechanisms have variable efficiencies of endocytosis, intracellular trafficking, release of the therapeutic agent into the cytoplasm, diffusion and translocation of the therapeutic agent to its susceptible target and partition into the nucleus or other organelles.

5.3.4.1 Cellular Phagocytosis

Phagocytosis involves the ingestion of materials up to 10 µm in diameter and can be accomplished by fairly few cell types of the reticuloendothelial system (RES), such as macrophages, neutrophils, and dendritic cells. It can be mediated by opsonins (immunoglobulins, complement system factors, fibronectins etc., and receptors (scavenger, mannose TLR, GLUT receptors etc). Phagocytic cells engulf opsonised nanocarriers to form phagosome, which fuse with lysosome that converts it into hydrolytic organelle, leading to digestion of particles by lysosmal enzymes to release drug in the cell.

5.3.4.2 Cellular Pinocytosis

Pinocytosis is an uptake mechanism that can be conducted by virtually all cell types, and normally involves ingestion of nano sized material and substances in solution. Larger microparticles provide selective access to phagocytic cells, while smaller nanoparticles provide access to virtually all cell types. This distinct capability of nanoparticles may be utilized for the delivery of therapeutic agents to a wide array of cellular types and targets.

5.3.4.3 Receptor-mediated Endocytosis

Receptor-mediated endocytosis offers the potential for even greater selectivity in cellular targeting. The cellular membrane possesses various receptors, which upon extracellular binding to their respective ligands (functionalized on nanocarriers), transduce specific signal to the intracellular space. This signal can trigger a multitude of biochemical pathways; which may cause internalization of the ligand and its appended nanoparticle *via* endocytosis. Cross-linking of receptors *via* ligands attached to nanoparticles results in penetration into cellular membrane to form an endosome. It has been shown that nanoparticles sized between 25 and 50 nm are a requisite for optimal endocytosis and intracellular localization. Furthermore, selective active targeting of nanocarriers to specific tissues may take advantage of the differential expression of receptors between cellular types. For example, it was recently reported that the attachment of lipomannan onto the surface of nanoparticles prompted superior cross-linking of the mannose receptors overexpressed on macrophage cells, with variable internalization depending on nanoparticle size (Zhu *et al.,* 2011).

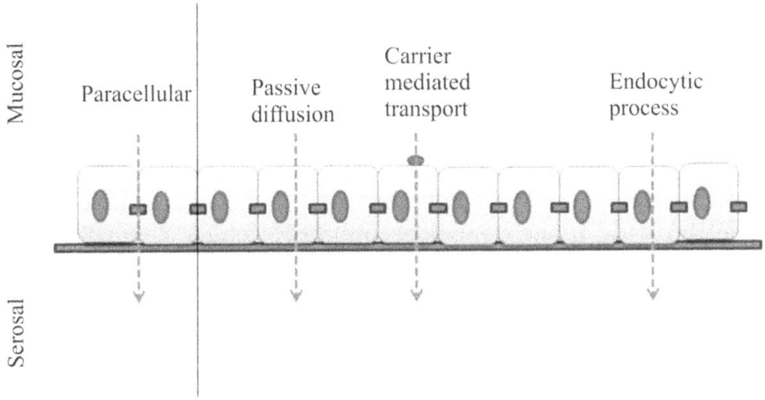

Fig. 5.2 Nanocarrier transport through epithelium.

5.3.5 Transport across Epithelium

Internal organs and cavities like buccal, oral, intestinal, nasal vaginal, rectal etc., are internally lined with one or more layers of epithelial cells, which are bound with each other by intracellular junctions. Various transport processes like passive diffusion, endocytosis and carrier mediated transport are involved in the transport of the soluble drug (Fig. 5.2). The transport of nanocarrier through highly cohesive epithelial membrane would be difficult using simple nanocarriers (without ligands or penetration enhancers). Targeting strategies to improve the penetration of nanoparticles into epithelium can be classified into those utilizing specific binding to ligands or receptors and those based on nonspecific adsorptive mechanism.

Blood brain barrier is one of the physiological barriers of the body which is characterized by the presence of tight junctions formed by the endothelial cells of the capillary which strictly prevents the entry of otherwise unknown molecules into the brain and this can be regarded as the mechanism of the body to safeguard the control room of the body i.e., brain. The blood brain barrier has active efflux transport systems and possesses enzymatic activity. Although the barrier limits the entry of the water soluble molecules it can also reduce the passage of the lipid soluble molecules as well. Hence it only permits specific molecules to pass through it which are essential for the normal functioning of the brain. Therefore the delivery to brain is a herculean task. Delivery of drug molecules can be performed through different strategies employing surface modified nanoparticles utilising the receptor mediated transport system present on the barrier. A number of such targeting ligands which can be tagged over the nanoparticles are available viz. transferrin receptor binding antibody (OX26), lactoferrin, cell penetrating peptides and polysorbate 80 etc. These have shown promising results to target the therapeutics to brain through the formulation of the nanoconstructs which can pass across barrier through receptor mediated endocytosis.

The buccal mucosa is a highly differentiated tissue which is readily accessible, has a rich vasculature, and bypasses hepatic first-pass metabolism Also, it has a relatively mild pH, which is suitable for drug delivery. The buccal cavity contains several drug-metabolizing enzymes such as oxidases, reductases, lipoxygenases, cyclo-oxygenases, phosphatases, carbohydrases, nucleases, esterases, and peptidases. Peptidases and proteases in the buccal cavity present a barrier to the buccal absorption of peptides and proteins even when the enzymatic activity is much lower than those of other mucosal barriers. These drugs encapsulated in nanocarriers can be an alternative. The use of nanoparticles for local delivery to the oral mucosa has been reported. Bioadhesive nanoparticles offer the same advantages as tablets but their physical properties enable them to make intimate contact with a larger mucosal surface area. These are typically delivered as an aqueous suspension or are incorporated into a paste or ointment or applied in the form of aerosols. Particulates have the advantage of being relatively small and more likely to be acceptable by the patients. Two types of nanoparticles have been reported for buccal delivery, idarubicin containing solid lipid nanoparticles and polystyrene nanoparticles (Fluo-Spheres®) (Holpuch *et al.,* 2010). The nanoparticles were investigated using monolayer-cultured human oral squamous cell carcinoma (OSCC) cell lines and normal human oral mucosal explants in a proof of concept study. The results demonstrated that cells internalized solid lipid nanoparticles. The observed penetration of nanoparticles through the epithelium and basement membranes into the underlying connective tissue suggested the possibility of oral transmucosal nanoparticles delivery for systemic therapy.

Nasal route is preferred due to its fast absorption and rapid onset of drug action also avoiding degradation of labile drugs in the GIT and insufficient transport across epithelial cell layers. The use of nanocarriers provides a suitable way for the nasal delivery of drug and vaccine candidate. Drug loaded nanocarriers has also proved to be useful in CNS drug delivery and migraine therapy (Zhang *et al.,* 2013). Antigen loaded nanoparticles are more lucrative as they provide improved protection and also facilitated transport of the antigen impart more effective antigen recognition by immune cells. These represent key factors in the optimal processing and presentation of the antigen and therefore in the subsequent development of a suitable immune response.

Nanotechnology based drug delivery system can be developed for the oral delivery of the drugs. Such systems can be targeted to specific sites of the gastrointestinal tract and hence effective protection of drugs can be practised which are vulnerable to the acid or some specific enzymes. The nanoparticles have also been used to enhance the bioavailability of the drugs such as cyclosporine-A by releasing the drug at specific pH through the pH sensitive nanoparticles of poly(methylacrylic acid and methacrylate).

In gastro-intestinal tract (GI tract) epithelium, surface of M-cells of Peyer's patches and enterocytes display cell-specific carbohydrates, which may serve as binding sites to nanocarriers containing appropriate ligands. Certain glycoproteins and lectins bind selectively to this type of surface structure by specific receptor-mediated mechanism. Lectins have been studied to enhance oral peptide absorption. Vitamin B-12 absorption from the gut under physiological conditions occurs *via* receptor-mediated endocytosis. The ability to increase oral bioavailability of various peptides (e.g., granulocyte colony stimulating factor, erythropoietin) and particles by covalent coupling to vitamin B-12 has been studied.

5.3.6 Extravasation

The migration by nanocarriers from a blood vessel lumen through vascular walls into the tissues is called as extravasation of nanocarriers (Fig. 5.3). Nanoparticles because of their small dimension interacts effectively with cells diffusing further into tissues and into and through individual cells. The biological features that control the extravasation of nanocarriers are: permeability of capillary walls, rate of blood supply, and normal physiopathological condition. Shape, size, and charge of nanocarrier also influence its extravasation. Nanocarrier extravasation is inversely proportional to size and small particles (fewer than 200 nm size) should be most effective for extravasating the tumor microvasculature. Blood capillaries can be divided into three types on the basis of morphology: continuous, fenestrated and sinusoidal. Continuous capillaries are common and widely distributed in body characterized by tight junctions and un-interrupted basement membrane. This shows extravasation through vesicular trafficking. Fenestrated capillaries show inter-endothilium gaps (20-80 nm) at regular interval. These capillaries show high extravasation. Sinusoidal capillaries have inter-endothilium gaps of 10 nm size. These capillaries are wider with irregular lumen. Variation in arterioles, venules and capillaries has an effect on the extravasation of nanocarriers. Endothelial cells of arterioles have tight junctions whereas capillaries have occluding junctions. Small nanoparticles are reported to get transported through trans-capillary pinocytosis and receptor mediated transport. Organs such as lungs which have large surface area have high permeability and large extravasation. Skeletal muscles, adipose tissues, liver, myocardial endothelium also shows extravasation.

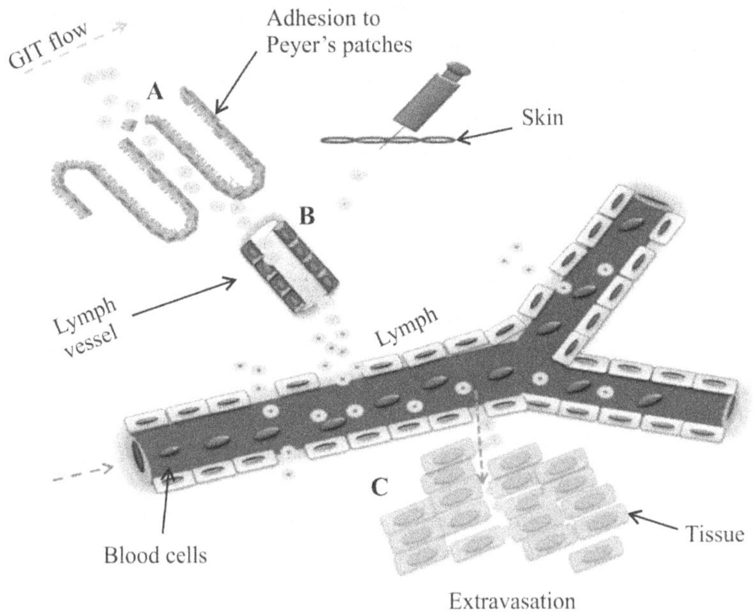

Fig. 5.3 (a) Transport through epithelium (b) Extravasation (c) Lymphatic uptake.

The changes in permeability of capillaries due to mediators like histamine, bradykinin etc., may also change extravasation phenomenon. Damaged capillaries also show increased permeability of capillaries. Nanoparticles smaller than 10 nm can be rapidly cleared by the kidneys or through extravasation while larger nanoparticles may have higher tendency to be cleared by cells of the mononuclear phagocyte system (also referred to as RES). Nanoparticles can be administered by the intraperitoneal route probably because their smaller size allow them to get into systemic circulation from the extracellular space and from there can be subjected to further extravasation. Drug-loaded nanoparticles carrying therapeutics to tumour sites undergo a multistep process to achieve their therapeutic goal, beginning with extravasation from leaky tumour vessels. It depends on the permeability of blood vessels/ capillaries which are thought to be more permissive to extravasation.

5.3.7 Lymphatic Uptake

The lymphatic system is the physiological system that maintains the body water balance. It also controls certain immunological responses. The lymphatic system originates as a network of fine capillaries in tissues, which coalesce to form vessels (afferent vessel) extending centrally to lymph nodes then unite to form efferent lymphatic vessels which further coalesce to venous supply. Due to the peculiarity of the anatomy of the lymphatic interstitial, the achievement of drug localization into the lymphatic system is limited. The nanocarriers smaller than 50 nm can pass through lymphatic system whereas nanoparticles larger than 50 nm are retained at interstitial sites and provide sustained release. Colloidal carriers biodegradable in nature such as liposomes, nanoparticles and nanoemulsions have also been utilised in the lymphatic targeting for effective anti cancer therapy wherein the metastasis of the tumor cells is prevented through effective localization of the drug in the lymphnodes (Fig. 5.3). These have also been used for effective targeting of the diagnostic agents in the similar region so as to have a close visualization of the lymphatic vessels prior to surgery. Polymeric nanospheres provide interesting opportunities for lymphatic drug delivery as well as for diagnostic imaging of the lymphatic vessels and their associated lymph nodes when injected interstitially. The degree of localization of the nanoparticles to a specific site depends on the size of the nanoparticles as well on the surface characteristics. This can be explained through an example that in contrast to the hydrophobic nanoparticles the hydrophilic nanoparticles with a size range of 30-100 nm have poor interaction with the interstitium and are drained rapidly into the lymphatics from where they are transported to the nodes. The particles are then taken up by the macrophages which in turn also depend upon the surface characteristics of the nanoparticles. It has also been known that the particles larger than 150 nm are retained at the sites and this particular trait can be utilised for the sustained drug delivery of the drugs and antigens. It has been_known that nanocarriers introduced into the circulation are taken up by RES. RES consists of cells that have the ability to phagocytose foreign material, cellular debris, pathogens and foreign substances. These cells reside mainly in the liver, spleen and bone marrow though their uptake also occurs in other organs such as the adrenal. The liver acts as a filter for the blood draining from the GI tract *via* the portal vein while the spleen has a similar function for the general circulation.

5.4 Pharmacokinetic and Pharmacodynamic Considerations

When a drug loaded nanocarrier is administered to a patient for example by intravenous administration, it is distributed systemically *via* the vascular and lymphatic systems. The amount of nanocarrier/drug available at target site(s) determines its efficacy whereas the amount available in non-target site(s) decides toxicity of the formulation. Target oriented nanocarriers as the name implies are designed to maximize therapeutic efficacy by delivering drug to intended target site. The main factors that determine the delivery of nanocarrier/drug to targeted sites include blood flow rate, distribution of nanocarriers to specific site, clearance/excretion and diffusion and transport of formulation/drug.

5.4.1 Blood Flow Rate

The distribution of a drug/nanocarrier in a tissue depends on blood flow passing through that tissue. Accordingly, tissues and organs with high blood flow (brain, liver, heart, intestines, lungs, kidneys and spleen) may be exposed to higher concentrations of a drug provided that the drug is able to penetrate into the particular tissue from the vasculature.

5.4.2 Distribution

The size range of the nanoparticles also effects its distribution based upon the extravasation of the particles from the vasculature. It has been found that the smaller particles of the range of 1-20 nm circulate for longer times with lesser extravasation. This leads to altered volume of distribution after intravenous administration. Injections to be used locally have to be designed keeping the size dependent extravasation in mind and hence if in such nanoparticulate based injection the size of the nanoparticles is kept in the range of 30-100 nm leakage into the capillaries will be prevented and on the other hand clearance via RES will also be avoided. In the similar way surface modification of the nanoparticles can also lead to such effects limiting clearance. Nanopaticles can also be prevented from such clearance through PEGylation thereby making them hydrophilic resulting in stealth nanosystems which in turn increases circulatory residence time and nanomaterials can become circulating depots of drug. The distribution properties of the drug ultimately depend on the kinetics of payload movement from the nanoparticle carrier; fast loss of the drug payload before the nanoparticle reaches its target may result in decreased drug efficacy. The surface of nanomaterials can be ligated to a biological marker, such as an RGD peptide, an antibody or an aptamer in order to increase the entrapment efficiency.

5.4.3 Clearance/Excretion

The natural clearance and excretion mechanisms of the human body provide a framework for the rational design of effective nanoparticles for use in medical therapies. Following systemic administration, the body normally distributes nutrients, clears waste and distributes drugs *via* the vascular and lymphatic systems. Intravenously injected particles are scavenged and cleared from circulation by the RES in a process that is facilitated by surface deposition of opsonic factors and complement proteins on the nanoparticles themselves. Both clearance and opsonization are influenced by the size and surface characteristics of injected nanoparticles. Particles greater than 200 nm in diameter activate the complement system more efficiently and are cleared more rapidly than very small nanoparticles. This may be a result of the geometry, charge and functional groups on the surface of these particles that mediate binding to proteins and blood opsonins. Nanoparticles must therefore evade the RES to be effective drug delivery agents. Many strategies to circumvent RES uptake may be implemented. As previously mentioned, PEGylation represents one approach to prepare stealth nanomaterials. Hydrophobic nanoparticles such as unmodified liposomes are rapidly cleared *via* the RES. The circulation times of these particles can be greatly increased simply by hydrophilic surface modification with PEG.

References

Aslan B, Ozpolat B, Sood A.K, and Lopez-Berestein G (2013). Nanotechnology in cancer therapy. *Journal of Drug Targeting* **21:** 904-913.

Bian J, Popovic Z.B, Benejam C, Kiedrowski M, Rodriguez L.L, and Penn M.S (2007). Effect of cell-based intercellular delivery of transcription factor GATA4 on ischemic cardiomyopathy. *Circulation Research* **100:** 1626-1633.

Chaurasia M, Chourasia M, Jain N.K, Jain A, Soni V, Gupta Y, and Jain S (2008). Methotrexate bearing calcium pectinate microspheres: a platform to achieve colon-specific drug release. *Current Drug Delivery* **5:** 215-219.

Chen W, Ayala-Orozco C, Biswal N.C, Perez-Torres C, Bartels M, Bardhan R, Stinnet G, Liu X.-D, Ji B, and Deorukhkar A (2013). Targeting pancreatic cancer with magneto-fluorescent theranostic gold nanoshells. *Nanomedicine* 1-14.

Chien M.P, Thompson M.P, Barback C.V, Ku T.H, Hall D.J, and Gianneschi N.C (2013). Enzyme-Directed Assembly of a Nanoparticle Probe in Tumor Tissue. Advanced Materials.

Chourasia M, and Jain S (2004). Design and development of multiparticulate system for targeted drug delivery to colon. *Drug Delivery* **11:** 201-207.

Gabizon A.A (1992). Selective tumor localization and improved therapeutic index of anthracyclines encapsulated in long-circulating liposomes. *Cancer Research* **52:** 891-896.

Gupta R, Mehra N.K, and Jain N.K (2013). Fucosylated multiwalled carbon nanotubes for kupffer cells targeting for the treatment of cytokine-induced liver damage. *Pharmaceutical Research* 1-13.

Gupta S, and Vyas S.P (2007). Development and characterization of amphotericin B bearing emulsomes for passive and active macrophage targeting: Research paper. *Journal of Drug Targeting* **15:** 206-217.

Hoang B, Ekdawi S.N, Reilly R.M, and Allen C (2013). Active Targeting of Block Copolymer Micelles with Trastuzumab Fab Fragments and Nuclear Localization Signal Leads to Increased Tumor Uptake and Nuclear Localization in HER2-Overexpressing Xenografts. *Molecular Pharmaceutics* **10:** 4229-4241.

Holpuch A.S, Hummel G.J, Tong M, Seghi G.A, Pei P, Ma P, Mumper R.J, and Mallery S.R (2010). Nanoparticles for local drug delivery to the oral mucosa: proof of principle studies. *Pharmaceutical Research* **27:** 1224-1236.

Jain S.K, Gupta Y, Ramalingam L, Jain A, Jain A, Khare P, and Bhargava D (2010). Lactose-Conjugated PLGA Nanoparticles for Enhanced Delivery of Rifampicin to the Lung for Effective Treatment of Pulmonary Tuberculosis. *PDA Journal of Pharmaceutical Science and Technology* **64:** 278-287.

Jing F, Li J, Liu D, Wang C, and Sui Z (2013). Dual ligands modified double targeted nano-system for liver targeted gene delivery. *Pharmaceutical Biology* **51:** 643-649.

Khare P, Jain A, Gulbake A, Soni V, Jain N.K, and Jain S.K (2009a). Bioconjugates: harnessing potential for effective therapeutics. *Critical Reviews™ in Therapeutic Drug Carrier Systems* **26**.

Khare P, Jain A, Jain N.K, Soni V, and Jain S.K (2009b). Glutamate-Conjugated Liposomes of Dopamine Hydrochloride for Effective Management of Parkinsonism's. *PDA Journal of Pharmaceutical Science and Technology* **63:** 372-379.

Lee S.J, Yhee J.Y, Kim S.H, Kwon I.C, and Kim K (2013). Biocompatible gelatin nanoparticles for tumor-targeted delivery of polymerized siRNA in tumor-bearing mice. *Journal of Controlled Release* **172:** 358-366.

Li H, Bian S, Huang Y, Liang J, Fan Y, and Zhang X (2013). High drug loading pH sensitive pullulan DOX conjugate nanoparticles for hepatic targeting. *Journal of Biomedical Materials Research Part A.*

Li S, and Huang L (2000). Nonviral gene therapy: promises and challenges. *Gene Therapy* **7:** 31-34.

Lindgren M, Hällbrink M, Prochiantz A, and Langel Ü (2000). Cell-penetrating peptides. *Trends in Pharmacological Sciences* **21:** 99-103.

Manoocheheri S, Darvishi B, Kamalinia G, Amini M, Fallah M, Ostad S.N, Atyabi F, and Dinarvand R (2013). Surface modification of PLGA nanoparticles via human serum albumin conjugation for controlled delivery of docetaxel. *Daru: Journal of Faculty of Pharmacy, Tehran University of Medical Sciences* **21:** 58.

Maya S, Kumar L.G, Sarmento B, Sanoj Rejinold N, Menon D, Nair S.V, and Jayakumar R (2013). Cetuximab conjugated O-carboxymethyl chitosan nanoparticles for targeting EGFR overexpressing cancer cells. *Carbohydrate Polymers* **93:** 661-669.

Moretton M.A, Chiappetta D.A, Andrade F, das Neves J, Ferreira D, Sarmento B, and Sosnik A (2013). Hydrolyzed galactomannan-modified nanoparticles and flower-like polymeric micelles for the active targeting of rifampicin to macrophages. *Journal of Biomedical Nanotechnology* **9:** 1076-1087.

Neekhra N, and Padh H (2004). An insight into molecular mechanism of endocytosis. *Indian Journal of Biochemistry & Biophysics* **41:** 69-80.

Sakhrani N.M, and Padh H (2013). Organelle targeting: third level of drug targeting. *Drug Design, Development and Therapy* **7:** 585-599.

Shrivastava P.K, Shrivastava A, Sinha S.K, and Shrivastava S.K (2013). Dextran Carrier Macromolecules for Colon-specific Delivery of 5-Aminosalicylic Acid. *Indian Journal of Pharmaceutical Sciences* **75:** 277-283.

Smith R.A, Porteous C.M, Coulter C.V, and Murphy M.P (1999). Selective targeting of an antioxidant to mitochondria. *European Journal of Biochemistry/FEBS* **263:** 709-716.

Tanaka M, Borgeld H.J, Zhang J, Muramatsu S, Gong J.S, Yoneda M, Maruyama W, Naoi M, Ibi T, Sahashi K, *et al.,* (2002). Gene therapy for mitochondrial disease by delivering restriction endonuclease SmaI into mitochondria. *Journal of Biomedical Science* **9:** 534-541.

Tiwari S, Chaturvedi A.P, Tripathi Y.B, and Mishra B (2011). Macrophage-specific targeting of isoniazid through mannosylated gelatin microspheres. *AAPS Pharm Sci Tech* **12:** 900-908.

Wirth M, Fuchs A, Wolf M, Ertl B, and Gabor F (1998). Lectin-mediated drug targeting: preparation, binding characteristics, and antiproliferative activity of wheat germ agglutinin conjugated doxorubicin on Caco-2 cells. *Pharm Res* **15:** 1031-1037.

Zhang X, Liu L, Chai G, Zhang X, and Li F (2013). Brain pharmacokinetics of neurotoxin-loaded PLA nanoparticles modified with chitosan after intranasal administration in awake rats. *Drug Development and Industrial Pharmacy* **39:** 1618-1624.

Zhu L, Chen L, Cao Q.R, Chen D, and Cui J (2011). Preparation and evaluation of mannose receptor mediated macrophage targeting delivery system. *Journal of Controlled Release* **152:** e190-e191.

Zwicke G.L, Mansoori G.A, and Jeffery C.J (2012). Utilizing the folate receptor for active targeting of cancer nanotherapeutics. *Nano Reviews 3.*

6

Pegylation and Long-Circulating Nanoparticles

Neha Gupta[1] and Prem N. Gupta[2]

[1]Sagar Institute of Pharmaceutical Sciences, Sagar-470003, India.

[2]Formulation & Drug Delivery Division, CSIR-Indian Institute of Integrative Medicine, Jammu-180001, India.

6.1 Introduction

Pegylation is the technique which has brought magnificent changes in pharmaceutical industry and many more to come yet. Pioneer work of pegylation was done by Davies and Abuchowski in 1970s, which was reported in two key papers on albumin and catalase modification (Abuchowski *et al.,* 1977a; Abuchowski *et al.,* 1977b). This was an important milestone, because at that time it was not conceivable to modify an enzyme so extensively and still maintain its activity. Proteins were in fact considered very delicate entities and only few gentle modifications with low molecular-weight products were carried out, mainly to study structure activity relationship. First time it came into limelight when FDA approved the Adagen (PEG-adenosine) in 1990. Enzon, established in 1981, was the first company to launch the product in market. From then till now many products have been launched and many are in pipeline.

Pegylation can be defined as method of attaching PEG (poly-ethylene-glycol) covalently to drug molecules to increase their therapeutic index and overcome the related problems. There were many problems related to proteins and many other drugs like short life time, instability, starvation by immune system, frequent dosing etc., which has been successfully overcome by conjugation with PEG polymer (Fig. 6.1). PEG brought the upheaval in the biopharmaceutical world. It is formed by linking repeating units of ethylene glycol to form polymer with linear or branched shapes of different molecular masses and its conjugation with drug of choice is called pegylation (Fig. 6.2). PEG is manufactured by the reaction of ethylene glycol with ethylene oxide in the presence of sodium hydroxide at elevated temperature and pressure.

$$HOCH_2CH_2OH + n(CH_2CH_2O) \longrightarrow HO(CH_2CH_2O)_{n+1}H$$

The materials with low molecular weights (200 to 600) are liquid at room temperature whereas high molecular weights (900 to 8000) are white, waxy solids at room temperature (Lachman L. *et al.,* 1990). The PEG molecules are readily soluble in water therefore pegylated drug act as though they are 5 to 10 times larger than a corresponding soluble protein of similar molecular mass. This can be confirmed by various techniques like size exclusion chromatography and gel electrophoresis (Kozlowski and Milton Harris, 2001). PEG makes the drug of choice stable over a range of pH and temperature changes (Monfardini *et al.,* 1995).

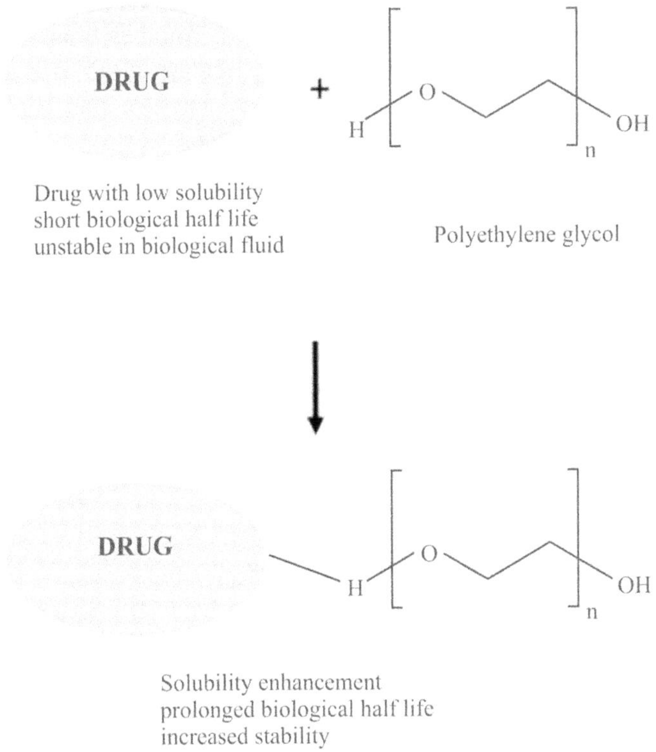

Fig. 6.1 Modified drug properties provided by pegylation.

Monomethoxy PEG (mPEG) is most useful for polypeptide modification. It is synthesized by anionic ring opening polymerization initiated with methoxide. But some molecules of diols are present in the commercially available mPEG. This is due to the presence of some water during polymerization. This can be eradicated by converting the PEGs to PEG-carboxylic acid that can then be purified by ion-exchange chromatography (Harris and Kozlowski, 1997). The branched PEG is also very functional for protein and peptide modification. The first branched PEG structure, 2,4-bis (methoxypolyethylene glycol)-6-chloro-s-triazine (mPEG2-chlorotriazine) was based on a triazine core (Matsushima, 1980). PEG2 turns out to be a very exciting protein pegylation reagent because of its unique characteristics when compared to linear PEGs. For example, PEG2 attached to proteins 'acts' much larger than a corresponding linear mPEG of the same molecular weight (Yamasaki *et al.,* 1988). This structure of PEG also has the advantage of adding two PEG chains per attachment site on the protein, therefore reducing the chance of protein inactivation. Furthermore, the PEG2 structure is more effective in protecting proteins from proteolysis, reducing antigenicity and immunogenicity (Veronese *et al.,* 1997). Another branched PEG is the forked PEG. Instead of having a single functional group at the end of two PEG chains, as with PEG2, forked PEG has two reactive groups at one end of a single PEG chain or branched PEG.

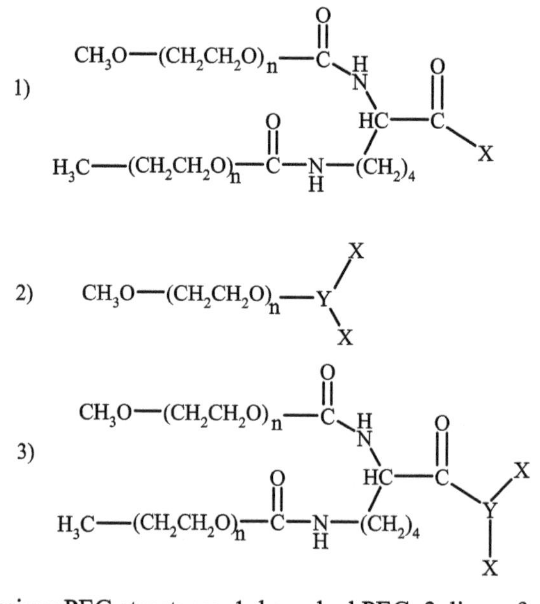

Fig. 6.2 Various PEG structures, 1. branched PEG, 2. linear fork PEG, 3. branched frok PEG.

6.2 Properties of Ideal Pegylating Agent

An ideal PEG reagent should have the following properties:

- Monodispersity or at least a dispersity index close to 1.00, in order to assure a reproducible higher quality
- Availability of one single terminal reactive group for the coupling reaction, in order to avoid cross-linking between drug molecules
- Non-toxic and non immunogenic, biochemically stable linker
- Branching for optimal surface protection
- Options for site-specific pegylation

With the advancement in technology, the polyPEG start replacing the PEG. PolyPEG molecules differ structurally from conventional PEGs in comprising a "comb-like" (Fig. 6.3) arrangement of short PEG chains attached to polymer backbone. It has 1-2 kDa molecular weights characteristically. These polymers can be synthesized, by proprietary living polymerization chemistry, with a chosen molecular weight and conjugating group for stable, site directed attachment to peptides and protein, or small molecules, using established or novel techniques. The polyPEG not only enjoys the indispensable properties of the conventional PEG but also augment therapeutic effect of biological molecules. It get easily degrade into small molecules that readily excreted over the time. Consequently they can be used in larger dose and devoid of any toxicological properties.

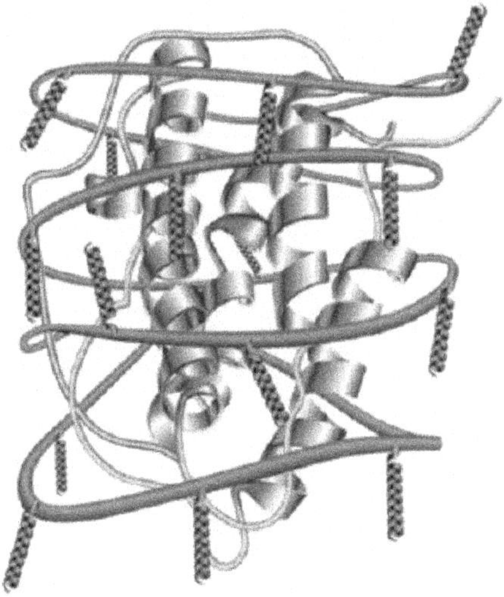

Fig. 6.3 PolyPEG conjugate protein showing the comb shape structure.

6.3 Types of Conjugates

Many revolutionary discoveries have been made in the area of gene and biotechnology. But they have some limitations because of their pharmacokinetic behaviour. These challenges were overcome by conjugation with PEG and it has been the trailblazing innovation of the last few years. The pharmacokinetic modifications produced in pegylated proteins, as compared with standard drug (Table 6.1), have led to the investigation of this technology for a number of therapeutic applications.

Table 6.1 Potential types of poly(ethylene glycol) conjugates (Zalipsky and Milton Harris, 1997)

Conjugate type	Properties and applications
Small molecule drugs	Improved solubility, controlled permeability through biological barriers, longevity in bloodstream, controlled release
Peptides	Improved solubility, conformational analysis, biologically active conjugates
Proteins	Resistance to proteolysis, reduced immunogenicity and antigenicity, longevity in bloodstream, tolerance induction
Saccharides	New biomaterials, drug carriers
Oligonucleotides	Improved solubility, resistance to nucleases, cell membrane permeability
Lipids	Used for preparation of PEG-grafted Liposomes
Liposomes and Particulates	Longevity in bloodstream, RES-evasion
Biomaterials	Reduced thrombogenicity, reduced protein and cell adherence
Diagnostic carrier	Better defined images
Hydrophopic compound (PLA, PLGA)	Reduce immunogenicity
n-Hexadecyl-cyanoacrylate nanoparticles	Transportation of drug across the blood brain barrier

6.4 Designing Pegylated Conjugates

The design of pegylation strategies predicts the pharmacokinetic and distribution behaviour of derivatives and for this knowledge of biological fate of polymer and protein is elementary. There are many parameters which control the fate, like systemic clearance by a number of mechanisms, including renal clearance, proteolysis and opsonisation and the binding affinity of the therapeutic protein to cellular receptors, resulting in changes in the bioactivity of the agent (Fung *et al.,* 1997). All these properties are affected by how the PEG is conjugated to the drug. The advantage of PEG conjugation to drug is depicted in the Fig. 6.4. Parameters affecting PEG conjugation include number of PEG molecule attached, site of attachment of the PEG, molecular weight and size of PEG reagent and strategy used to attach PEG to conjugate (Roberts *et al.,* 2012).

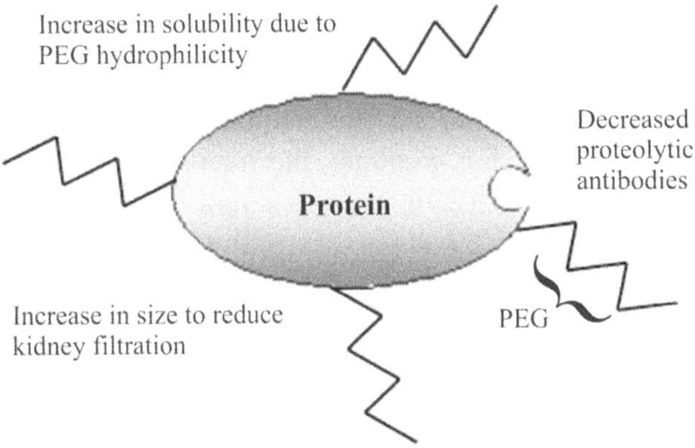

Fig. 6.4 Pegylation alters *in vivo* protein behaviour.

Polymeric conjugates must be carefully designed for their individual use, taking into account the nature of the individual drug payload and the location of each molecular pharmacological target. Typical PEG conjugates contain the polymer, a linker and the bioactive agent. The following are important considerations:

- The molecular mass and physico-chemical properties of the polymer are most important drivers governing biodistribution, elimination and metabolism of the conjugate, therefore the choice of a suitable PEG is important.
- The water-soluble biocompatible polymeric carrier must be suitable for repeated administration. PEG polymers have been typically limited to < 30 kDa in relation to their viscosity radius in order to ensure eventual glomerular elimination.

- In the case of non-biodegradable high molecular weight polymers, the linker to the molecule is an important design feature. The *in vivo* protein stability of most polypeptides is limited and therefore needs to be attached to a polymer of high molecular weight. However, pegylation of high molecular weight non-biodegradable polymers can alter the structure of the drug and reduce bioactivity when compared to the original protein. Drug-polymer conjugates or complexes need to be stable in the blood prior to the drug being liberated at the site of action. In principle, the polymer-bound drug can be released by non-specific hydrolysis by enzymes, by reduction, or by pH-dependent metabolism. Tissue-specific expression of enzymes and altered local pH, as well as cellular endocytotic pathways, offer several options for designing conjugates that can be preferentially cleaved at the preferred site of delivery. For example, the microenvironment of tumors can be acidic in both animal models and human patients. Low pH in endosomes and lysosomes, as well as the presence of lysosomal enzymes present in tumor cells, can be exploited for releasing the drugs bound to polymers through acid-sensitive linkers.

6.5 Bioactivity of Pegylated Conjugates

Kidney is the route for ultra-filtration for hydrophilic protein, polymer and polymer-protein conjugates and the behaviour of conjugate affect this. To impede the renal filtration, PEG of about 40 to 50 kDA is to be attached to small drug molecule (Bailon and Berthold, 1998). The apparent molecular weight of the PEG conjugate is more than the actual weight due to easy hydration of PEG molecules. The *in vivo* degradation of polymer conjugates is not so fast by all the reported pathways. But dosing in small amount will not cause accumulation of PEG in high quantity because of slow kidney elimination and excretion through bile (Brenner *et al.,* 1978).

The PEG polymer conjugates bottle up the protein immunogenicity and antigenicity. This was first shown by Abuchowski and is now confirmed by many studies (Abuchowski *et al.,* 1977b; Davis *et al.,* 1991). This is due to PEG molecules ability to abate the immunological response by steric masking of potential antigenic sites. Equally there are many more advantages of Pegylation (Table 6.2) which makes it so successful. Increasing understanding of the mechanism of action of polymer-drug conjugates is helping to design second generation conjugates and optimize clinical protocols for their evaluation. Conjugation of hydrophobic chemotherapy to hydrophilic polymers markedly improves solubility, and the synthesis of macromolecular prodrugs dramatically alters drug biodistribution. Conjugate pharmacokinetics and the rate and location of drug liberation are the most important factors that define therapeutic index (Duncan, 2006).

The effects of pegylation on the pharmacokinetic and pharmacodynamic properties of several therapeutic proteins have been summarized in Table 6.3. Pegylation of interleukin-6 (IL-6) produced a 100-fold increase in half-life, resulting in a 500-fold increase in thrombopoietic potency, and a decrease in immune response as evidenced by reduced plasma IgG1 and adverse effects compared with the native compound in mice. A marked decrease in uptake of IL-6 by the reticuloendothelial system was also demonstrated. The same investigators also showed that pegylation of tumor necrosis factor increased antitumour potency and decreased toxic effects in the murine fibrosarcoma model (Tsutsumi *et al.,* 1996). In other animal models, pegylated analogues of growth hormone releasing factor produced an increase in the area under the growth hormone concentration-time curve and a prolonged duration of action compared with the native compound, presumably because of a decrease in clearance. These changes represent the potential for a decrease in dosage of up to 20-fold in mice and to 50-fold in pigs (Campbell *et al.,* 1997).

Table 6.2 Advantages of pegylation

Benefit	Example
Reduced antigenicity and immunogenicity	Peg-asparaginase, reduce to 10 fold
Increased half life	PEG-l-asparaginase, increase plasma half life
Solubility enhancement	PEG-modified-antibbody
Proteolytic resistance (e.g., trypsin, chymotrypsin)	Reduced degradation of asparaginase by trypsin
Reduced toxicity	Tumour necrosis factor, antitumour potency increased 4 to 100 times
Thermal and mechanical stability enhancement	Branched chain PEG conjugates

Table 6.3 Influence of pegylation on pharmacokinetics and/or pharmacodynamics of therapeutic proteins

PEG conjugate	Pharmacokinetic effect	Pharmacodynamic effect
Interferon-α-2a	Sustained absorption	*In vitro* antiviral activity increased 12- to 135-fold, antitumour activity increased 18-fold
Interleukin-6	$t_{1/2}$ ↑ 100-fold	Thrombopoietic potency increased 500-fold
Tumour necrosis factor	$t_{1/2}$ ↑ 14- to 43-fold	Antitumour potency increased 4- to 100-fold
Megakaryocyte growth and development factor	$t_{1/2}$ ↑ 10-fold	*In vitro* activity increased 20-fold
Brain-derived neurotrophic factor	$t_{1/2}$ ↑ 5-fold CL ↓ 2.6-fold Vd ↑ 1.7-fold	
Asparaginase	$t_{1/2}$ ↑ 18-fold Vd unchanged AUC ↑ 26-fold	
Superoxide dismutase	$t_{1/2}$ ↑ > 150-fold	
Lactoferrin	$t_{1/2}$ ↑ 5- to 20-fold	
Streptokinase	$t_{1/2}$ ↑ 1.7- to 5-fold	Decreased antigenicity
Interleukin-2	$t_{1/2}$ ↑ up to 6-fold CL ↓up to 10-fold	

AUC = area under the plasma concentration-time curve; CL = systemic clearance; $t_{1/2}$= terminal elimination half-life; Vd = volume of distribution.

To couple PEG to a molecule it is necessary to activate the PEG by preparing a derivative of the PEG having a functional group at one or both termini. The functional group is chosen based on the type of available reactive group on the molecule that will be coupled to the PEG. For proteins, typical reactive amino acids include lysine, cysteine, histidine, arginine, aspartic acid, glutamic acid, serine, threonine, tyrosine, N-terminal amino group and the C-terminal carboxylic acid. In the case of glycoproteins, vicinal hydroxyl groups can be oxidized with periodate to form two reactive formyl moieties. The linkage between PEG moiety and the drug should be stable in order to retain PEG-induced pharmacological changes. The amino group on the protein and an active carbonate, active ester, aldehyde or tresylate derivative of PEG, at large are involved in the formation of linkage to yield a pegylated protein (Zhao and Milton Harris, 1997). The modification of the terminal hydroxyl groups of the native PEG moiety may lead to chemically reactive groups (Fig. 6.5) (Zalipsky and Milton Harris, 1997). The methoxy-PEG has a single hydroxyl group for activation and its methoxy group is inert to standard chemical processes (Katre, 1993).

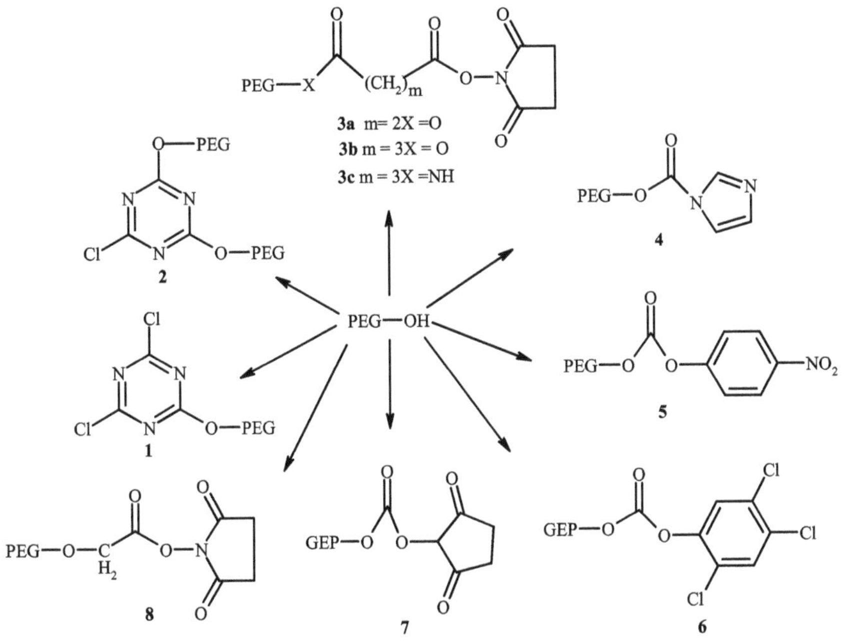

Fig. 6.5 Methods for the activation of PEG molecules.

6.6 Rational of Long Circulation

The rapid recognition of intravenously injected colloidal carriers, such as liposomes and polymeric nanoparticles from the blood by Kupffer cells, has initiated a surge of development for "Kupffer cell evading" or long-circulating particles. Such carriers have myriad of applications in vascular drug delivery, site-specific targeting and transfusion medicines.

6.6.1 Passive Targeting

The nanoparticles exhibit passive targeting following *in vivo* administration and this characteristic can be explored for selective drug delivery to tumours *via* enhanced permeability and retention (EPR) effect. The unique structural changes associated with a given vascular pathophysiology could provide opportunities for the use of long-circulating particles. For example, particle escape from the circulation is normally restricted to sites where the capillaries have open fenestrations as in the sinus endothelium of the liver (Roerdink *et al.,* 1984) or when the integrity of the endothelial barrier is perturbed by inflammatory processes (e.g., rheumatoid arthritis) or by tumours (Jain, 1989). There is evidence in support of liposomal extravasation to hepatic parenchyma as well as increased capillary permeability to liposomes and polymeric nanospheres (in the size range of 50-200 nm) during inflammation (Dams *et al.,* 1999) and in specific cancers (Yuan *et al.,* 1994). As a result of prolonged residence in blood, long-circulating carriers with the appropriate sizes have a better chance of reaching the above-mentioned targets, resulting in improved treatment or diagnosis.

6.6.2 Active Targeting

The drugs and gene therapeutics targeting to non-macrophage cells within the vasculature has been one of the highly desirable goals in clinical therapeutics. A lot of efforts have been devoted in achieving "active targeting" to deliver drugs or other bioactive moieties to the intended cells, based on molecular recognition processes. Active targeting uses the over-expression of surface receptors on cancer cells by providing targeting ligands that can engage these receptors. Ligands may be proteins (antibodies), nucleic acids (aptamers), and small molecules (vitamins, peptides or carbohydrates). However still there are concerns regarding the efficacy of such systems based on circulation time of the ligand appended carrier in blood. In order to get the maximum benefits of ligand receptor interaction (i.e., active targeting) the carrier systems should remain in circulation for a prolonged period of time. This problem can be alleviated by attachment of specific ligands onto the surface of long circulatory carriers (developed using pegylated technique) that provides enough time for the carrier to remain in systemic circulation for a longer period of time to perform the requisite functions. One example is the abnormal lymphocyte differentiation antigens on leukemia cells, which could serve as target molecules for ligand directed targeting of long circulatory carriers containing anticancer agents. Another important target is vascular endothelial cells. The vascular endothelium is remarkably heterogeneous; endothelial cells from different tissues of the body differ in expression of surface antigens and receptors (Kumar *et al.,* 1987).

6.6.3 Circulating Drug Reservoir in the Blood Compartment

Long circulatory particles provide a drug reservoir for prolonged release of therapeutic agents into the vascular compartment. The therapeutic candidate may be one with short elimination half-lives (e.g., cytokines, growth factors). With the use of such systems the stay of these therapeutic candidates can be enhanced leading to elicitation of optimum activity.

6.6.4 Artificial Oxygen Delivery Systems

Long-circulating particles may serve as a carrier for oxygen. The desired attributes of an artificial colloidal blood substitute includes compatibility with all blood types and better shelf life than blood itself. The artificial blood substitutes will reduce the risk of transmittable diseases from the donated blood and they can be used to temporarily augment oxygen delivery in patients at risk for acute tissue oxygen deficit in the condition like transient anemia or ischemia.

6.6.5 Blood-Pool Imaging

Long-circulating delivery systems can be explored as a carrier of radiopharmaceuticals and/or contrast agents for use in blood-pool imaging, detection of vascular malformations, and gastrointestinal bleeding. Red blood cell labelled with technetium-99m are commonly used in nuclear medicine for blood-pool imaging, however, poor binding of technetium-99m with the red cell results in the dissociation and clearance of free technetium through the kidney and bladder. The dissociation of technetium-99m interferes with the detection of sites of bleeding in the lower abdomen. In order to overcome this limitation synthetic long-circulatory particles can be developed for the use in nuclear medicine.

6.7 Clearance of Nanoparticles from Body

The size and surface characteristics of intravenously administered colloidal drug carriers profoundly influence their clearance behaviour and tissue distribution in the body. These physicochemical characteristics can influence the level of particle self-association in the blood and opsonisation behaviour. Following introduction into plasma, the size of a particle may substantially change. Thus the size of particles and their aggregates in the blood should be small enough in order to avoid removal from the circulation by simple filtration in the first capillary bed encountered (e.g., rat or mouse lung following tail vein injection). The particles of differing surface characteristics, size, and morphology following administration may attract opsonins and plasma proteins, the content and conformation of which may influence the rate and site of particle clearance from the vasculature.

6.8 Stealth Nanoparticles

There has been a surge in development of long circulating carriers during last few decades and various strategies for the design and engineering of long circulating carriers have been described. The surface stabilization of nanocarriers with a range of nonionic surfactants or polymeric macromolecules has proved to be one of the most promising approaches for their prolonged circulation in the blood (Moghimi and Hunter, 2000). The surface attachment of nanocarriers with nonionic surfactants can be achieved by physical adsorption or by covalent attachment to any reactive surface groups. The macrophage-resistant property of polymer-grafted particles is attributed to the suppression of surface opsonization by serum or plasma proteins (Moghimi *et al.,* 1993). Therefore, polymer-grafted particles exhibit prolonged residency times in the blood. Some examples of the colloidal carriers and the effect of surface coating on the *in vivo* behaviour are shown in Table 6.4.

Polymeric carriers are recognized by the cells of the mononuclear phagocyte system (MPS) through the process of opsonization and cleared from systemic circulation by phagocytosis. An opsonin is a proteinaceous molecule that facilitates the process of phagocytosis. Phagocytic cells express surface receptors for opsonin molecules. In order to improve the long circulation behaviour of nanoparticles, there is a trend to engineer nanocarrier with a surface coating that can limit or avoid opsonin adsorption and the subsequent removal by phagocytic cells. For example, nanoparticles modified by surface coating of poly(ethylene glycol) (PEG) have demonstrated a diminished uptake by cells of the phagocytic system and an improved circulation time to efficiently target diseased cells. The hydrophilic PEG molecules on the nanocarrier surface can decrease the adsorption of opsonins by the "steric repulsion effect".

Table 6.4 Surface coating of colloidal delivery systems (Allen, 1994; Gregoriadis *et al.,* 1993; Illum *et al.,* 1987; Müller and Wallis, 1993; Tröster *et al.,* 1992)

Colloidal carrier	Surface coating	Size (nm)	*In vivo* behaviour
Polystyrene nanoparticles	Poloxamer-188	60	MPS avoidance observed
	Poloxamer-338	60, 100	MPS avoidance observed
	Poloxamine-908	250	MPS avoidance observed
Poly(methyl methacrylate) nanoparticles	Poloxamer-188	130	MPS avoidance observed
	Poloxamer-407	130	MPS avoidance observed
	Poloxamine-908	130	MPS avoidance observed
	Poloxamine-1508	130	MPS avoidance observed
	Polysorbate 80	130	MPS avoidance observed
	Hydroxylpropyl cellulose	130	MPS avoidance not observed
Poly(butyl-2-cyanoacrylate) nanoparticles	Poloxamer-338	130	MPS avoidance observed
	Poloxamine-908	130	MPS avoidance observed
Poly(P-hydroxy-butyrate)	Poloxamer-338 and -407	90 or 250	Not reported
Poly(lactic acid-co-glycolic acid)	Polyethylene glycol,	140	MPS avoidance observed
Liposomes	Polyethyleneglycol, phosphatidylinositol, dextran, pullulan	-	MPS avoidance observed

6.8.1 Poly(ethylene glycol) Anchored Stealth Nanoparticles

PEG has been widely used in the field of formulation and development and was introduced two decades ago to modify the liposomes' surface for improved pharmacokinetics following intravenous delivery. This hydrophilic polymer provides a steric barrier on nano-carrier's surface and minimizes opsonization. The recognition of circulating nanocarrier by binding to plasma protein is the main mechanism of phagocytic system to recognize the circulating nanocarrier, resulting in major loss of the administered dose (> 50%) within a few hours after intravenous delivery. Liver, spleen and bone marrow are primary organs for clearance of polymeric nanocarriers.

Pegylation technology is receiving wide recognition for improving the pharmacokinetics of a number of nanocarrier. The PEG coated nanocarriers are also known as "stealth" nanoparticles, because they escape the recognition by RES better than the non-pegylated delivery systems. The nanocarriers in the size range of 100-200 nm are good candidate for site specific delivery to cancer cells because of the EPR effect, which allows accumulation of nanocarriers in tissues with leaky blood vessels (i.e., tumor and inflamed tissues) following intravenous delivery. The inefficient lymphatic system in the cancer tissue also contributes to the accumulation of nanocarriers that penetrate through the angiogenic vasculature from the systemic circulation. The widened capillary gaps (> 400 nm) in the cancer tissue vasculature permits transport of nanoparticles. Nanocarriers that are not rapidly cleared from the systemic circulation will have a chance to encounter the leaky vasculature in tumor tissue. Therefore the use of long circulatory nanocarriers is promising strategy for site specific delivery to tumor vasculature.

6.8.2 Circulation Kinetics of Stealth Particles

Nanocarriers (i.e., liposomes, nanoparticles etc.) are rapidly cleared from the systemic circulation following intravenous administration by elements of the phagocytic system. On the other hand, stealth nanoparticles circulate for prolonged period with half-lives in the range varying from 2 to 24 hr in mice and rats and can be as high as 45 hr in humans depending on the nanoparticle size and coating characteristics (Allen, 1994). It is interesting to note that a common but often ignored observation following injection of long-circulating nanocarrier is rapid hepatic and splenic accumulation of a fraction of the administered dose. Despite the presence of the hydrophilic polymeric barrier, some PEG-grafted phospholipid vesicles are rapidly cleared by macrophages of the liver and the spleen. This observation may imply surface heterogeneity among the injected carriers, with a small population bearing insufficient or no protective PEG molecules. In accordance to this, a research study demonstrated that at very low lipid doses (20 nmol/kg bodyweight), PEG2000-decorated phospholpid vesicles are rapidly cleared from the systemic circulation by macrophages of the phagocytic system (Laverman *et al.,* 2001). The phagocytic clearance of low doses of PEG coated nano-vesicles is mediated by a pool of blood opsonins. Hence, it appears to be a limited pool of an opsonin protein in the systemic circulation that can interact with PEG coated phospholipid vesicles resulting in rapid clearance by macrophages. These observations indicated opsonization of even stealth vesicles following intravenous administration. Therefore, an important factor influencing prolonged circulatory behaviour of large doses of pegylated vesicles may be the limited concentration of the unidentified opsonin molecules.

6.8.3 Toxicity of the Long Circulating Pegylated Nanoparticles

The long circulatory behaviour provides the particles with the attributes of site specific delivery, however, it also result in enhanced drug exposure to other tissues leading to new adverse effects. For example, the cardiotoxicity of doxorubicin is significantly reduced by formulating the drug into the pegylated liposomes; however, extended half-life of this pegylated system introduces a new side effect termed as hand-foot syndrome and mucositis that limits the maximum tolerated dose. Moreover, repeated injections of pegylated liposomes in mouse induced the immune system to develop PEG-specific IgM antibodies, which significantly reduced the half-life of the subsequently injected stealth vesicles. A similar observation was observed in another study involving nucleic acid containing nanocarries (Tagami *et al.,* 2010) and it is hypothesized that the PEG specific antibody was generated due to the prolonged contact of the stealth nanocarrier with the immune cells which were also activated by the nucleic acid in the delivery systems. The observations suggesting a fine line between long circulatory behaviour and systemic over-exposure of the nanocarrier, which are likely to cause side effects including drug related immunotoxicity. The attributes of an ideal drug carrier includes efficient drug delivery to the target tissue, and elimination from the blood in a reasonable period of time for minimal adverse effects.

6.9 Conclusion

The numbers of studies are burgeoning involving pegylation technology for the product development. Pegylation technology based few products are already approved by the FDA demonstrating the potential of pegylation in the improvement of therapeutic value of drugs. The most significant attributes that pegylation technology offers includes prolonged circulation in blood which in turn allows less frequent dose administrations, the improved stability towards enzymes (proteases or nucleases) and the reduced immunogenicity.

An ideal delivery system carries the payload to the target site efficiently (> 10% injected dose in 4 hr) (i.e., potent) and is cleared from the systemic circulation in a short period of time (in 4-10 hr) (i.e., safe).

The research trend in drug delivery is no longer to develop a vehicle that is capable of circulating in the blood indefinitely but to employ a smart mechanism allowing efficient distribution to the diseased tissue and also with a rapid elimination from the circulation (90% injected dose elimination in 4-10 hr). For a drug that is membrane permeable, it is desirable to release it locally in the tumor tissue for improved tumor penetration and intratumoral distribution. Ideally, the release kinetics should match with the pharmacokinetics of the nanoparticles to attain local drug release without significant loss of the dose in the circulation, which probably requires a pulse release mechanism after the nanoparticles have extravasated in the target tissue with a minimal dose in the circulation. This is very difficult to achieve if the drug release is solely dependent on the formulation design; however, in the presence of external (e.g., heat, and ultrasound) or internal (e.g., pH and enzyme) triggering mechanisms, local drug release (or pulse release) can be attained. In addition to the degree of Pegylation and kinetics of de-pegylation, the chain length of the PEG block might have profound impact on the particle size, stability, activity and toxicity. Pegylation is required for nanoparticles to exhibit prolonged circulation half-life and de-pegylation is needed to facilitate the clearance of the particles from the body or to enhance the drug release at the target site. A balance between pegylation and de-pegylation is needed to produce a nanoparticle formulation that is potent and safe.

References

Abuchowski A, McCoy J.R, Palczuk N.C, van Es T and Davis F.F (1977a). Effect of covalent attachment of polyethylene glycol on immunogenicity and circulating life of bovine liver catalase. *J. Biol. Chem.* **252:** 3582-3586.

Abuchowski A, Van Es T, Palczuk N and Davis F.F (1977b). Alteration of immunological properties of bovine serum albumin by covalent attachment of polyethylene glycol. *J. Biol. Chem.* **252:** 3578-3581.

Allen T.M (1994). Long-circulating (sterically stabilized) liposomes for targeted drug delivery. *Trends Pharm. Sci.* **15:** 215-220.

Bailon P and Berthold W (1998). Polyethylene glycol-conjugated pharmaceutical proteins. *Pharm. Sci. Tech. Today* **1:** 352-356.

Brenner B, Hostetter T and Humes H (1978). Glomerular permselectivity: barrier function based on discrimination of molecular size and charge. *American J. Physiol - Renal Physio.***234:** F455-F460.

Campbell R.M, Heimer E.P, Ahmad M, Eisenbeis H.G, Lambros T.J, Lee Y, Miller R.W, Stricker P.R and Felix A.M (1997). Pegylated peptides. V. Carboxy-terminal pegylated analogs of growth hormone-releasing factor (GRF) display enhanced duration of biological activity *in vivo*. *J. Peptide Res.* **49:** 527-537.

Dams E.T, Becker M.J, Oyen W.J, Boerman O.C, Storm G, Laverman P, de Marie S, van der Meer J.W, Bakker-Woudenberg I.A and Corstens F.H (1999). Scintigraphic imaging of bacterial and fungal infection in granulocytopenic rats. *J. Nuclear Med.* **40:** 2066-2072.

Davis F, Kazo G, Nucci M and Abuchowski A (1991). Reduction of immunogenicity and extension of circulating half-life of peptides and proteins. *Peptide Protein Drug Deliv.* 831-864.

Duncan R (2006). Polymer conjugates as anticancer nanomedicines. *Nat. Rev. Cancer* **6:** 688-701.

Fung W, Porter J and Bailon P (1997). Strategies for the preparation and characterization of polyethylene glycol (PEG) conjugated pharmaceutical proteins. *Polym Prepr.* **38:** 565-566.

Gregoriadis G, McCormack B, Wang Z and Lifely R (1993). Polysialic acids: potential in drug delivery. *FEBS Letters* **315:** 271-276.

Harris J.M and Kozlowski A (1997). Polyethylene glycol and related polymers monosubstituted with propionic or butanoic acids and functional derivatives thereof for biotechnical applications, US. Patent WO 1997003106 A1.

Illum L, Jacobsen L, Müller R, Mak E and Davis S (1987). Surface characteristics and the interaction of colloidal particles with mouse peritoneal macrophages. *Biomaterials* **8:** 113-117.

Jain R.K (1989). Delivery of novel therapeutic agents in tumors: physiological barriers and strategies. *J. Natl. Cancer Inst.* **81:** 570-576.

Katre N.V (1993). The conjugation of proteins with polyethylene glycol and other polymers: altering properties of proteins to enhance their therapeutic potential. *Adv. Drug Deliv. Rev.* **10:** 91-114.

Kozlowski A and Milton Harris J (2001). Improvements in protein pegylation: pegylated interferons for treatment of hepatitis C. *J. Control. Rel.* **72:** 217-224.

Kumar S, West D.C and Ager A (1987). Heterogeneity in endothelial cells from large vessels and microvessels. *Differentiation* **36:** 57-70.

Lachman L, Libermen H and J K (1990). The Theory and practice of industrial Pharmacy. Varghese publishing house, pp.366.

Laverman P, Boerman O.C, Oyen W.J.G, Corstens F.H.M and Storm G (2001). *In vivo* applications of PEG liposomes: unexpected observations. *Crit. Rev.Ther. Drug Carrier Syst.* **18:** 551-566.

Matsushima A (1980). Modification of *E. coli* asparaginase with 2,4-bis (O-methoxypolyethylene glycol)-6-chloro-s-triazine (activated PEG2); disappearance of binding ability towards anti-serum and retention of enzymic activity. *Chem Lett* **7:** 773-776.

Moghimi S, Muir I, Illum L, Davis S and Kolb-Bachofen V (1993). Coating particles with a block co-polymer (poloxamine-908) suppresses opsonization but permits the activity of dysopsonins in the serum. *Biochim. Biophys. Acta-Mol. Cell Res.* **1179:** 157-165.

Moghimi S.M and Hunter A.C (2000). Poloxamers and poloxamines in nanoparticle engineering and experimental medicine. *Trends Biotech.* **18:** 412-420.

Monfardini C, Schiavon O, Caliceti P, Morpurgo M, Harris J.M and Veronese F.M (1995). A branched monomethoxypoly(ethylene glycol) for protein modification. *Bioconj. Chem.* **6:** 62-69.

Muller R and Wallis K (1993). Surface modification of iv injectable biodegradable nanoparticles with poloxamer polymers and poloxamine 908. *Int. J. Pharm.* **89:** 25-31.

Roberts M, Bentley M and Harris J (2012). Chemistry for peptide and protein pegylation. *Adv. Drug Del. Rev.* **54:** 459-476.

Roerdink F, Regts J, Van Leeuwen B and Scherphof G (1984). Intrahepatic uptake and processing of intravenously injected small unilamellar phospholipid vesicles in rats. *Biochim. Biophys. Acta* **770:** 195-202.

Tagami T, Nakamura K, Shimizu T, Yamazaki N, Ishida T and Kiwada H (2010). CpG motifs in pDNA-sequences increase anti-PEG IgM production induced by PEG-coated pDNA-lipoplexes. *J. Control. Rel.* **142:** 160-166.

Troster S.D, Wallis K.H, Muller R.H and Kreuter J (1992). Correlation of the surface hydrophobicity of C-poly (methyl methacrylate) nanoparticles to their body distribution. *J. Control. Rel.* **20:** 247-260.

Tsutsumi Y, Kihira T, Tsunoda S, Kamada H, Nakagawa S, Kaneda Y, Kanamori T and Mayumi T (1996). Molecular design of hybrid tumor necrosis factor-alpha III: polyethylene glycol-modified tumor necrosis factor-alpha has markedly enhanced antitumor potency due to longer plasma half-life and higher tumor accumulation. *J. Pharmacol. Exp. Therapeutics* **278:** 1006-1011.

Veronese F.M, Caliceti P and Schiavon O (1997). Branched and linear poly (ethylene glycol): influence of the polymer structure on enzymological, pharmacokinetic and immunological properties of protein conjugates. *J. Bioactive Compatible Poly.* **12:** 196-207.

Yamasaki N, Matsuo A and Isobe H (1988). Novel Polyethylene Glycol Derivatives for Modification of Proteins (Biological Chemistry). *Agri. Biol. Chem.* **52:** 2125-2127.

Yuan F, Leunig M, Huang S.K, Berk D.A, Papahadjopoulos D and Jain R.K (1994). Microvascular permeability and interstitial penetration of sterically stabilized (stealth) liposomes in a human tumor xenograft. *Cancer Res.* **54:** 3352-3356.

Zalipsky S and Milton Harris J (1997). Introduction to chemistry and biological applications of poly (ethylene glycol). Paper presented at: ACS Symposium series (ACS Publications).

Zhao X and Milton Harris J (1997). Novel degradable poly (ethylene glycol) esters for drug delivery. Paper presented at: ACS Symposium Series (ACS Publications).

7

Nanoparticles and Targeted Systems for Cancer Diagnosis and Therapy

S. Asthana[1], Nitin K. Jain[2] and Manish K. Chourasia[1]
[1]Pharmaceutics Division, CSIR-Central Drug Research Institute, Lucknow-226031, India.
[2]Department of Biotechnology, Ministry of Science & Technology, New Delhi-400003, India.

7.1 Introduction and Background

7.1.1 Cancer

Human cancer is a complex disease caused by somatic gene mutations and accumulation of multiple molecular alterations that result in the transformation of a normal cell into a malignant tumor cell.

Eventually, the tumor cell phenotype progresses along three major steps. First step involves uncontrolled growth with increased proliferation rate and/or decreased apoptosis (programmatic death), causing an increase of tumor cell mass. This is followed by invasion of surrounding tissues and switch on of angiogenesis. This is a critical step that differentiates *in situ,* non-invasive, tumors with no metastatic potential from invasive tumors with metastatic and life-threatening potential. Although there is considerable variability, tumors with angiogenic potential become vascularized when the cell load reaches an order of 107 cells, equivalent to a nodule of ~2 mm diameter. The third step involves progress in metastases, i.e., abnormal migration of tumor cells from the primary tumor site *via* blood vessels or lymphatics to distant organs, with formation of secondary tumors. This is most commonly the process that causes death of the host due to disruption of the function of vital organs or systems (i.e., brain, lung, liver, kidney, bone marrow, coagulation, intestinal passage, and others).

7.1.1.1 TNM Cancer Staging

The most common cancer staging method is called the TNM system

- **T: Tumor (1-4)** indicates the size and direct extent of the primary tumor and is normally given as T_0 through T_4. T_0 stage demonstrates that there are no signs of tumor invasion to local tissues and this stage is generally referred as "*In situ*". On the contrary, stage T_1 to T_4 express size and/or extension of the primary tumor, where T_4 characterizes the extension and spread of large primary tumor to adjacent tissues which is not able to be operated.
- **N: Lymph Node (0-3)** indicates the degree to which the cancer has spread to nearby regional lymph nodes. Stage N_0 indicates absence of tumor cells in regional lymph nodes. Whereas, N_1 indicates tumor spread to closest or little number of regional lymph nodes and N_3 means tumor spread to more distant or abundant regional lymph nodes resulting in greater enlargement of the involved nodes.
- **M: Metastasis (0-1)** indicates whether the cancer has metastasized to other organs in the body. Stage M_0 demonstrates absence of metastases while M_1 represents distant organs metastasis beyond regional lymph nodes.

7.1.2 The Challenge of Cancer Therapy

Conventional anticancer agents do not differentiate between cancerous and normal cells, and distributed nonspecifically in the body where they affect both cancerous and normal cells, thereby limiting the dose achievable within the tumor and also resulting in suboptimal treatment due to excessive toxicities to normal cells. Additionally, cancer is often diagnosed and treated too late, when the cancer cells have already invaded and metastasized into other parts of the body. Limited ability to monitor therapeutic responses and development of multiple drug resistance are also problematic issues.

Current problems and unmet needs in translational oncology include:

(a) Advanced technologies for tumor imaging and early detection

(b) New methods for accurate diagnosis and prognosis

(c) Strategies to overcome the toxicity and adverse side effects of chemotherapy agents

(d) Basic discovery in cancer biology leading to new knowledge for treating aggressive and lethal cancer phenotypes such as bone metastasis.

Advances in these areas will form the major cornerstone for a future medical practice of personalized oncology in which cancer detection, diagnosis, and therapy are tailored to each individual's tumor molecular profile and also for predictive oncology in which genetic/molecular markers are used to predict disease development, progression, and clinical outcomes.

7.1.3 Cancer Nanotechnology

Nanotechnology is beginning to change the scale and methods of drug delivery that can have enormous positive impact on human health. For successful treatment of a complicated disease (cancer), in addition to therapeutic agents, early detection of disease is also necessary. Nanomaterials, which measure 1-1000 nm, allow unique interaction with biological systems at the molecular level. The potential applications of nanoparticles are predominantly in detection, diagnostics (disease diagnosis and imaging), monitoring and treatment of human cancers (Fig. 7.1). Nanotechnology's greatest advantage over conventional therapies may be the ability to combine more than one function (multifunctionality). Multifunctional nanoparticle system may consists of biologically programmed layers that can effectively target, enter, diagnose and treat specific cells within a multiple cells in a population.

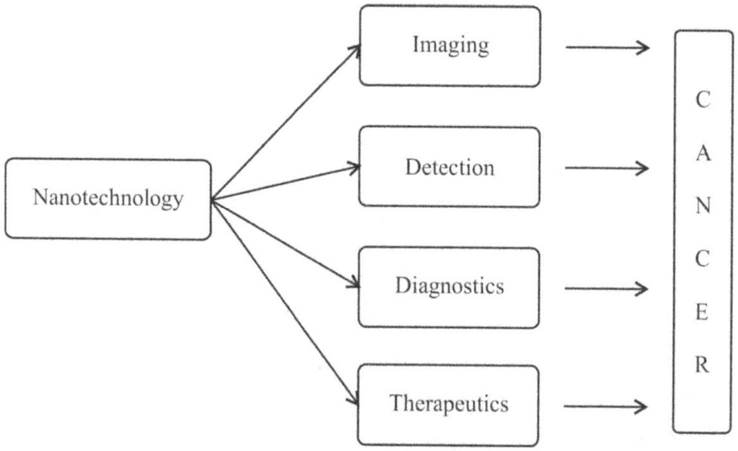

Fig. 7.1 Schematic diagram showing nanotechnology applications in cancer through molecular tumor imaging, early detection, molecular diagnosis and targeted therapy.

7.2 Types of Nanoparticles as Delivery Systems

The basic rationale is that metal, semiconductor, polymeric structure (nanoparticles, micelles or dendrimers) and lipids vesicles (liposomes) have novel optical, electronic, magnetic, and structural properties that are often not available in individual molecules or bulk solids. Recent research has developed functional nanoparticles encapsulating therapeutic or diagnostic agents that are covalently linked to biological molecules such as peptides, proteins, nucleic acids, or small-molecule ligands.

7.2.1 Polymer-based Drug Carriers

Polymeric nanocarriers possess several merits for nano-oncology applications, such as biocompatibility, biodegradability, process ability, and high drug-loading capacity, which render them attractive candidates as drug delivery devices. Drug can be either physically entrapped in or covalently bound (polymer-drug conjugates) to the polymer matrix. The resulting system may have the structure of sphere (polymeric nanoparticles), amphiphilic core/shell (polymeric micelles), or hyperbranched macromolecules (dendrimers; Fig. 7.2). Polymers used for drug delivery can be of natural or synthetic polymeric group. Polymers such as albumin, chitosan, and heparin occur naturally and have been a material of choice for the delivery of drugs as well as oligonucleotides. Among synthetic polymers some of the examples are N-(2-hydroxypropyl)-methacrylamide copolymer (HPMA), polystyrene-maleic anhydride copolymer, polyethylene glycol (PEG), poly(lactide-co-glycolide) (PLGA), poly(lactide) (PLA), poly(ε-caprolactone) (PCL) and poly-L-glutamic acid (PGA).

7.2.1.1 Polymeric Nanoparticles

Nanoparticles are solid and spherical structures of 10 nm-1000 nm size range. The drug of choice is dissolved, entrapped, adsorbed, attached or encapsulated into the nanoparticle matrix. Depending on the method of preparation, nanoparticles ("nanospheres" or "nanocapsules", Fig. 7.2 A, B) can be obtained with different properties and release characteristics for the encapsulated therapeutic agent. Nanospheres are matrix systems in which the drug is physically and uniformly dispersed throughout the particles and nanocapsules are vesicular systems in which the drug is confined to a cavity surrounded by a unique polymer membrane. The advantages of using nanoparticles for drug delivery result from two main basic properties viz. small size responsible for high surface area as well as easy re-dispersibility and use of biodegradable materials. They have ability to get sterilized by filtration. Nanoparticles can be tailor-made to achieve both controlled drug release and disease specific localization by tuning the polymer characteristics and surface chemistry.

7.2.1.2 Polymeric Micelles

Polymeric micelles are nanostructures generated from spontaneous self-assembly of amphiphilic block copolymers with two or more polymer chains of different hydrophobicity. In aqueous environments, these block copolymers spontaneously self-assemble into core-shell nanostructures, with a hydrophobic core and a hydrophilic shell (Fig. 7.2 C). The hydrophobic core region serves as a reservoir for hydrophobic drugs, whereas the hydrophilic shell region stabilizes the hydrophobic core and renders the polymers water-soluble, making the particle an appropriate candidate for i.v. administration. They are considered to be potent candidates for targeted drug delivery and controlled drug release. One example of polymeric micelle composed of PLA-PEG (Genexol®-PM), for delivery of paclitaxel, was first approved for cancer therapy in South Korea in 2007 and is being evaluated in a clinical Phase II trial in the United States for the treatment of metastatic pancreatic cancer.

7.2.1.3 Dendrimers

Dendrimers are hyperbranched polymeric macromolecules with controlled three-dimensional architecture. These well-defined macromolecules have a globular architecture with multiple branches that emerge radially from the central core by a series of polymerization reactions (Fig. 7.2 D). Properties associated with these dendrimers such as their monodisperse size, modifiable surface functionality, multivalency, water solubility, and available internal cavity make them attractive for drug delivery. Their specific molecular structure enables dendrimers to carry various therapeutic drugs *via* covalent conjugation to the multivalent surfaces or encapsulation in the cavities of the cores through hydrophobic interaction, hydrogen bond, or chemical linkage. The rigidity and the density of the branched units of dendrimers affect release kinetics of drug. By use of pH or enzyme-sensitive linkages, stimulus-responsive dendrimers can be generated for effective delivery and site specific release of drug. One example, folate-conjugated, methotrexate-loaded poly(amidoamine) (G5) dendrimer, which has demonstrated a 10-fold reduction in tumor size and exhibited less systemic toxicity, compared to free methotrexate (Kukowska-Latallo *et al.,* 2005).

7.2.2 Lipid-based Drug Carriers

7.2.2.1 Liposomes

Liposomes are self-assembling closed colloidal structures composed of lipid bilayers and have a spherical shape in which an outer lipid bilayer surrounds a central aqueous space (Fig. 7.2 E). They have superior biocompatibility owing to their composition that is similar to the cell membranes. A unique feature of liposomes is that they possess distinct hydrophilic and hydrophobic regions, which enable them to simultaneously encapsulate both water insoluble and water-soluble materials. Currently, several kinds of cancer drugs have been applied to this lipid-based system using a variety of preparation methods. Various liposomal formulations are commercially available in market for the treatment of cancer (Table 7.1).

Table 7.1 List of commercial liposomal formulations for treatment of cancer

Liposomal formulation	Trade name	Company	Indication
Liposome-PEG doxorubicin	Doxil/Caelyx	Alza Corporation	HIV-related Kaposi's sarcoma, metastatic breast and ovarian cancer
Liposomal cytarabine	Depocyt	Pacira (formerly SkyePharma)	Malignant lymphomatous meningitis
Liposomal daunorubicin	DaunoXome	Gilead Sciences	HIV-related Kaposi's sarcoma
Liposomal doxorubicin	Myocet	Zeneus	Combination therapy with cyclophosphamide in metastatic breast cancer

7.2.3 Carbon Nanotubes

Carbon nanotubes are carbon allotropes of cylindrical nanostructure and composed of benzene rings (Fig. 7.2 F). Carbon nanotube technology has extensive potential to alter drug delivery and biosensing methods that presents ideal nanomaterials for drug delivery carriers. These nanotubes possess exclusive electronic, mechanical and structural properties along with excellent chemical stability and hold enormous hopes for cancer imaging and treatment. Generally, carbon nanotubes have complete insolubility in all solvents and sometimes elicits health related toxic manifestations. However, chemical modification of carbon nanotubes can render them water soluble property. Specific drug targeting of cancerous cells using carbon nanotubes can be provided by functionalization strategy where a wide variety of target specific active molecules such as peptides, proteins, nucleic acids, and therapeutic agents can be incorporated into the architecture of the carbon nanotubes. Additionally, nanotubes possess extraordinary property of adsorbing materials on their surface and heating up upon absorbing near-infrared light wave responsible for quick release of excess energy as heat (~70 °C), which can kill cancer cells.

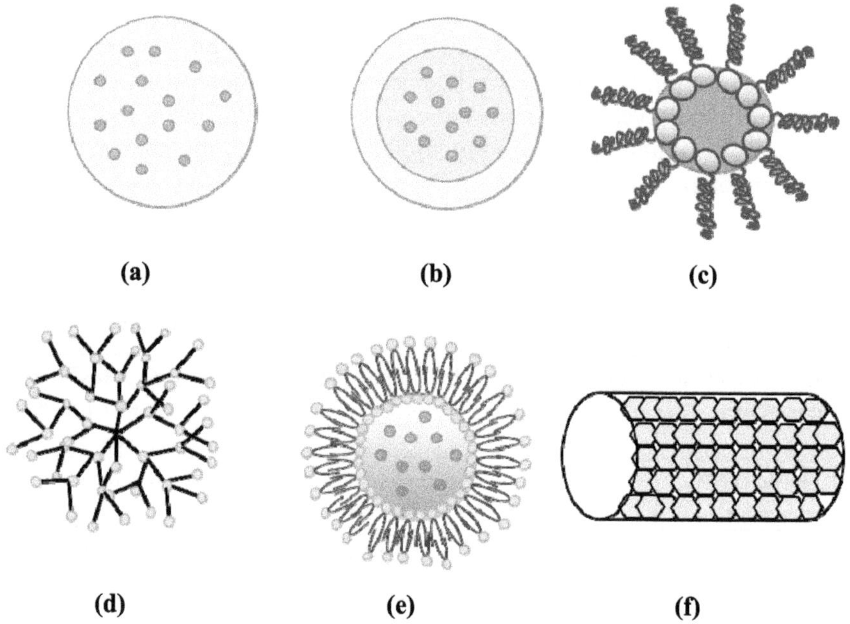

Fig. 7.2 Types of nanoparticles for drug delivery. (a) polymeric nanosphere (b) polymeric nanocapsule (c) polymeric micelles (d) dendrimers (e) liposomes (f) carbon nanotubes.

7.3 Targeted Delivery of Nanoparticles

For effective cancer treatment after administration firstly, anticancer drugs should be able to reach the desired tumor tissues through the penetration of barriers in the body with minimal loss of their volume or activity in the blood circulation. Secondly, after reaching the tumor tissue, drugs should have the ability to selectively kill tumor cells without affecting normal cells with a controlled release mechanism of the active form. These two basic strategies are also associated with improvements in patient survival and quality of life by increasing the intracellular concentration of drugs and reducing dose-limiting toxicities simultaneously.

Nanotechnology offers a more targeted approach and has the potential to satisfy both of these requirements for effective drug carrier systems and could thus provide significant benefits to cancer patients. In fact, the use of nanoparticles for drug delivery and targeting is likely one of the most exciting and clinically important applications of cancer nanotechnology.

7.3.1 Size and Surface Characteristics of Nanoparticles

For potentially effective tumor tissue targeted chemotherapeutics, drug loaded nanoparticles must stay or be retained in the bloodstream for longer time period without being removed by reticuloendothelial system (RES). Conventional nanoparticles with unmodified surface, are quickly captured form circulation by the RES organs (such as liver and spleen) or circulating macrophages, depending on their unique size and surface characteristics (Moghimi *et al.*, 2001), and restrict them to reach their desired destination, i.e., tumor sites. The *in vivo* circulating characteristics of nanoparticles can be directed by regulating their size and surface characteristics.

7.3.1.1 Size

Nanoparticles offer the flexibility of size manipulation as per need lending advantages as far as drug delivery is concerned. For cancer therapeutics, desirable size characteristic of nanoparticles should be in the range that they should be small enough to escape arrest by fixed macrophages of RES organs, but large enough to avert quick leakage back into blood capillary after reaching the cancerous sites. The fenestra in case of Kupffer cells of liver and sinusoid present in spleen are reported to have size in the range of 150 to 200 nm (Wisse *et al.,* 1996) while the leaky tumor vasculature has 100 to 600 nm wide gap junction between endothelial cells (Yuan *et al.,* 1995). These particular facts reflect that formulation has to encounter the two vascular barriers in order to reach tumor site which necessitates that size of the nanoparticles intended to achieve tumor directed delivery should be up to 100 nm.

7.3.1.2 Surface Characteristics

In addition to their size, the surface characteristic of nanoparticles is also an important factor determining their life span and fate during circulation relating to their capture by macrophages of RES. Nanoparticles should ideally have a hydrophilic surface to escape macrophage capture (Moghimi and Szebeni, 2003). This can be achieved in two ways: coating the surface of nanoparticles with a hydrophilic polymer, such as polyethylene glycol (PEG). The coating of PEG chains to the surface of nanoparticles results in an increase in the blood circulation half-life by several times of magnitude. By creating a hydrophilic protective layer around the nanoparticles, steric repulsion forces repel the absorption of opsonin proteins, thereby blocking and delaying the opsonization process protects them from opsonization by repelling plasma proteins; alternatively, nanoparticles can be formed from block copolymers with hydrophilic and hydrophobic domains (Adams *et al.,* 2003).

7.3.2 Passive Targeting by Nanoparticles

7.3.2.1 Enhanced Permeability and Retention Effect

Fast-growing cancer cells demand the recruitment of new vessels (neovascularization) or rerouting of existing vessels near the tumor mass to supply them with oxygen and nutrients. This neovasculature differs greatly from that of normal tissues in microscopic anatomical architecture. The resulting imbalance of angiogenic regulators makes tumor vessels highly disorganized and dilated with numerous pores showing enlarged gap junctions as large as 600 to 800 nm between poorly aligned or disorganized endothelial cells. Also, the basement membrane or the pericyte smooth-muscle layer is frequently absent or abnormal in the vascular wall. This defective vascular architecture is responsible for enhanced permeability. Additionally, impaired lymphatic drainage from cancerous area is responsible for enhanced retention of matter. This anatomical defectiveness, along with functional abnormalities, results in extensive leakage or extravasation of blood plasma components, such as macromolecules, nanoparticles and lipidic particles, into extra vascular spaces which accumulates inside tumor tissues through gaps. Moreover, the slow venous return in tumor tissue and the poor lymphatic clearance mean that macromolecules are retained in the tumor. This passive phenomenon termed as "Enhanced Permeability and Retention (EPR) effect" (Fig. 7.3) and is the basis for the selective targeting of macromolecular drugs to the site of solid tumors.

The abnormal vascular architecture is responsible for EPR effect in tumor and the effect can be summarized as follows:

1. Extensive angiogenesis- new vessel formation
2. Lack of smooth-muscle layer, pericytes, irregular blood flow → induced hypertensive state due to passive accumulation of angiotensin-II in vessel→ more leakage
3. Inefficient lymphatic clearance → enhanced retention of macromolecular drugs in the interstitium of tumors

The unique pathophysiological characteristics of tumor vessels enable macromolecules, including nanoparticles, to selectively accumulate into the tumor interstitium through leaky tumor capillary fenestrations (Maeda, 2001). For such a passive targeting mechanism to work exploiting EPR effect, the size and surface properties of drug delivery nanoparticles must be controlled as described above, to avoid capture by the RES so that they can circulate for longer times in the bloodstream and a greater chance of reaching the targeted tumor tissues. To maximize circulation times and targeting ability, the particle should be of 20-200 nm and the surface should be hydrophilic to circumvent clearance by macrophages.

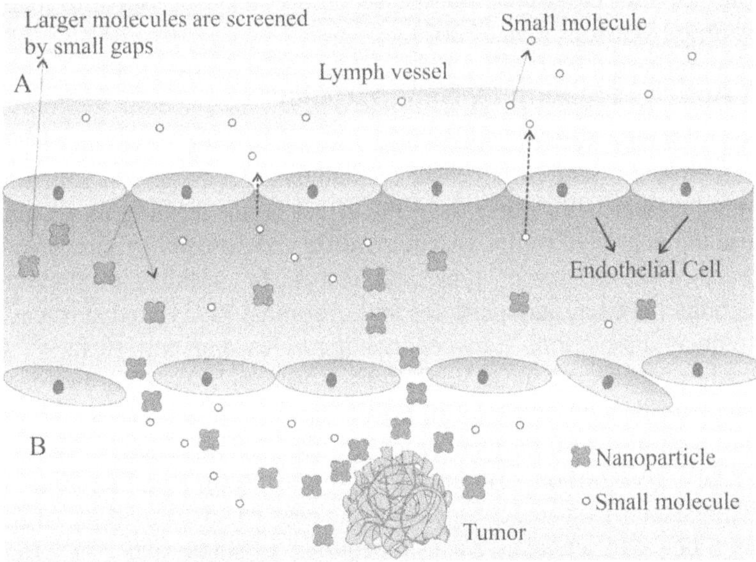

Fig. 7.3 Schematic representation of passive tissue targeting by extravasation of nanoparticles through increased permeability of the tumor vasculature and ineffective lymphatic drainage (EPR effect).

7.3.2.2 Tumor Microenvironment

The microenvironment surrounding tumor cells is entirely different when compared to the environment around normal cells and is contributing to passive targeting. Hyperproliferative cancer cells display dramatically increased metabolic rate that results in tumor microenvironment with insufficient oxygen and nutrient supplies, especially glucose. Consequently, tumor cells have high glycolytic rate to obtain extra energy to counter hypoxic (low-oxygen) condition. During this process abundant lactic acid is produced in tumor areas resulting in more acidic environment compared to normal tissues (Pelicano *et al.,* 2006). Usually, average extracellular tumor pH found in between 6.0 and 7.0 which depends on tumor area. Whereas extracellular pH value of normal tissues and blood is around 7.4. Therefore, nanoparticles with pH-sensitive behavior may provide targeted drug delivery towards tumor cells as they remain stable at physiologic pH of 7.4 but degraded to release drug in acidic environment of tumor cells. In addition, tumor cells express their malignant potency in form of unique enzymes such as matrix metalloproteinases, which control invasion and survival of tumor cells. These matrix metalloproteinases can be used as target for tumor activated prodrug having cleavable matrix metalloproteinases specific peptide linked drug (Mansour *et al.,* 2003).

7.3.3 Active Targeting by Nanoparticles

A drug delivery system comprising a drug bearing nanoparticles that depends only on passive targeting mechanisms faces several limitations. Targeting cancer cells using the EPR effect is not feasible in all tumors because the degree of tumor vascularization and porosity of tumor vessels can vary with the tumor type and status. In addition to preventing interactions between nanoparticles and opsonins, PEGylated surfaces can also reduce interactions between nanoparticles and cell surfaces. One approach to overcome these limitations is to attach targeting moieties to the nanoparticle surface. A lot of efforts have been devoted in achieving "active targeting" to deliver drugs to the desirable cells, based on molecular recognition processes. Active targeting exploits the overexpression of surface receptors on cancer cells by providing targeting ligands that can engage these receptors. Ligands may be proteins (antibodies), nucleic acids (aptamers), and small molecules (vitamins, peptides or carbohydrates). Specific ligand targeting proteins or receptors expressed on cancer cell membranes or endothelial cells lining the newly generated blood vessels into the tumor are among the possible options to achieve active targeting that provides preferential accumulation of nanoparticles in the tumor bearing organ, in the tumor itself, individual cancer cells, or intracellular organelles inside cancer cells. This approach is based on specific ligand-receptor interactions. The recent development and introduction of a wide variety of liposomes and polymers as drug delivery carriers increases the potential number of drugs that can be conjugated to targeted nanoparticles without compromising their targeting affinity.

Cell-surface receptors are required to possess certain properties that make them predominantly appropriate tumor-specific targets (Allen, 2002). Firstly, receptors should be expressed entirely on tumor cells with no expression on normal cells. Moreover, receptors should be expressed homogeneously on entire tumor cells which are intended to be targeted. Furthermore, cell-surface receptors should be efficiently bound to the tumor cells and should not be detached and enter into blood circulation. Examples of relevant targets are the folate receptor, herceptin or the integrin surface receptor. Other examples include galactolipids that bind to the asialoglycoprotein receptor of the human hepatoma HepG2 cells.

7.3.3.1 Folate Receptors

Folic acid is a vitamin that is essential for the biosynthesis of nucleotides. It is consumed in elevated quantities by proliferating cells and is transported across the plasma membrane using the folate receptor (FR). FR is frequently overexpressed on tumor cells as a consequence of increased folate requirements, and, furthermore, its expression level increases with advancing stage of the disease including ovary, brain, kidney, breast, and lung malignancies. When, folate-targeted conjugate binds with FR on the cell surface, the invaginating plasma membrane envelopes complex of receptor and ligand to form an endosome *via* receptor mediated endocytosis (Fig. 7.4). Newly formed endosomes are transferred to target organelles. As the pH value in the interior of the endosome becomes acidic and lysozymes are activated, the drug is released from the conjugate and enters the cytoplasm, provided the drug has the proper physicochemical properties to cross the endosomal membrane. Released drug is then trafficked by its target organelle depending on the drug. Meanwhile, the FR released from the conjugate returns to the cell membrane to start a second round of transport by binding with new folate-targeted conjugates. Interest in exploiting folate receptor targeting in cancer therapy and diagnosis has rapidly increased, as attested by many conjugated systems, including proteins, liposomes, imaging agents. For example folate targeted liposomes with encapsulated doxorubicin and daunorubicin have been found to efficiently deliver the entrapped drug into cancer cells, thus increasing cytotoxicity (Ni *et al.*, 2002; Pan *et al.*, 2003).

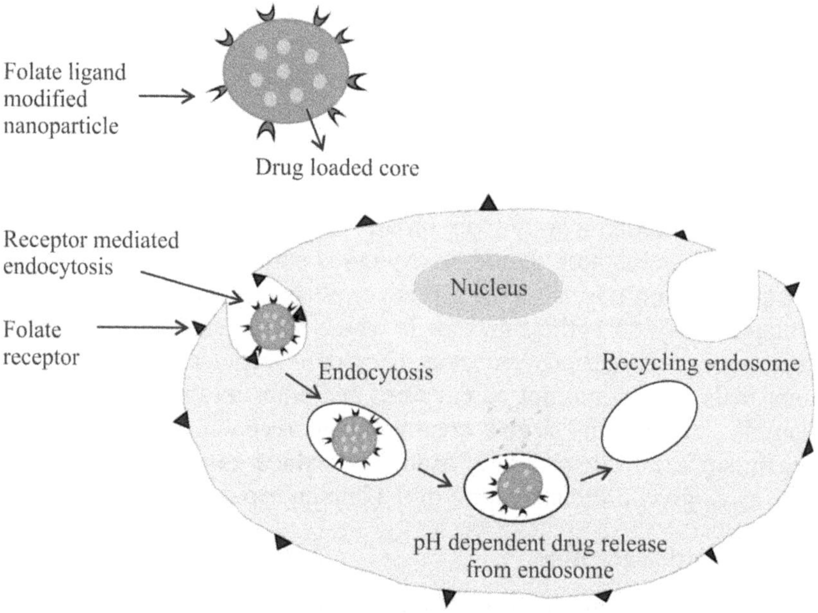

Fig. 7.4 Illustration showing nanoparticle with tumor-targeting and therapeutic functions (*upper panel*) and delivery of the nanoparticle drugs by receptor-mediated endocytosis and controlled drug release inside the cytoplasm (*lower panel*).

7.3.3.2 Targeting through Angiogenesis

Robust angiogenesis is a hallmark of cancer which underlies aggressive growth of tumors. Angiogenesis is not only essential for tumor growth, but it is also implicated in the initial progression from a pre-malignant lesion to a fully invasive cancer, and in the growth of dormant micro-metastases into clinically detectable metastatic lesions. Angiogenesis is a process of new blood vessels formation from existing ones. For solid tumors (1-2 mm^3), oxygen and nutrients can reach the center of the tumor by simple diffusion process. Because of their non-functional or non-existent vasculature, non-angiogenic tumors are highly dependent on their microenvironment for oxygen and nutrients supply. When tumor size reaches 2 mm^3, cellular hypoxia condition begins, initiating angiogenesis. Angiogenesis is regulated through a complex set of mediators. In the angiogenesis process, five phases are distinguishable:

1. Endothelial cell activation,
2. Basement membrane degradation,
3. Endothelial cell migration,
4. Vessel formation, and
5. Angiogenic remodeling.

Advantages of the tumoral endothelium targeting

1. There is no need of extravasation of nanocarriers to arrive to their targeted site
2. The binding to their receptors is directly possible after intravenous injection
3. Most of endothelial cells markers are expressed whatever the tumor type, involving an ubiquitous approach and an eventual broad application spectrum.

Targeting angiogenesis has become a promising strategy for cancer treatment, and a wide variety of therapies directed at interfering with this process are under development. Angiogenesis is regulated through a complex set of mediators such as integrin $\alpha_v\beta_3$ and vascular endothelial growth factors (VEGFs), integrins, and matrix metalloproteinases (MMPs), which play important regulator roles. Therefore, selective targeted of $\alpha_v\beta_3$ integrin, VEGFs and MMPs is effective anti-angiogenesis strategy for treating a wide variety of solid tumors.

VEGF molecule is a highly conserved, disulfide-bonded homodimeric glycoprotein of 34 to 45 Kd, that belongs to the platelet-derived growth factor (PDGF) superfamily of growth factors. VEGF receptors are extensively studied and represent important targets for cancer chemotherapy. VEGF receptor-1 plays an important role in physiologic and developmental angiogenesis, while VEGF receptor-2 is crucial towards mitogenic, angiogenic and vascular permeability-enhancing properties of VEGF. Overexpressed one or more targets in the VEGR/VEGF receptor pathway can be selectively targeted by specific ligand modified nanoparticles.

Integrin is a family of cell-cell adhesion molecules, abundantly expressed on angiogenic endothelial cells. Integrins play an important role in regulation of cellular functions crucial to endothelial cell growth, proliferation, migration, and apoptosis. Extensively investigated $\alpha_v\beta_3$ integrin type is significantly upregulated in activated endothelial cells throughout angiogenesis. Generally, $\alpha_v\beta_3$ integrin interacts with the arginine-glycine-aspartic acid (RGD) peptide sequence. RGD antagonists and monoclonal antibodies (Vitaxin) can be used to obstruct this interaction responsible for angiogenesis inhibition and induction of endothelial apoptosis and tumor regression (Cai and Chen, 2006). In addition, we can target angiogenic blood vessels overexpressing $\alpha_v\beta_3$ integrin by RGD-anchored nanoparticles encapsulating anticancer drug which can potentially inhibit the tumor growth and proliferation.

The MMPs are classified as the matrix in subfamily of zinc-dependent endopepetidase enzyme family. Common MMPs are interstitial collagenase, stromelysins, metalloelastase, gelatinases, and membrane-associated MMPs. Generally, MMPs play an important role in the degradation and remodeling of the extracellular matrix and basement membranes of vascular endothelium. MMPs participate in tumor invasion and metastasis; remodel the surrounding microenvironment to facilitate new vessel formation. Tumor cells express many MMPs which can be used as tumor marker for angiogenesis specific targeted delivery (Furumoto *et al.,* 2003). Thus, surface modification of nanoparticles with peptides that bind specifically to the $\alpha_v\beta_3$ integrin, the VEGF receptor and MMPs, may be a fruitful strategy for selective delivery of anticancer agents.

7.3.3.3 Targeting to Specific Organs or Tumor Types

Tumor-selective delivery of anticancer agents is desirable to increase the cell-kill effect, while protecting the healthy tissues from exposure to a cytotoxic agent, thereby reducing systemic toxic effects, and nanoparticles could be used for this purpose. Two targeting strategies, active and passive targeting can be utilized. Much preclinical research has been done on the use of nanoparticles as a means of targeted therapy in oncology. We will focus on the use of nanoparticles formulations in the treatment and targeting of breast cancer and liver cancer.

7.3.3.3.1 Breast Cancer

Breast cancer continues to be one of the most common cancers and a major cause of death among women worldwide. Breast cancer cells overexpress various receptors or tumor markers may originate by a tumor (tumor-derived), or the host (tumor-associated) that differentiates neoplastic from normal tissue.

7.3.3.3.1.1 *Human Epidermal Growth Factor Receptor 2 (HER-2)*

HER2 is a HER2/neu oncogene-encoded growth factor receptor and is a member of epidermal growth factor receptor family. This gene gets amplified and overexpressed during breast cancer progression. During normal condition HER-2/neu pathway promotes cell growth and division, while its overexpression leads to strengthen and constant proliferative signaling. HER-2 protein overexpression can be used an excellent breast tumor biomarker for targeted chemotherapy.

7.3.3.3.1.2 *Estrogen Receptor (ER) and Progesterone Receptor (PR)*

Endocrine receptors (ER or PR) are clinically used as breast cancer biomarkers. Presence of estrogen receptors represents ER-positive breast cancer, while progesterone receptors occurrence represents PR-positive breast cancer. Breast cancer cells expressing these receptors depend on estrogen and progesterone hormones to grow. Testing of ER and PR is a standard part of diagnosis and results are used to guide prognosis and treatment preparation for women with breast cancer.

7.3.3.3.1.3 *Alpha-fetoprotein (AFP) and Carcinoembryonic Antigen (CEA)*

These tumor marker oncofetal antigens are generally produced at the time of embryonic development and disappear when immune system is fully developed. These oncofetal antigens are non-specifically expressed by various types of cancer cells. AFP is a marker and can be indicative of liver, testicular, ovarian and breast cancers.

7.3.3.3.1.3.1 Cancer Antigen (CA) 27.29

CA 27.29 is a tumor marker antigen which is elevated during breast, ovarian and lung cancer. This antigen is indicator of early detection of breast cancer recurrence (the return of cancer after treatment).

These mentioned receptors and tumor biomarkers can be utilized for active targeted delivery of anticancer agent *via* nanoparticles. Following are some of the examples of breast cancer targeted delivery of nanoparticles:

Liposomal Anthracyclines

Anthracyclines are some of the most active agents in the treatment of breast cancer and are widely used in all stages of disease. However, the use of anthracyclines is limited by cardiac toxic effects, which occurs with high cumulative doses of these agents. Liposomal anthracycline formulations improve the therapeutic index of conventional anthracyclines, while maintaining their widespread antitumor activity. Three liposomal anthracyclines, all of which are nanoparticles measuring about 100 nm, are being assessed in human cancers: liposomal daunorubicin, approved for the treatment of Kaposi's sarcoma; liposomal doxorubicin, which, in combination with cyclophosphamide, is approved for the treatment of metastatic breast cancer and PEGylated liposomal doxorubicin, approved for both Kaposi's sarcoma and ovarian cancer. Liposomal anthracyclines associated with less cardiac toxic effects than conventional doxorubicin.

Breast cancer cells have overexpression of HER2 receptor. Herceptin, a monoclonal antibody that targets HER2, improves treatment of this aggressive form of breast cancer (Yezhelyev *et al.,* 2006). So the combination of liposomal formulation encapsulating anthracycline with herceptin warrants effective breast cancer therapy.

Paclitaxel

The taxanes, paclitaxel and docetaxel are some of the most important agents in the treatment of solid tumors, and are widely utilized in all stages of breast cancer. Both drugs are highly hydrophobic, and have to be delivered in synthetic vehicles (polyethylated castor oil for paclitaxel and polysorbate-ethanol for docetaxel). The toxic effects associated with both taxanes are increasingly recognized to be cause by these synthetic vehicles, and not the agents themselves. Marketed formulation of paclitaxel, Taxol® has limited clinical application because of toxicity of added Cremophor® EL surfactant in formulation.

Alternatively, solvent and surfactant free albumin-bound nanoparticles of paclitaxel (Abraxane®) has been developed and approved. Abraxane® also known as nab-paclitaxel, is currently used in metastatic breast cancer after failure of combination chemotherapy for metastatic disease or relapse within 6 months of adjuvant chemotherapy. Albumin is a plasma protein with a molecular weight of 66 kDa. Because albumin is found in the plasma of the human body, it is non-toxic and well tolerated by immune system. Albumin has attractive phamacokinetics owing to its long half-life which is particularly interesting to design a drug carrier for passive targeting. Albumin seems to help endothelial transcytosis of protein bound and unbound plasma constituents *via* the binding to a cell surface receptor (gp60). It has shown excellent efficacy in breast cancer which results in improved tumor penetration, pharmacokinetics with an overall decrease in toxic effects, compared with conventional paclitaxel (Yezhelyev *et al.,* 2006).

Tamoxifen

Tamoxifen remains widely used in all stages of breast cancer, in both premenopausal and postmenopausal women. It undergoes substantial metabolism, and an inability to get active drug into breast tumors that might hinder its effectiveness. The use of tamoxifen-loaded poly(ethylene oxide)-modified poly(epsilon-caprolactone) nanoparticles offers the promise of improved tumor penetration, with selective tumor targeting, and a subsequent decrease in toxic effects (Shenoy and Amiji, 2005).

7.3.3.3.2 Liver or Hepatic Cancer

Hepatocellular carcinoma is the most common cancer to strike the liver, which arises from the main cells of the liver (the hepatocytes). This type is usually confined to the liver, although occasionally it spreads to other organs. It is more common in men and occurs mostly in people with liver cirrhosis. The second type of primary liver cancer is cholangiocarcinoma or bile duct cancer, is so called because it starts in the cells lining the bile ducts. Liver transplantation remains the most effective therapeutic option for hepatocellular carcinoma; however, due to the lack of donors and the relatively high cost, a substantial number of patients die. The disadvantages of most anticancer drugs that are currently available include low bioavailability, poor selectivity because they can act on both tumor cells and healthy cells, and immunosuppression that can cause complications and even patient death. However, targeted therapy to liver may be useful because it is relatively less expensive compared to the current therapies and it also produces fewer side effects.

Hepatocytes express asialoglycoprotein receptor (ASGPR) on the membrane of cells facing the sinusoids, with specificity for glycoproteins with galactose or acetyl galactosamine at the end. Each hepatocyte cell membrane contains approximately two million binding sites for ASGPR. For targeted delivery of anticancer agent, nanoparticles can be modified by galactose ligand. The binding of the galactose modified nanoparticle with ASGPR will induce liver-targeted drug transfer through receptor mediated endocytosis.

A pyrimidine anticancer drug, 5-fluorouracil (5-FU) is highly effective in the management of liver cancer. 5-FU can also accumulate in cancerous as well as normal cells including normally proliferating tissues, leading to bone marrow suppression and gastrointestinal reactions. One example showing reduced side effects and immunosuppressive action of 5-FU, is by encapsulation of this anticancer drug in galactosylated chitosan nanoparticles mediated by active targeting to ASGPR receptor of hepatocyte (Cheng *et al.,* 2012).

7.4 Cancer Diagnosis

Early detection of cancer can greatly improve the odds of successful treatment and survival. There is a wide array of procedures to diagnose cancer, detect tumor location and organs affected by it.

7.4.1 Biopsy

Biopsy, a medical test involves surgical removal of tissue sample for examination under a microscope to observe the presence of tumor cells. When tumor is filled with fluid then needle biopsy is used. Thin needle is inserted directly into the suspicious area to aspirate fluid samples.

7.4.2 Endoscopy

Endoscopy is a medical technique which involves using of a flexible plastic tube with a terminal tiny camera. It is inserted into the interior of organ or cavity of the body, allows difficult-to-access to be illuminated and viewed providing important information related to progress of disease. Sometimes it is very difficult to diagnose the disease condition, however with the use of endoscopy it can be viewed with substantial important information helping to diagnose the problem and also helps in treatment planning. To view particular affected areas of the body, specially designed endoscopes are available, i.e., colonoscope to view inside the colon, and laparoscope to examine the abdominal cavity.

7.4.3 Blood Tests

Some tumors release substances called tumor markers, which can be detected in the blood. A blood test for prostate cancer determines the amount of prostate specific antigen (PSA). Higher than normal ($\leq$ 4.0 ng/mL) PSA levels can indicate cancer. However, blood tests by themselves can be inconclusive, and other methods should be used to confirm the diagnosis.

7.4.4 Diagnostic Imaging

Several techniques are used to produce an internal picture of the body and its structures. Generally, X-rays, positrons, photons or sound waves energy are utilized to derive the visual information. An ideal imaging modality should be non-invasive, sensitive, and provide objective information on cell survival, function and localization. Types of imaging modalities include:

7.4.4.1 Ultrasound

In this technique high-frequency sound waves determine if a suspicious lump is solid or fluid. These sound waves are transmitted into the body and are converted into a computerized image.

7.4.4.2 X-rays

It is the most common way to make pictures of the inside of the body and to spot abnormal areas that may indicate the presence of cancer.

7.4.4.3 X-ray-based Computer-assisted Tomography or CT Scan

Light or sound scattering-based imaging techniques have limited tissue penetration depths and can therefore be challenging in applications requiring deep tissue imaging. Standard clinical imaging modalities, such as CT and magnetic resonance imaging (MRI) with micrometer resolution, can have advantages for deep tissue *in vivo* diagnostics with the presence of appropriate contrast agents. CT utilizes radiographic beams to create detailed computerized pictures taken with a specialized X-ray machine. It is more precise than a standard X-ray, and provides a clearer image.

7.4.4.4 Radionuclide Imaging

Radionuclide-based imaging techniques such as positron emission tomography (PET) and single-photon emission computed tomography (SPECT) are imaging techniques that provide physiologic information.

7.4.4.4.1 Positron Emission Tomography (PET)

PET is a test that uses a special type of camera and a tracer (radioactive chemical) to look at organs in the body. The tracer usually is a special form of a substance (e.g., 18F-Fludeoxyglucose) that collects in cells that are using a lot of energy, such as cancer cells which have a much higher metabolic rate than other cells.

During the test, the tracer liquid is administered intravenously. The tracer moves through body, where much of it collects in the specific organ or tissue. The tracer gives off tiny positively charged particles (positrons). The camera records the positrons and turns the recording into pictures on a computer. A PET scan can distinguish between benign and malignant disorders. PET is dependent on metabolic and not structural changes.

7.4.4.4.2 Single-Photon Emission Computed Tomography (SPECT)

A special type of CT scan in which a small amount of a radiotracer is injected into a vein and a scanner is used to make detailed 2D images of areas inside the body where the radioactive material is taken up by the cells. SPECT can give information about blood flow to tissues and chemical reactions (metabolism) in the body.

7.4.4.5 Magnetic Resonance Imaging (MRI)

MRI is a medical imaging technique used in radiology to visualize internal structures of the body in detail. MRI makes use of the property of nuclear magnetic resonance (NMR) to image nuclei of atoms inside the body which create images of organs and other internal structures.

Overall, nuclear imaging by PET or SPECT offers greater sensitivity ($> 5 \times 10^3$ cells) but is limited by the lack of anatomical context, whereas MRI provides accurate anatomical detail but no data on cell viability and shows poor sensitivity ($> 10^5$ cells). Although none of these modalities is ideal, MRI is the preferred option for cellular tracking. MRI provides good contrast between the different soft tissues of the body, which makes it especially useful in imaging the brain, muscles, the heart, and cancers compared to other medical imaging techniques such as CT or X-rays, without the use of harmful ionizing radiations (the case with CT, PET or SPECT). In addition, MRI offers a longer tracking window in comparison to PET and SPECT, which are limited by the decay of the short-lived radioactive isotopes.

7.4.4.6 Fluoresce Optical Imaging

Optical imaging techniques of the breast such as diffuse optical tomography (DOT), diffuse optical imaging, and diffuse optical spectroscopy are being investigated as an adjunct technique. Electrical impedance spectroscopy (EIS) and microwave imaging spectroscopy (MIS) are also being explored for potential use in breast cancer detection.

Optical imaging is a novel imaging technique that uses near-infrared (NIR) light to assess optical properties of tissues, and is expected to play an important role in breast cancer detection. When fluorescent probes are excited by NIR light, they emit photons at predefined wavelength ranges, detectable by an optical imaging system.

Intrinsic contrast of carcinoma alone is probably not sensitive enough for lesion detection. Optical tumor imaging using a fluorescent contrast agent may improve lesion contrast and can potentially detect changes in breast tissue earlier. The fluorescent probes can either binds specifically to certain targets associated with cancer or can nonspecifically accumulate at the tumor site, mostly by extravasations through leaky vessels (Fig. 7.1).

Major advantages of optical imaging include exclusion of any radioactive components (as in PET and SPECT), very high sensitivity (nanomolar to picomolar concentration range) compared to MRI, relatively inexpensive, and easily accessibility. However, this technique is still in a very early phase of development. Characteristics and performance of common imaging techniques is shown in Table 7.2.

Table 7.2 Characteristics and performance of common imaging techniques

Imaging technique	Signal measured	Cost	Imaging time
CT	X-rays	High	Minutes
PET, SPECT	Positron from radionuclides	Very high	Minutes
MRI	Alteration of magnetic field	Very high	Minutes to hours
Fluorescence imaging	Light, usually near infra-red	Low	Seconds to minutes

7.5 Nanoparticulate Contrast Agents for Imaging

Currently use of contrast agents in the field of diagnosis is very common. These contrast agents are used to enhance image contrast of structures within the body that would otherwise be inaccessible. Nanoformulated contrast agents have received massive attention, presenting the advantage of greater biocompatibility and reduced toxicity compared to conventional contrast agents (Table 7.3).

The majority of **nanoparticles** in **development** for this role include followings:

7.5.1 Inorganic Nanoparticles for Imaging

Most inorganic nanoparticles share the same basic structure- a central core that defines the fluorescence, optical, magnetic, and electronic properties of the particle, with a protective organic coating on the surface (Fig. 7.5). This outside layer protects the core from degradation in a physiologically aggressive environment.

7.5.1.1 Fluorescent Nanoparticles for Optical Imaging

Optical imaging in conjunction with nanoparticles incorporating fluorescent dyes (indocyanine green) or quantum dots can facilitate imaging *in vitro* or *in vivo* (in small animals) without the requirement for sophisticated or expensive instruments. The imaging performance of dyes can be enhanced by encapsulation in polymeric nanoparticles, improving contrast and boosting signal to noise ratios (this favourable result comes from a significant local dye concentration enhancement in the nanoparticle structure). However, it is important to optimize the nanoparticle design to avoid quenching effects. To allow for signal detection through the skin (and other tissues), dyes with an excitation and emission wavelength range of 600 nm to 900 nm are employed, i.e., in the near infra-red region.

7.5.1.1.1 Quantum Dots

These are inorganic fluorescent semiconductor nanoparticles with sizes of 2-10 nm that contain a core of hundreds to thousands of atoms of group II and VI elements (e.g., cadmium, technetium, zinc, and selenide) or group III (e.g., tantalum) and V elements (e.g., indium) (Medintz *et al.,* 2005). Quantum dots containing a cadmium selenide core and a zinc sulphide shell, surrounded by a coating of a coordinating ligand and an amphiphilic polymer, are most commonly used for biological application (Fig. 7.5 A).

Quantum dots display size dependent fluorescence spectra and size-dependent fluorescent life time. Moreover, quantum dots show several advantages over conventional fluorescent dyes: they have narrower emission spectra, larger stokes shift, higher quantum yield, and higher photostability. In addition, the broad excitation spectrum of quantum dots facilitates their use in multicolor imaging applications. Quantum dots can be tuned to emit at between 450 nm and 850 nm (i.e., from ultraviolet to near infrared) by changing the size or chemical composition of the nanoparticles. This so-called quantum confinement effect produces many quantum-dot colours, which can be visualized simultaneously with one light source. Quantum dots emit narrow symmetrical emission peaks with minimum overlap between spectra, allowing unique resolution of their spectra and measurement of fluorescent intensity from several multicolour fluorophores by real-time quantitative spectroscopy. The high fluorescence quantum yield of the quantum dots, their resistance to photobleaching and their unique physical, chemical and optical properties make them good candidates for fluorescent tagging for *in vivo* molecular and cellular imaging. These key advantages make it possible to label multiple molecular targets simultaneously by use of quantum dots both *in vitro* and *in vivo*. However, use of quantum dots in imaging and therapeutics *in vivo* is limited by the toxic effects of the heavy-metal core. On excitation, the quantum dot can sometimes release toxic cadmium *via* photolysis-a clearly undesirable outcome. To avoid the release of toxic metal, the quantum dot can be coated with biocompatible polymers, improving colloidal stability. The surface of quantum dots can be engineered or modified to improve solubility, sensitivity, specificity and visualization in target tissue.

7.5.1.2 Magnetic Nanoparticles

Magnetic nanoparticles have proven its use as cell magnetic separators, transport of antitumor molecules, for hyperthermal treatment and as contrast agent to improve the sensitivity of MRI, among other biomedical applications. Magnetic nanoparticles contain a metal core (e.g., iron, cobalt, or nickel) that is magnetically active. Key advantages of the magnetic nanoparticles are biocompatibility, low toxic effects and high level of accumulation in the target tissue. Magnetic particles, when coated with an organic outer layer, can also be conjugated to biomolecules and used as site-specific drug-delivery agents for cancer treatment (Fig. 7.5 B). Iron-oxide-based magnetic materials have been used widely in clinical practice as magnetic resonance agents and in studies of gene expression, angiogenesis imaging, and cellular trafficking. Metal nanoparticles in combination with fluorescent active molecules can be used for combined optical and magnetic imaging.

7.5.1.3 Raman Probes

Surface-enhanced Raman scattering (SERS) is another sensitive method for spectroscopic detection of multiple targets on cancer cells. Modern surface-enhanced Raman scattering probes typically contain a metal core of gold or silver for optical enhancement, a reporter molecule (spectroscopic encoding chromophores adsorbed on the surface of colloidal gold such as crystal violet, nile blue, basic fuchsin or cresyl violet) for spectroscopic signature, and a silica shell for protein conjugation (Fig. 7.5 C). When illuminated with a laser beam, the reporter dye molecule produces a unique shift in the electromagnetic spectrum, which manifests as several sharp peaks and give the characteristic fingerprint of the reporter (Moore *et al.*, 2004). Silica-based gold nanocarriers have been tested as targeted-therapy probes for human breast, prostate, brain and liver cancers. Colloidal gold nanoparticles with a size range of 55-60 nm can be optimised for surface enhancement at 632-647 nm excitation.

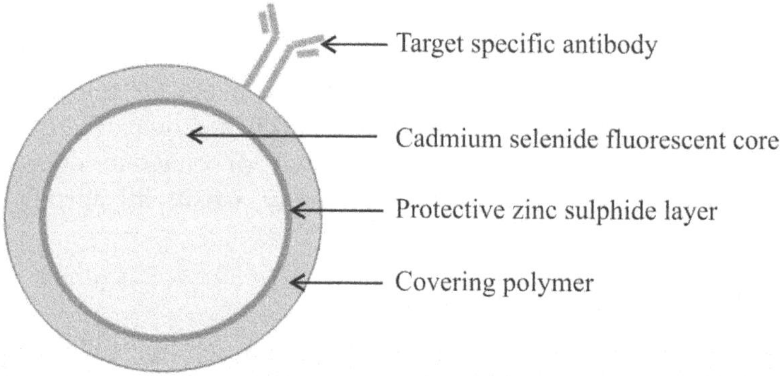

(A)

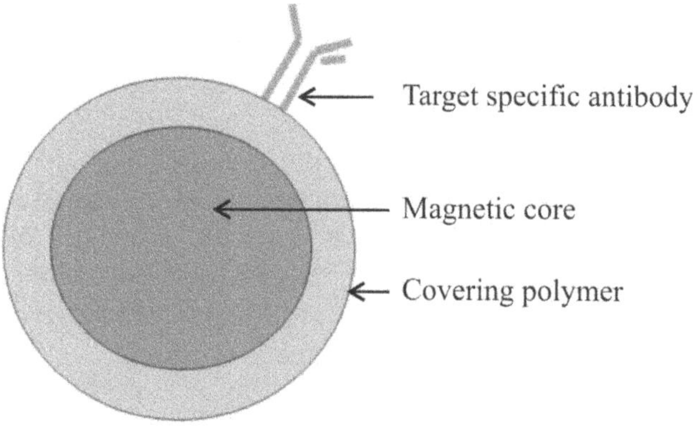

(B)

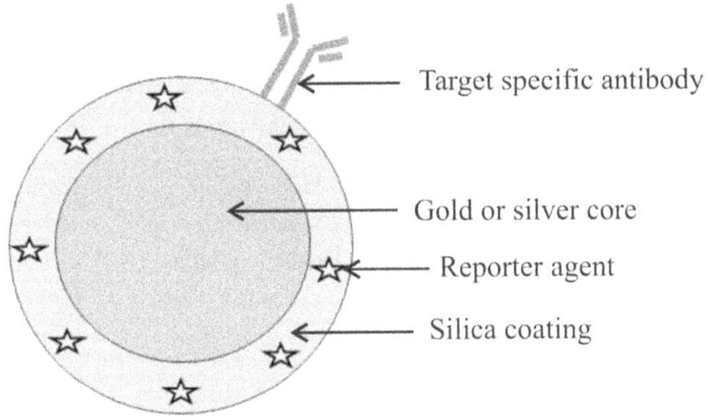

(C)

Fig. 7.5 Imaging probes: (a) Quantum dots (b) Magnetic nanoparticle (c) Raman probe.

7.5.1.4 Colloidal Gold Nano-Rods/Particles

The light absorption and emission characteristics of gold nanocarriers have become a key advantage in diagnosis of cancer, both the location and type of cancer. Since each type of cancer has a unique protein on its cell surface, the gold nanocarriers orient differently, depending on which type of cancer cells they have been attached to. This results in each type of cancer having its own unique pattern of scattered light, thus both the location and type of cancer can be determine.

Quantum dots have toxicity concern and burn out after extended exposure to light. While gold nanocarriers, on the other hand, have little or no long-term toxicity and not burn out after extended light exposure, allowing them to illuminate cancerous cells for much longer periods of time than the quantum dots. Gold nanoparticles luminescence is also a more highly sensitive technique, permitting to use fewer chemical markers in order to obtain the same information (Huang *et al.,* 2007). Gold nanocarriers in shape of spheres greatly increase the rate of cell penetration by the nanoparticles when compared to the larger and less agile 'nanorods'.

Table 7.3 Contrast agent and advantages as well as disadvantages of different imaging techniques

Imaging technique	Contrast agent/probe	Advantages	Limitations
CT	Iodine compounds, gold nanoparticles, barium sulfate nanoparticles	High spatial resolution, excellent bone imaging	Radiation, limited soft-tissue discrimination, high concentration of molecular contrast agent
PET, SPECT	Nanoparticles incorporating radioisotopes (e.g., ^{64}Cu ($t_{1/2}$: 12.7 hr), ^{89}Zr (78 hr), ^{18}F (1.82 hr), ^{68}Ga ($t_{1/2}$: 1.13 hr), ^{111}In ($t_{1/2}$: 2.8 days), 99mTc ($t_{1/2}$: 6.0 hr), I^{123} ($t_{1/2}$: 13.3 hr)	Very high sensitivity, quantitative, very low concentration required	Radiation, relatively low spatial resolution, need cyclotron or radioelement source
MRI	Paramagnetic: Gadolinium and Manganese-based nanoparticles Super-paramagnetic: Iron oxide, iron platinum particles	High spatial resolution, very high soft tissue discrimination, combined anatomic and functional imaging	Low sensitivity, long scan, high mass of probe, possible toxic side effect for gadolinium
Fluorescence imaging	Quantum dots, dye-doped nanoparticles, carbon-based nanomaterials	High sensitivity, multiplexed imaging, immense catalogue of probes	Poor depth penetration, relatively low spatial resolution

7.5.2 Targeting Tumor Vasculature for Imaging

Significant opportunities exist at the interface between cancer biomarkers and nanotechnology for molecular cancer diagnosis. In particular, nanoparticle probes can be used to quantify a panel of biomarkers on intact cancer cells and tissue specimens. Conjugation of nanoparticle to multiple ligands, leads to enhanced binding affinity and exquisite specificity through a multivalency effect. The development of tumor-targeted contrast agents based on a nanoparticles formulation may offer enhanced sensitivity and specificity for *in vivo* tumor imaging using currently available clinical imaging modalities (Fig. 7.6).

Tumor angiogenesis is important for tumor growth and development. Current imaging techniques can be adapted to provide functional information regarding the status of the tumor vasculature (Fig. 7.6). A targeted approach relies on binding of labeled molecules to highly expressed markers on the endothelium of tumor vasculature. As we have discussed above that overexpressed VEGF, integrins, and MMPs are potential targets for active targeting mechanism mediated delivery of anticancer agents encapsulated nanoparticles and these targets can also be utilized for imaging and have been the basis for several molecular imaging agents. We can modify various imaging nanoparticles with target specific ligand to obtain specific and enhanced imaging. The RGD peptide which bind specifically to $\alpha_v\beta_3$ integrin, can be labeled, for instance with ^{18}F, to synthesize a PET-capable integrin-targeted imaging agent of angiogenesis (Chen *et al.,* 2004). Use of quantum dots that emit in the near-infrared spectrum is an alternative approach for the imaging of tumor structures *in vivo*. The use of quantum dots allows differentiation of tumor vasculature from perivascular cells and tumor matrix. Fluorescent emission peaks of these nanoparticles are in the 800-1000 nm range, distant from the typical spectrum of tissue autofluorescence (400-600 nm). This unique feature of near-infrared quantum dots makes probes easily recognisable under near-infrared light, even in the tissues with high fluorescent background (Stroh *et al.,* 2005).

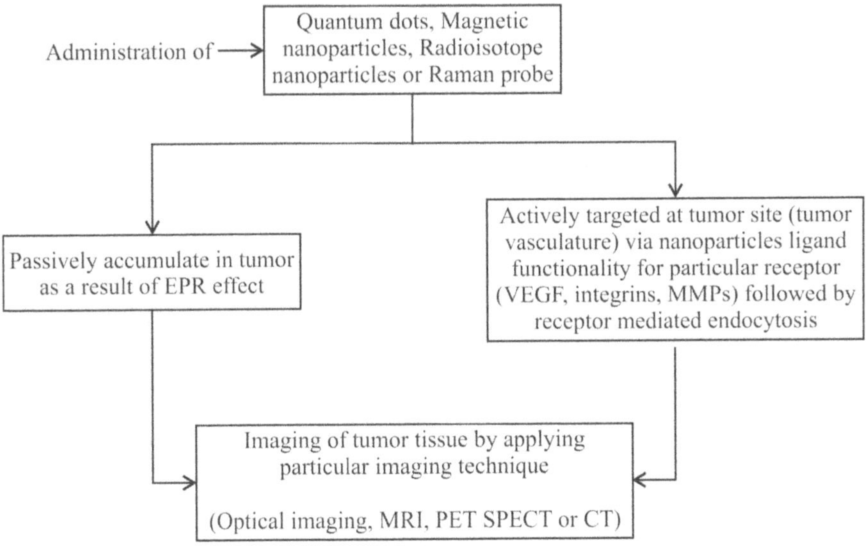

Fig. 7.6 Flow chart demonstrating contrast enhanced imaging of tumor.

Advantageously, binding sites can be created for targeted delivery in tumor, particularly when they are within the vascular space (Fig. 7.7). After administration of gold nanorods, it get passively accumulate in the tumor as a result of EPR effect. After laser irradiation, nanorods activate tumor cells. The gold nanorods absorb laser energy, heating the surrounding tissue. This localized rise in temperature increases tissue permeability and induces expression of receptor proteins on the surface of the tumor cells. These overexpressed proteins can be targeted by various suitable ligand modified nanoparticles.

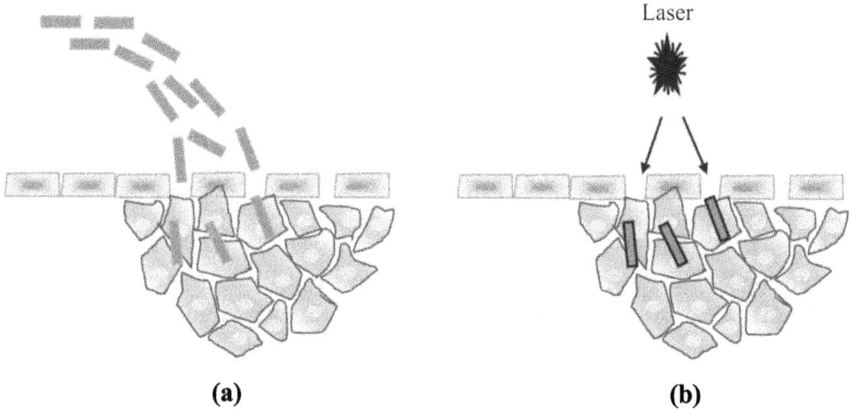

Fig. 7.7 This scheme illustrates a method to induce cooperative nanoparticle behaviour that results in more effective delivery of treatments to tumors. (a) Passive accumulation of circulating nanorods in the tumor as a result of leakiness of the tumor vasculature, the EPR effect. (b) Activation of tumor cells by laser irradiation of nanorods.

References

Adams M.L, Lavasanifar A, and Kwon G.S (2003). Amphiphilic block copolymers for drug delivery. *J Pharm Sci* **92:** 1343-1355.

Allen T.M (2002). Ligand-targeted therapeutics in anticancer therapy. *Nat Rev Cancer* **2:** 750-763.

Bianco A, Kostarelos K, Partidos C.D, and Prato M (2005). Biomedical applications of functionalised carbon nanotubes. *Chem Commun (Camb)* 571-577.

Cai W, and Chen X (2006). Anti-angiogenic cancer therapy based on integrin alphavbeta3 antagonism. *Anticancer Agents Med Chem* **6:** 407-428.

Chen X, Park R, Shahinian A.H, Tohme M, Khankaldyyan V, Bozorgzadeh M.H, Bading J.R, Moats R, Laug W.E, and Conti P.S (2004). 18F-labeled RGD peptide: initial evaluation for imaging brain tumor angiogenesis. *Nucl Med Biol* **31:** 179-189.

Cheng M.R, Li Q, Wan T, He B, Han J, Chen H.X, Yang F.X, Wang W, Xu H.Z, Ye T, *et al.,* (2012). Galactosylated chitosan/5-fluorouracil nanoparticles inhibit mouse hepatic cancer growth and its side effects. *World J Gastroenterol* **18:** 6076-6087.

Furumoto S, Takashima K, Kubota K, Ido T, Iwata R, and Fukuda H (2003). Tumor detection using 18F-labeled matrix metalloproteinase-2 inhibitor. *Nucl Med Biol* **30:** 119-125.

Huang X, Jain P.K, El-Sayed I.H, and El-Sayed M.A (2007). Gold nanoparticles: interesting optical properties and recent applications in cancer diagnostics and therapy. *Nanomedicine* (Lond) **2:** 681-693.

Kukowska-Latallo J.F, Candido K.A, Cao Z, Nigavekar S.S, Majoros I.J, Thomas T.P, Balogh L.P, Khan M.K, and Baker J.R, Jr (2005). Nanoparticle targeting of anticancer drug improves therapeutic response in animal model of human epithelial cancer. *Cancer Res* **65:** 5317-5324.

Maeda H (2001). The enhanced permeability and retention (EPR) effect in tumor vasculature: the key role of tumor-selective macromolecular drug targeting. *Adv Enzyme Regul* **41:** 189-207.

Mansour A.M, Drevs J, Esser N, Hamada F.M, Badary O.A, Unger C, Fichtner I, and Kratz F (2003). A new approach for the treatment of malignant melanoma: enhanced antitumor efficacy of an albumin-binding doxorubicin prodrug that is cleaved by matrix metalloproteinase 2. *Cancer Res* **63:** 4062-4066.

Medintz I.L, Uyeda H.T, Goldman E.R, and Mattoussi H (2005). Quantum dot bioconjugates for imaging, labelling and sensing. *Nat Mater* **4:** 435-446.

Moghimi S.M, Hunter A.C, and Murray J.C (2001). Long-circulating and target-specific nanoparticles: theory to practice. *Pharmacol Rev* **53:** 283-318.

Moghimi S.M, and Szebeni J (2003). Stealth liposomes and long circulating nanoparticles: critical issues in pharmacokinetics, opsonization and protein-binding properties. *Prog Lipid Res* **42:** 463-478.

Moore B.D, Stevenson L, Watt A, Flitsch S, Turner N.J, Cassidy C, and Graham D (2004). Rapid and ultra-sensitive determination of enzyme activities using surface-enhanced resonance Raman scattering. *Nat Biotechnol* **22:** 1133-1138.

Ni S, Stephenson S.M, and Lee R.J (2002). Folate receptor targeted delivery of liposomal daunorubicin into tumor cells. *Anticancer Res* **22:** 2131-2135.

Pan X.Q, Wang H, and Lee R.J (2003). Antitumor activity of folate receptor-targeted liposomal doxorubicin in a KB oral carcinoma murine xenograft model. *Pharm Res* **20:** 417-422.

Pelicano H, Martin D.S, Xu R.H, and Huang P (2006). Glycolysis inhibition for anticancer treatment. *Oncogene* **25:** 4633-4646.

Shenoy D.B, and Amiji M.M (2005). Poly(ethylene oxide)-modified poly(epsilon-caprolactone) nanoparticles for targeted delivery of tamoxifen in breast cancer. *Int J Pharm* **293:** 261-270.

Stroh M, Zimmer J.P, Duda D.G, Levchenko T.S, Cohen K.S, Brown E.B, Scadden D.T, Torchilin V.P, Bawendi M.G, Fukumura D, *et al.,* (2005). Quantum dots spectrally distinguish multiple species within the tumor milieu *in vivo*. *Nat Med* **11:** 678-682.

Wisse E, Braet F, Luo D, De Zanger R, Jans D, Crabbe E, and Vermoesen A (1996). Structure and function of sinusoidal lining cells in the liver. *Toxicol Pathol* **24:** 100-111.

Yezhelyev M.V, Gao X, Xing Y, Al-Hajj A, Nie S, and O'Regan R.M (2006). Emerging use of nanoparticles in diagnosis and treatment of breast cancer. *Lancet Oncol* **7:** 657-667.

Yuan F, Dellian M, Fukumura D, Leunig M, Berk D.A, Torchilin V.P, and Jain R.K (1995). Vascular permeability in a human tumor xenograft: molecular size dependence and cutoff size. *Cancer Res* **55:** 3752-3756.

8

Transdermal Drug Delivery Systems

D. Mishra[1] **and P. Bhatnagar**[2]

[1] College of Pharmacy, IPS Academy, Indore-452012, India.

[2] Sri Aurobindo Institute of Pharmacy (S.A.I.P.), SAIMS Campus, Indore-453111, India.

8.1 Introduction

In order to achieve a desirable therapeutic benefit there should be proper selection of three major pillars i.e., the drug, delivery system and route of administration. In above stated pillars each has its own importance but the latter two plays a vital role. Since, historically the oral route of drug administration has remained the choice of preference undisputedly. Oral route is mainly preferred over others because of its leading advantages like no need of supervision, ease of administration and noninvasive nature etc., but as a matter of fact it has various limitations like slow onset of action, first pass metabolism, gastric irritation, poor bioavailability, non-targeted delivery and fluctuation in serum drug concentration.

To overcome these difficulties there is a need for the development of a new drug delivery system; which will improve the therapeutic efficacy and safety of drugs by more precise (i.e., site specific), spatial and temporal placement within the body thereby reducing both the size and number of doses. Since then, after tedious research work it has been found that the '*human skin*' can be explored as a potential site for drug delivery and led to the development of transdermal drug delivery systems (TDDS). It was the Merriam Webster who coin the term *"Transdermal"* in 1944.

In the above context TDDS emerged as a better and effective substitute for oral drug delivery. TDDS means the drug permeate through the skin to dermis then to systemic circulation in a sequence and undistorted manner. TDDS is *"a system capable of delivering drugs to the systemic circulation via the skin"* and is able to provide the drug at a controlled rate so as to minimize the fluctuation in serum-drug concentration reduces the number & frequencies of doses, improves the patient's compliance, avoid dysphasia and trespasses defense mechanism of body. Thus, by recognizing the unbeatable potentials of TDDS, in 1979 FDA approved the first transdermal patch (TDP) i.e., Transderm-Scop® for the treatment of motion sickness. Till date we are flourished with ample numbers of patches (around 35) in the market which are used to cure various diseases and their symptoms (Brown *et al.,* 2006).

8.1.1 Transdermal Drug Delivery System (TDDS)

TDDS is defined as that system in which the drug penetrates through the skin and reaches systemic circulation and elicits desired therapeutic response. Drug delivery *via* skin portal system include multifarious dosage forms ranging from conventional (syringe or needle) to the novel (transdermal patches & films). TDDS can be defined as a system that "*can deliver the drugs through the skin portal to systemic circulation at a predetermined rate and maintain clinically the effective concentrations over a prolonged period of time*".

The possible *in-vivo* fate of drug that can challenge the formulation and development of TDDS is shown in Fig. 8.1.

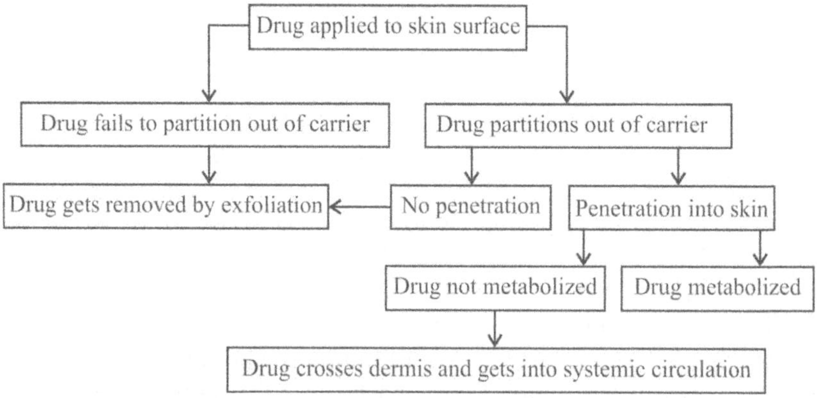

Fig. 8.1 Possible *in-vivo* fate of drug after transdermal application.

8.1.1.1 Merits of TDDS

The leading edge merits of TDDS over conventional dosage forms are as follows:

- Simple and non-invasive technique in comparison to parenteral.
- Avoidance of first pass metabolism of drugs e.g., scopolamine, ketoprofen, diclofenac and naproxen.
- Reduction of fluctuations in plasma levels of drugs e.g., nitroglycerine, clonidine and leuteinizing hormone releasing hormone.
- Most suitable for drug candidates having short half-life and low therapeutic index e.g., ketoprofen and diclofenac.
- Reduction of dosing frequency and delivery of drug over an extended period of time improves the patient compliance.
- It can minimize the daily intake of dose in comparison to oral administration e.g., diclofenac.
- It can minimize the side effects e.g., minimizes the liver damage by delivery of estrogen through TDDS.

The therapy can be simply terminated by removal of system from skin especially in case of transdermal patch.

8.1.1.2 Demerits of TDDS

As like any other system the TDDS also subjected to some limitations like (Thomas and Finnin, 2004)

- The possibility of local irritation which may develop at the site of application. Erythema, itching, and local edema can be caused by the drug, the adhesive, or other excipients in the patch formulation.
- The skin's low permeability may limit the number of drugs that can be delivered in this manner.
- A constant concentration gradient is to be made for the successful delivery of drug, but practically it is not possible resulting in "drug loss".
- Damage to drug reservoir may lead to improper release of drug.
- Upon exposure to atmosphere there may be chances of drug degradation or poor adhesiveness and may lead to removal of TDDS.

8.1.2 Ideal Requirements of Drug for Transdermal Delivery

In order to develop an effective TDDS which is capable of managing the diseases and its symptoms, there should be proper selection of drug. For developing TDDS the drug candidate should have properties reported in Table 8.1.

Table 8.1 Ideal properties of drug candidate to be delivered *via* TDDS

S. No.	Ideal properties	Requirements
1	Toxicity profile	Drug should be non-toxic, non-irritant and non-sensitizing
2	Dose	It should be of low dose
3	Half Life (in hours)	Short
4	Molecular weight	Should be less than 500 Dalton
5	Partition coefficient	1-4
6	Skin permeability coefficient	$> 0.5 \times 10^3$ cm/h
7	Oral bioavailability	Low
8	Therapeutic window	Narrow
9	Stability profile	Drug should be photostable and stable at skin temperature
10	Compatibility	Drug should be compatible with skin secretions and skin pH
11	Adhesiveness	Should adhere to skin for desired period of time
12	Ease of removal	Should be easily remove from skin without leaving a stain or causing any damage to skin

8.1.3 Topical *v/s* Transdermal Delivery

In general topical and transdermal terminology is used synonymously, but there is a major difference between them. Topical administration means the dosage form is applied on restricted area of skin in order to achieve a localized effect e.g., creams, gels, pastes, and powders are applied to treat the fungal and bacterial infections (Osborne, 2008). While in case of transdermal drug administration; drug is delivered *via* skin in order to achieve systemic therapeutic effect e.g., *Catapres-TTS*® patch containing clonidine is used for the management of hypertension and *Transderm-Nitro*® patch containing nitroglycerin is used for the treatment of angina (Brown *et al.,* 2006). They can also be used for local effect e.g., local anesthetic effect. At present in market there are basically three types of TDDS i.e., reservoir type, matrix with rate controlling membrane and matrix without rate controlling membrane. The drugs which can be given by transdermal route are scopolamine, nitroglycerine, fentanyl, clonidine, diclofenac, indomethacin, nicotine, estradiol etc.

8.2 Anatomy and Physiology of Human Skin

The skin is the largest organ of body and comprises about 10% of the total body weight of an average healthy human body. It is vital interface between external atmosphere and visceral organs. It acts as a barrier for harmful radiations, pathogens, dust, chemical allergens, and also prevents the loss of water, endogenous metabolites and nutrients.

Human skin is about 0.5 mm thick and can be broadly classified into two distinct layers i.e., outermost epidermis and inner dermis. In-spite of that skin consists of various appendages (hairs, glands, nails, etc.). Cross-sectional view of skin can be depicted as in Fig. 8.2. Epidermis is outermost layer of body and is of avascular (no blood vessels) nature. It is basically composed of stratified keratinized squamous epithelial cells, which is also known as "Stratum Corneum" (SC). This SC; act as major barrier in drug diffusion process. The cells of SC are non-nucleated dead squamous cells in which cytoplasm is replaced by the deep deposition of "Keratin" protein which provides a barrier function. Apart from that, it also contains another protein "Melanin" which imparts color to skin. Apart from SC there are four more layers namely (in descending order) stratum lucidum, stratum granulosum, stratum spinosum, stratum basale finally touching dermis.

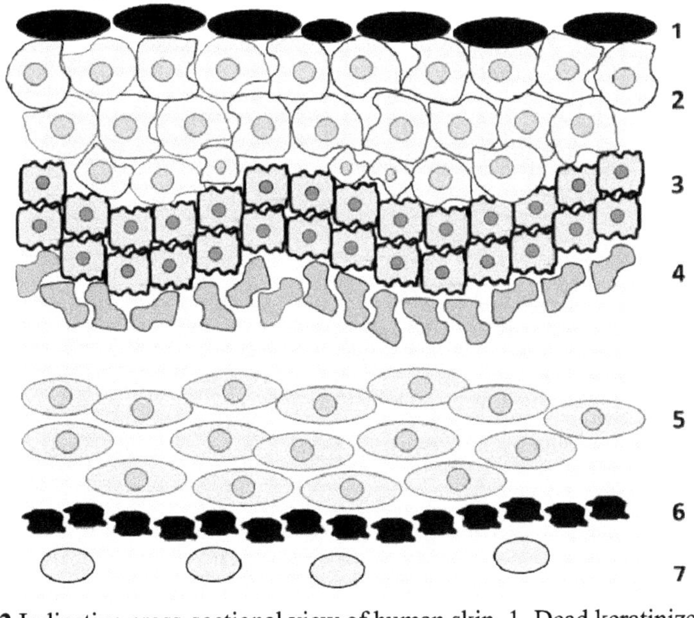

Fig. 8.2 Indicative cross-sectional view of human skin. 1. Dead keratinized cells, 2. Stratum corneum, 3. Stratum lucidium, 4. Stratum granulosum, 5. Stratum spinosum, 6. Stratum baselae, 7. Dermis

Dermis is a highly vascular (supplied with blood vessels) and the bulk forming layer of the skin. It is about 1-2 mm thick and is made up of connective tissue elements. It is metabolically less active as compared to epidermis. It is made up of blood vessels, lymph vessels, sebaceous glands, sweat glands, sensory nerve endings, adipose tissue, mast cells, arrector pili and some leukocytes. The prime function of dermis is to nourish and anchor it to deeper tissues.

The three major skin appendages i.e., hair, sweat glands, and sebaceous glands arises from dermis. Sebaceous glands are associated with hair follicles and secrete sebum which ultimately lubricates the skin (Elias, 1983).

8.2.1 Subcutaneous Tissue (ST)

It resides below the dermis and is composed of fat cells arranged in lobular fashion. The main function of this tissue is to act as heat insulator and shock absorber. It is the blood vessels and nerves which connect the skin to ST (Hadgraft, 2004).

8.2.2 Functions of Human Skin

Human skin plays a vital role in day to day life and performs various indispensible functions like protection, maintenance of body temperature and water level etc. (Menon, 2002). These functions are effectively summarized (Chien, 2003) in Fig. 8.3.

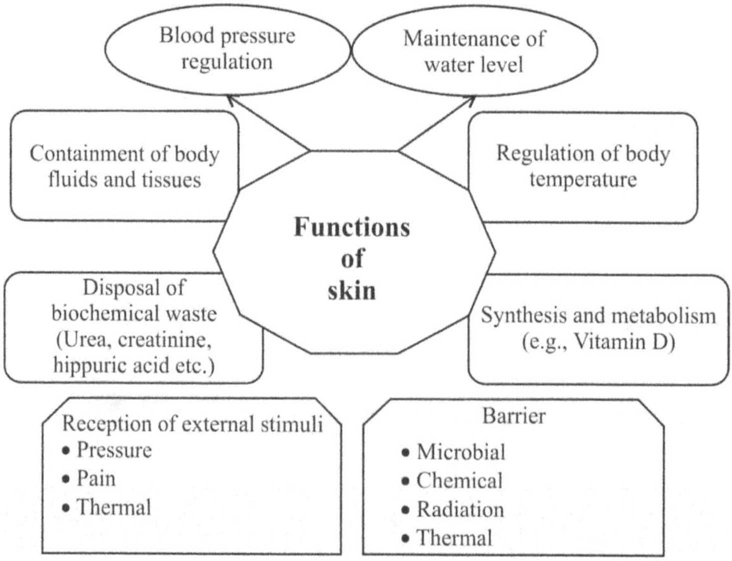

Fig. 8.3 Functions of human skin.

8.2.3 Possible Drug Delivery Channels *via* Skin

Delivery of drug across the skin to systemic circulation is a crucial matter of concern and debate. After a thorough study and extensive research, it has been concluded that the three major possible channels by which a drug can reach systemic circulation *via* skin are SC, transfollicular and glandular pathway. SC plays a vital role in the diffusion of drugs through skin. SC is around 12-15 μm thick layer composed of dead keratinized cells arranged in a brick fashion with natural tortuosity. Drug basically follows two pathways i.e., paracellular or transcellular. In *paracellular* pathway drug moves around the periphery of cells (does not traverse) and reaches systemic circulation; while in *transcellular* pathway the drug readily traverse across the cells and reaches blood stream and elicits a therapeutic response (Barry, 2001). This drug permeation can be effectively visualized as shown in Fig. 8.4.

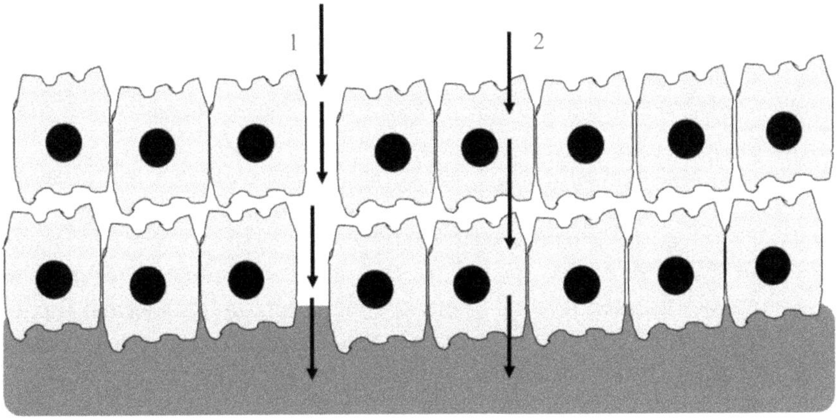

Fig. 8.4 Possible drug delivery channels operating in skin. 1. Paracellular path, 2. Transcellular path

8.3 Factors Affecting TDDS

Drug delivery *via* skin depends upon innumerable factors which governs the effectiveness and performance of a delivery system. The factors which directly or indirectly affect the TDDS can be broadly classified into three major categories i.e., biological factors, dosage form related factors, and physiochemical properties of enhancers (Fig. 8.5).

8.3.1 Physiological Factors

- ***Stratum corneum***: In normal conditions it is semipermeable in nature and acts as a barrier of impervious nature to xenobiotics. But with the application of electric field, magnetic field, ultrasonic sounds etc., the structure of layer can be distorted which may gear up the drug diffusion process.

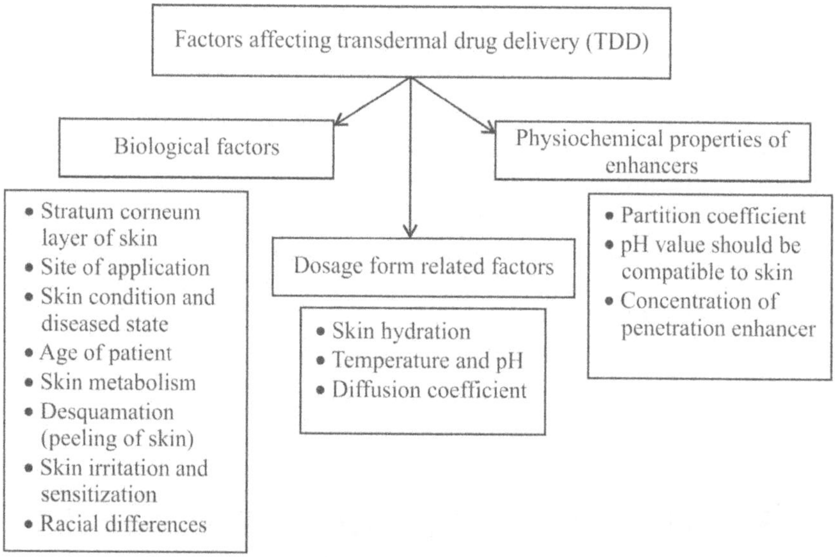

Fig. 8.5 Factors affecting transdermal drug delivery.

- ***Skin Condition:*** In general as the structural integrity of skin is altered or erupted it leads to marked increment in transdermal flux of drug. In chronic stage of psoriasis and eczema, the most commonly encountered skin diseases there is ascertainable loss of intra-void lipids and transepidermal water loss (TEWL) ultimately generating enhanced transdermal drug permeation. But the skin barrier condition is well restored as soon as the diseased condition is healed up. Many solvents and chemicals including methanol, ethanol, dimethyl sulfoxide (DMSO) may alter the skin structure thus can promote the drug permeation.

- ***Age of patient:*** Skin of neonates and children is more permeable thus allow easy access of drug across the skin. While with the gradual process of ageing there is a heavy deposition of keratin in the cells that transform the cell to an impervious and dead structure.

- ***Site of application:*** The nature, thickness, and density of SC greatly vary from site to site. These factors ultimately affect the drug permeation. For example the drug can be easily passed through skin of hands and legs as compared to the skin of palm and sole.

- ***Skin metabolism:*** Epidermis is equipped with plentiful of enzymes of various natures like neucleotidase, esterase, phosphatase, protease, and lipase. They are capable of metabolizing drugs with different functional groups. The drug that lost functional group may lose its therapeutic activity.

8.3.2 Dosage Form Related Factors

- ***Skin hydration:*** Long term exposure of skin to water may alter the permeability of skin. Generally hydration increases the drug diffusion process.
- ***Temperature and pH of application site:*** Usually a rise in temperature gear up the drug diffusion and pH of application site plays a vital role in determining the concentration of unionized drug. It is the concentration of unionized drug which determine the concentration gradient thus facilitates the drug diffusion.
- ***Diffusion coefficient:*** Drug permeation mainly depends upon the diffusion coefficient which in turn depends on properties of drug, diffusion medium and interaction between two.
- ***Drug concentration:*** The driving force for the diffusion is concentration of drug on either side of skin. The drug diffusion increases with increase in concentration gradient.
- ***Molecular size and shape:*** Drug diffusion strictly obeys Fick's first law of diffusion which ultimately suggests that the diffusion is inversely proportional to molecular weight and shape. Thus the drug molecule with small size and low molecular weight readily crosses the skin.

8.3.3 Physiochemical Properties of Enhancers

- ***Partition coefficient of enhancers:*** The partition coefficient plays a crucial role in deciding the fate of TDDS. Ample research in the field of TDDS revealed a fact that the log P value should be in a range of 2-3 in order to cross the skin barrier. The drug and penetration enhancers should possess optimal lipophilicity.
- ***pH compatibility:*** The pH of enhancers and drug should be compatible to that of skin otherwise may lead to the precipitation of drug with consequent reduction in absorption.
- ***Concentration of penetration enhancers:*** The diffusion of drug is directly proportional to the concentration of penetration enhancers.

8.4 Approaches for TDDS

The basic approaches which are applied for the development of TDDS are depicted in Fig. 8.6.

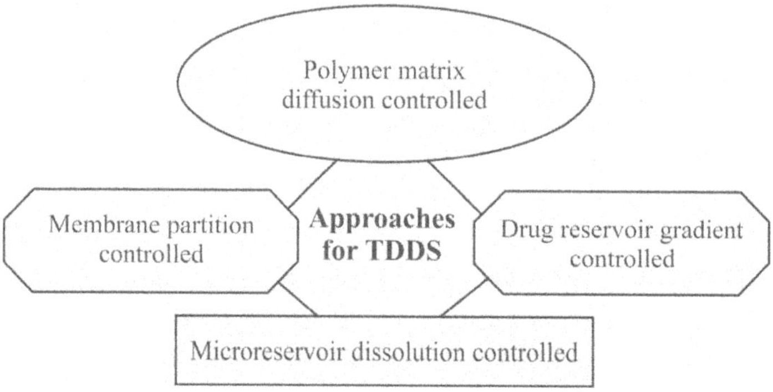

Fig. 8.6 Various approaches for TDDS.

8.4.1 Membrane Permeation Controlled TDDS

The system comprises of drug reservoir which is sandwiched between drug impermeable backing membrane and rate controlling release liner. The drug is only allowed to permeate through release liner in a unidirectional way. The release liner is either microporous or nonporous in nature. On the outermost surface of release liner there is a relatively thin pressure sensitive adhesive layer (Fig. 8.7). Marketed approved membrane permeation controlled TDDS include Transderm-Nitro® containing nitroglycerine for the treatment of angina, Transderm-Scop® containing scopolamine for the treatment of motion sickness and Catapres-TTS® containing clonidine for the management of hypertension.

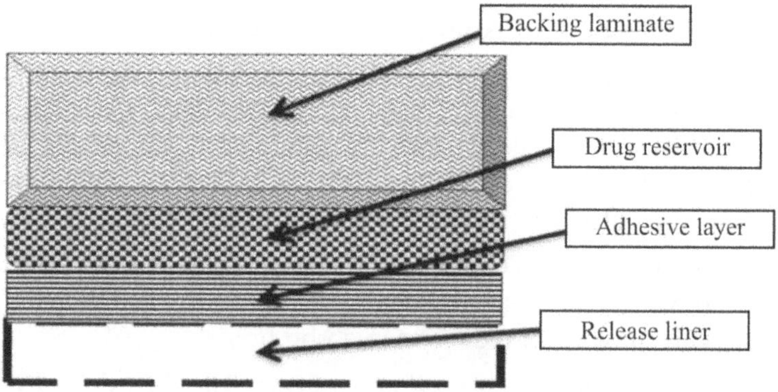

Fig. 8.7 Membrane permeation controlled TDDS.

The drug release kinetics for membrane permeation controlled TDDS can be represented by following equation:

$$\frac{dQ}{dt} = \frac{K_{\frac{a}{m}} K_{\frac{m}{r}} D_a D_m}{K_{\frac{m}{r}} h_a D_m + K_{\frac{a}{m}} D_a h_m} C_R$$

Where,

dQ/dt = Rate of drug diffusion

$K_{a/m}$ = Partition coefficient of drug from membrane to adhesive

$K_{m/r}$ = Partition coefficient of drug from reservoir to membrane

D_a = Diffusion coefficient in adhesive layer

D_m = Diffusion coefficient in membrane

h_a = Thickness of adhesive layer

h_m = Thickness of membrane

C_R = Drug concentration in reservoir compartment

8.4.2 Polymer Matrix Diffusion Controlled TDDS

In this, the drug is homogeneously and uniformly dispersed in hydrophilic and lipophilic polymeric mixture and casted over a disc of definite area. The system is then entangled in an occlusive base whose circumference has adhesive covering (Fig. 8.8). The example of marketed polymer matrix diffusion controlled TDDS is Nitro-Dur® for the treatment of angina.

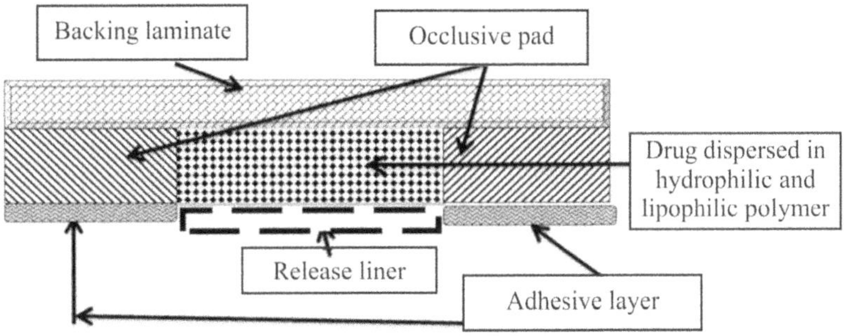

Fig. 8.8 Polymer matrix diffusion controlled TDDS.

The release kinetics of polymer matrix diffusion controlled TDDS can be summarized as follows:

$$\frac{dQ}{dt} = \sqrt{\left(\frac{L_d C_P D_P}{2t}\right)}$$

Where,

dQ/dt = Rate of drug diffusion

L_d = Initial drug loading dose

C_p = Solubility of drug in polymer

D_p = Diffusivity of drug in polymer

t = Time

8.4.3 Drug Reservoir Gradient Controlled TDDS

It is simply prepared by dispersing drug in polymeric adhesive layer which will allow drying for some time. Finally the medicated adhesive film is supported by backing laminate and the drug is allowed to cross through release liner in a unidirectional pattern (Fig. 8.9). The marketed example of drug reservoir gradient controlled TDDS is Deponit® and Nicotrol®.

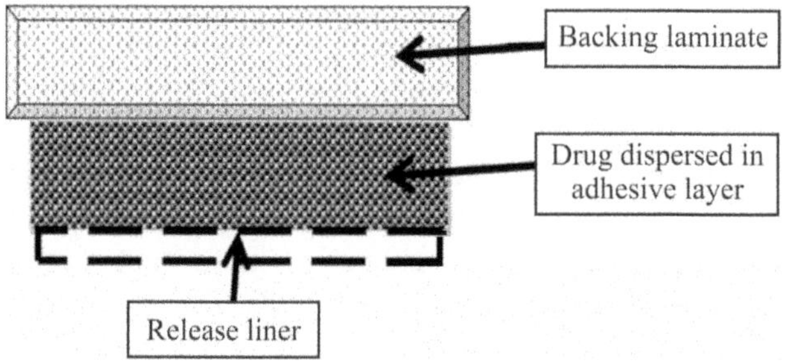

Fig. 8.9 Drug reservoir gradient controlled TDDS.

The release kinetics of drug reservoir gradient controlled TDDS can be summarized as follows:

$$\frac{dQ}{dt} = \frac{K_{\frac{a}{r}} D_a}{h_a (t)} L_d h_a$$

Where,

dQ/dt = Rate of drug diffusion

$K_{a/r}$ = Initial drug loading dose

D_a = Solubility of drug in polymer

h_a = Diffusivity of drug in polymer

t = Time

L_d = Initial drug loading dose

8.4.4 Microreservoir Dissolution Controlled TDDS

It is the unique combination of matrix and reservoir type system. In this the drug is dispersed in aqueous polymeric solution. The drug is in micronized form and is supported over an occlusive pad (Fig. 8.10). It is highly thermodynamically unstable system. The Nitro-Disc® is one such commercially available formulation based on this concept.

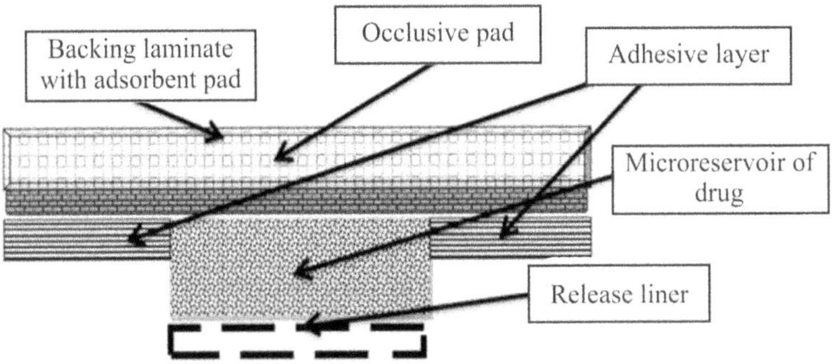

Fig. 8.10 Microreservoir dissolution controlled TDDS.

The release kinetics can be summarized as follows:

$$\frac{dQ}{dt} = \frac{D_P\, D_S A K_P}{h_d\, D_P + K_P\, AD_S\, h_P}\left(\frac{BSP - D_l S_l (1-B)}{h_l}\right)\left(\frac{1}{K_l} + \frac{1}{K_m}\right)$$

Where,

dQ/dt = Rate of drug diffusion

A = h'/B', h' is the ratio of drug concentration in the bulk of elution solution to drug solubility in same medium and B' is the ratio of drug concentration at the outer edge of polymer coating membrane to drug solubility in the same polymer composition

K_l, K_m, and K_p = Partition coefficients for the interfacial portioning of drug from polymer matrix to polymer coating membrane, and polymer coating membrane to the elution solution (or skin) respectively

D_l, Dp and D_s = Drug diffusibilities in liquid compartment and in the polymer matrix respectively

S_l and S_p = Solubility of drug in liquid compartment and in the polymer matrix, respectively.

8.5 Transdermal Patches (TDP)

They are the most popular and unique dosage form in itself. They are basically consisting of medicated drug reservoir film sandwiched between impermeable backing laminate and rate controlling release liner. They are applied on skin and drug diffuses in a sequential manner in order to reach systemic circulation to provide therapeutic response. The first TDP was a plastic piece dipped in ethanol solution of drug and was applied to patient to achieve intended effect. ***Transderm-Scop®*** containing scopolamine for the treatment of motion sickness and ***Transderm-Nitro®*** containing nitroglycerine for the treatment of angina were approved by FDA in 1981. With the gradual evolution in the field of TDP we are now equipped with the fourth generation of TDP.

8.5.1 How a TDP Works?

The basic hypothesized mechanism for the working of TDP is represented in Fig. 8.11.

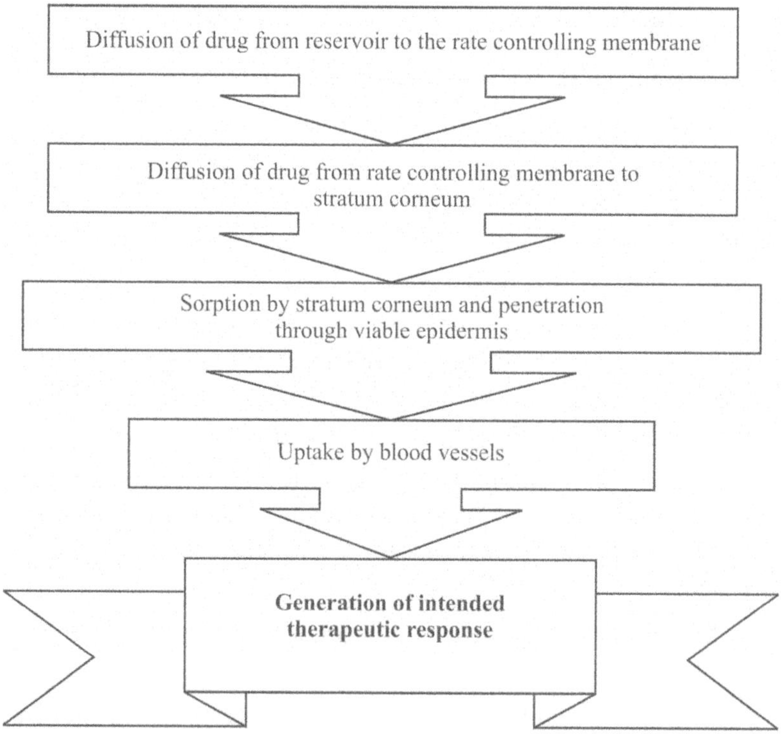

Fig. 8.11 Possible mechanism of working of TDP.

8.5.2 Conditions in which TDP can be used

The conditions in which a TDP can be used for treatment or cure of diseases are as follows:

- When patient is suffering from intolerable effect (stomach ache or severe constipation) or has problem in swallowing the drug (dysphasia).
- The delivery route is beneficial for patients in unconscious state or those requiring a constant medication for a prolonged period of time (hormonal therapy/hypertension management).
- When the patient is suffering from a severe cognitive disorder and not in a position of self-medication e.g., amnesia or schizophrenia.

8.5.3 Conditions in which TDP is not used

The use of TDP is precluded in conditions where rapid onset of action is required or when the dose of drug to be administrated is very high.

8.5.4 What Care should be taken while Applying a TDP?

Prior to the administration of TDP to the skin, following points should be considered in order to improve the transdermal therapy:

- The site at which the TDP is to be applied should be properly cleaned.
- TDP to be applied should not be cut/damaged/tear otherwise may lead to dose dumping or improper drug release profile.
- While applying a TDP care should be taken, otherwise it may come in contact with the skin of person who is applying.
- While removing a TDP it should be ensure that, it does not cause any type of irritation or skin disease at the site of application, or does not leave any kind of stain.
- After application of TDP, it should be ensured that it is properly attached to skin.

8.5.5 Types of TDP

After extensive studies and research, we are able to classify the fabricated TDP into six broad classes either on the basis of layer or on the basis of drug entrapped or on the basis of performance (Fig. 8.12).

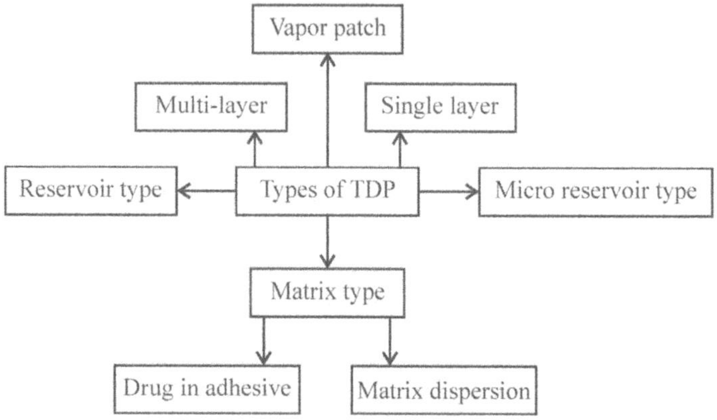

Fig. 8.12 Types of TDP.

(a) Single layer type: In this type the drug is uniformly distributed in an adhesive layer. The medicated adhesive layer is solely responsible for controlled release of drug. This layer is supported by an impermeable backing laminate and frontally covered by a release liner.

(b) Multi-layer type: This type of TDP is unique combination of two consecutive layers of medicated adhesive system. One is for immediate release of drug and another layer delivers the drug at a predetermine rate in order to maintain blood spike concentration. Both medicated adhesive layers are sandwiched between impermeable backing laminate and release liner.

(c) Vapor patch: This patch is comprised of medicated adhesive which simultaneously serves two purposes at a time. It helps to adhere the patch to site of application and releases the drug in vapor form to elicit a therapeutic effect. Most of the essential oils are delivered in such a way to treat decongestion. Some time it is also used in cigarette smoking cessation therapy.

(d) Reservoir type: These types of patches are prepared by dispersing, solubilizing, gel forming, or making suspension of drug in polymer matrix. This act as drug reservoir and is entrapped between backing laminate and rate controlling release liner. The drug is only passes through this release liner.

(e) **Matrix type:** These types of patches are further sub classified into two categories:

- ***Drug in adhesive type:*** Drug is dispersed in molten adhesive which is then casted over backing laminate. Finally covered by an unmedicated adhesive layer for protection.
- ***Matrix dispersion type:*** The drug is uniformly dispersed in molten mixture of hydrophilic and lipophilic mixture of molten polymer. It is then fixed in an occlusive pad with adhesive at its circumference.

(f) **Micro-reservoir type:** It is basically a reservoir type system which is capable of delayed drug release. It consists of drug solution containing microreservoir globules entangled in a crosslinked matrix. At lab scale it is prepared by suspending the drug in the aqueous solution of hydrophilic polymer and then the drug-polymer solution is uniformly dispersed in molten lipophilic carrier with assistance of high speed shearing. The overall process leads to the fabrication of small thermodynamically unstable micro-globules system which is stabilized by immediate addition of suitable crosslinking agent. Finally, the whole system is casted on a suitable mould and modified to be dispensed as patch.

8.6 Generations of TDP

Since historically skin was explored as a site of administration of various drugs and cosmaceuticals. It was Merriam Webster, who coined the term "Transdermal", for the delivery of drug across the skin. Since, then we are equipped with plentiful of TDP. The first TDP was a piece of plastic which was dipped in ethanolic solution of drug and used for therapy. No matter it has achieved success or failure; it has led to the development of a new therapy known as transdermal drug delivery technology. Gradually with the progress we have classified the TDP into three generations (Prausnitz and Langer, 2008) as shown in Fig. 8.13.

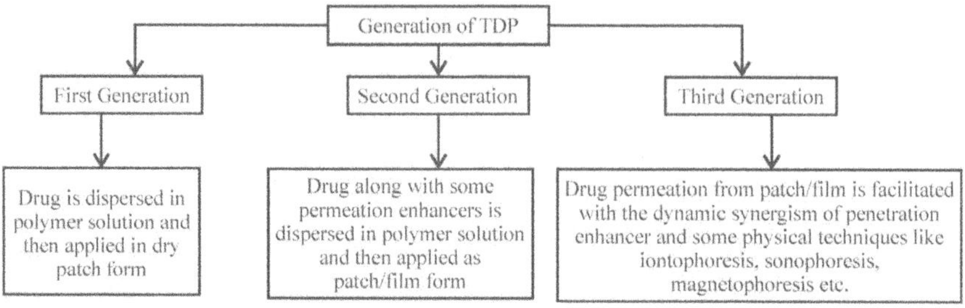

Fig. 8.13 Generations of TDP.

8.7 Components of TDP

The basic components of a TDP can be listed as follows

- Drug
- Polymer matrix/drug reservoir
- Permeation enhancer
- Pressure sensitive adhesive (PSA)
- Backing laminate
- Release liner
- Plasticizer
- Miscellaneous excipients

8.7.1 Drug

The drug candidate for which a TDP is to be proposed should be of low dose (10-30 mg) and low molecular weight (< 500 Da). It should be potent and compatible to skin secretions. It should be stable at wide variety of pH on skin with optimum partition coefficient value (log P; 2-3). The drugs which are good candidates for TDP include nicotine, scopolamine, fentanyl, diclofenac, indomethacin, scopolamine and estradiol.

8.7.2 Polymer Matrix

Drug is mainly dispersed in polymer matrix followed by support on backing laminate and release liner. It is primarily polymer matrix which dictates the drug release profile and final performance of patch. It can be made from *natural* polymers like pectin, sodium alginate, gelatin, chitosan etc., *semi-synthetic* polymers like cellulose derivatives and *synthetic* polymers like polyvinyl chloride, polyvinyl alcohol and eudragit.

8.7.3 Permeation Enhancers

They are the chemical substances which play a crucial role in drug diffusion across the skin. Usually water act as a natural penetration enhancer which hydrates the skin and alters its permeability for drug and allow its easy access to blood circulation. But now a day there is a long list of chemical agents which can be used as penetration enhancers. They may be either natural (terpens, terpenoids, fatty acid and alcohols) or synthetic (sulfoxide, glycols and cyclodextrin) in origin (Hori *et al.*, 1990). Various classes of penetration enhancers are shown in Table 8.2.

Table 8.2 Classification of penetration enhancers.

S. No.	Classes	Examples
1	Terpenes	Nerodil, menthol, 1,8 cineol, limonene, carvone
2	Pyrrolidones	N-methyl-2-pyrrolidone, azone
3	Fatty acids and esters	Oleic acid, linoleic acid, lauric acid, capric acid
4	Sulfoxide	DMSO, N,N dimethyl formamide
5	Alcohols, glycols and glycerides	Ethanol, propylene glycol
6	Miscellaneous	Phospholipids, cyclodextrins, amino acids

8.7.4 Pressure Sensitive Adhesive (PSA)

They are mainly used for perfect adherence of TDP to skin. When pressure is applied to them, they are attached to the skin firmly and allow the drug to diffuse out slowly. They should be non-toxic, non-irritant, and non-sensitizing in nature. They should be easily removed from skin and should not leave any kind of stain on skin after removal. They are broadly classified into three groups i.e., acylates, polyisobutylene, and polysiloxane.

8.7.5 Backing Laminate

They are generally made up of impervious materials like aluminum foil, polyethylene and ethyl vinyl acetate. They are applied in order to maintain the physical and chemical integrity of patch during shelf life as well as during its therapy period. It acts as shelter for the drug reservoir and maintains its release by protecting it from harmful effects of external environment.

8.7.6 Release Liner

They are used to maintain the unidirectional flow of drug from reservoir to adhesive and then from adhesive to skin in a controlled manner over a longer period of time at a predetermined rate. They are either microporous or nonporous in nature. They should be easily peeled off without damaging the TDP. They are generally made up of vinyl acetate derivatives, silicone derivatives and perfluorocarbon polymers.

8.7.7 Plasticizers

They are added to TDP in order to provide flexibility and strength to TDP. They readily eliminate brittleness of system and reduce the chances of wear and tear of TDP. The examples of plasticizers include aliphatic esters, phthalate esters, propylene glycol, polyethylene glycols and glycerin.

8.8 Methods of Preparation of TDP

There are various possible methods of preparations of TDP which are discussed below.

8.8.1 Asymmetric Membrane TPX Method

It is prepared by dry or wet inversion method. It can be demonstrated as shown in Fig. 8.14.

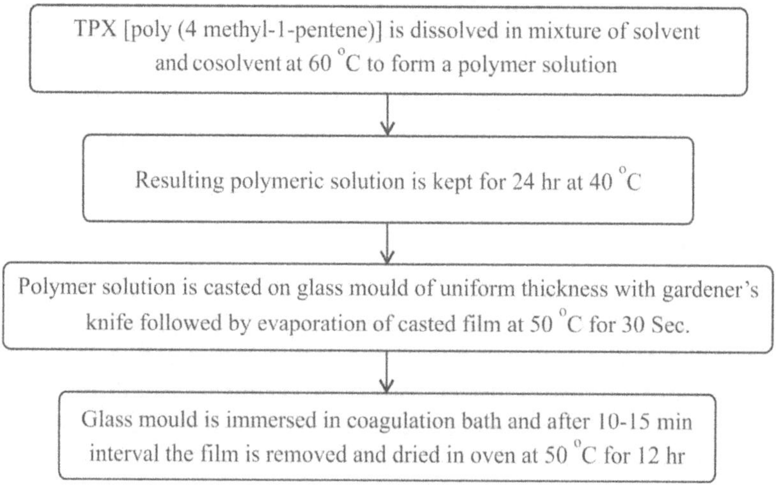

Fig. 8.14 Asymmetric TPX method.

8.8.2 Circular Teflon Mould Method

The overall method is schematically represented in Fig. 8.15.

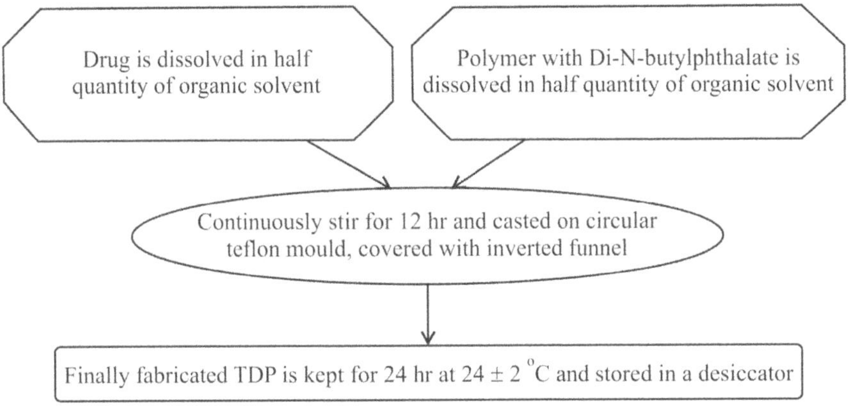

Fig. 8.15 Flow diagram of circular teflon mould method.

8.8.3 IPM Membrane Method

This particular method is most suitable for hydrophilic drugs. The drug is dissolved in water containing propylene glycol and carbopol 940 and allowed to stir for 12 hr. The medicated polymeric solution is neutralized by triethanolamine solution and finally casted over isopropyl myristate (IPM) membrane. The process is schematically presented in Fig. 8.16.

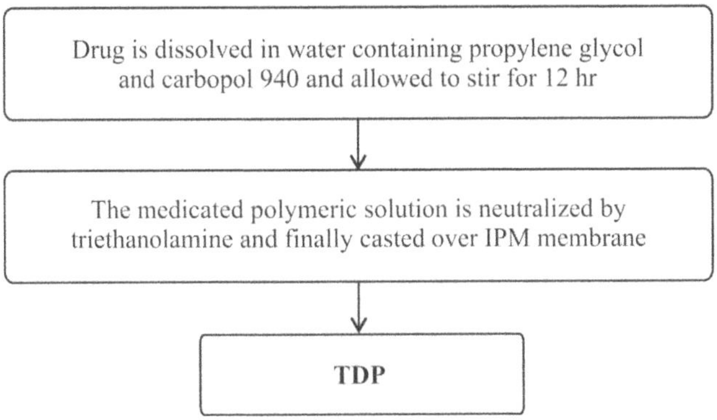

Fig. 8.16 Flow diagram of IPM membrane method.

8.8.4 EVAC Membrane Method

Drug is dissolved in a mixture of water, propylene glycol and ethylene-vinyl acetate (EVAC) polymer solution and finally the prepared gel is neutralized with 5% NaOH solution. The medicated gel is placed over backing laminate and from other side it is heat sealed by placing a rate controlling membrane. The entire process is summarized in Fig. 8.17.

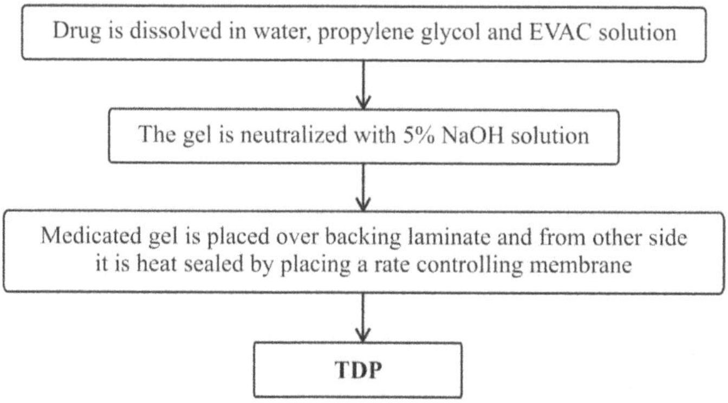

Fig. 8.17 Flow diagram of EVAC membrane method.

8.9 Evaluation of TDP

Fabricated TDP is to be evaluated in order to ensure its better performance at site of application. TDP can be evaluated on following parameters (Pathak and Thassu, 2009) mentioned in Fig. 8.18.

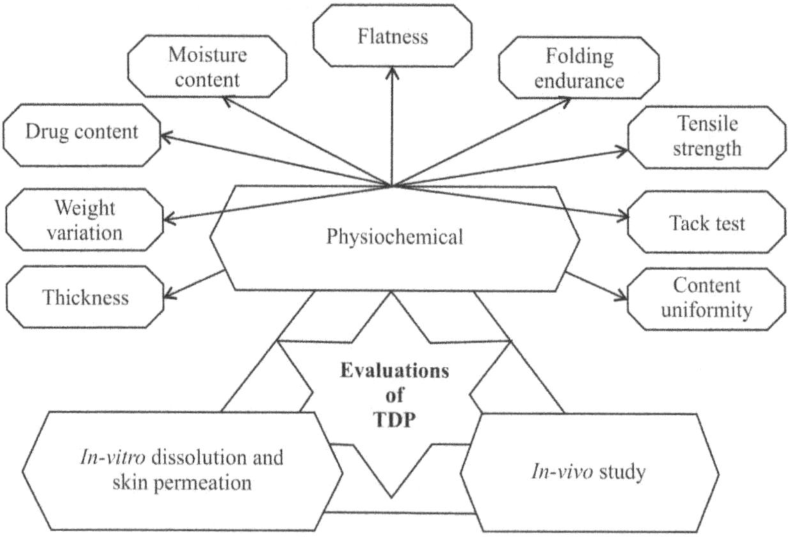

Fig. 8.18 Evaluation parameters for TDP.

8.9.1 Moisture Content Study

The prepared film is weighed individually and is placed in a desiccator containing activated desiccant at room temperature for at least 24 hours.

Afterwards the film is weighed again, until constant weight is achieved. Finally the moisture content of subjected TDP can be determined by following formula

$$\% \text{ Moisture Content} = \frac{\text{Initial Weight}}{\text{Final Weight}} \times 100$$

8.9.2 Tensile Strength Test

In this test the polymeric films are sandwiched separately by corked linear iron plates. One end of the films is fixed with the help of an iron screen and other end is connected to a freely movable thread over a pulley. The weights are added in the pan in a gradual fashion. A pointer on the thread is used to measure the elongation of the film. The weight just sufficient to break the film is noted. The tensile strength can be calculated using the following formula

$$\text{Tensile strength} = \text{F/ab}\ (1 + \text{L}/l)$$

Where,

- F is the force required to break;
- a is width of film;
- b is thickness of film;
- L is length of film;
- *l* is elongation of film at break point

The other tests can be summarized as shown in Table 8.3.

Table 8.3 Evaluation parameters of TDP

S. No.	Parameters	Instruments used	Process
1	Thickness	Travelling microscope, screw gauge and dial gauge	Thicknesses of at least five different sites of same patch are determined and mean with standard deviation is reported.
2	Weight variation	Digital balance	Randomly 10 patches are selected, weighed and mean with standard deviation is calculated.
3	Drug content	UV Spectrophotometer/ HPLC	100 mg of patch is added to 100 ml of solvent and is shaken for 24 hr followed by sonication and filtration. The solution is appropriately diluted and drug content is estimated using either UV Spectrophotometer or HPLC.

Table 8.3 *Contd...*

S. No.	Parameters	Instruments used	Process
4	Folding endurance	———	It is used to determine the folding capacity of the films which is subjected to frequent extreme conditions of folding. It is determined by repeatedly folding the film at the same place until it breaks. The number of times the film could be folded at the same place without breaking is folding endurance value.

8.9.3 *In-vitro* Release Study

The cumulative release of TDP can be determined by paddle over disc or cylindrical modified or reciprocating disc type apparatus. The test is conducted at 37 ± 2 °C and samples are withdrawn at regular intervals followed by analysis with suitable analytical method.

8.9.4 Skin Permeation Study

It is used to determine the amount of drug release from a fixed area of patch also known as flux. Test is conducted at 37 ± 2 °C using Franz diffusion cell/flow through cell and samples are withdrawn at regular intervals followed by analysis with suitable analytical method.

8.9.5 *In-vivo* Study

It provides a suitable platform for determination of various hidden factors which cannot be explored during *in-vitro* study. This study takes into account various factors like skin heterogenicity, racial difference, inter and intra subject variability etc. The study can be carried out in animal and human models.

- ***Animal models:*** Prior to the application of TDP to human, considering about the economy and safety values involved in; it is always better to carry *in-vivo* study on animal models. Animals which can be used for study are mouse, hairless rat, hairless dog, hairless rhesus monkey, rabbit and guinea pig. In order considering the skin resemblance and minimizing the heterogenicity barrier, *"Rhesus monkey"* is the model of preference.
- ***Human models:*** It is mainly the final stage of evaluations which involve huge amount of money, man power and effective resources with considerable amount of longer duration. Test like skin irritation, skin toxicity, skin sensitization, etc., are carried out in various stages

of clinical trials, i.e., from Phase I to Phase III. At each and every step the parameters are effectively documented as *Drug master file* and *Common Technical Document.* The recorded data is submitted along with *Investigational New Drug (IND)* application or with *Abbreviated New Drug Application (ANDA)* for grant of market launch. Finally after-market launch post market surveillance is carried out to ensure the public safety (Phase IV trial). If no issue is detected regarding any adverse effect, the TDP is allowed to flourish in market.

8.10 Clinical Trial Overview of TDP

The dynamic journey of TDP is not end yet. Day by day various new chemical entities are being given by means of TDP in order to provide safe and effective treatment against multifarious disease. They are enlisted in Table 8.4.

Table 8.4 TDP of various drugs in clinical phase

S. No.	Drug	Indication	Clinical Phase
1	Acyclovir	Herpes labialis	II
2	Heat labile enterotoxin of *E. coli*	Diarrhea	II
3	Parathyroid hormone	Osteoporesis	II
4	Influenza vaccine	Influenza	Pre-registration
5	Granisetron	Nausea and vomiting	Pre-registration
6	Buprenorphine	Pain	III
7	Human growth hormone	Dwarfism	I

8.11 Marketed TDP

With the advancement of research, time and continuous efforts of formulation scientists, some of the drugs are now available in market in form of TDP. Table 8.5 shows the list of the drugs commercially available in form of TDP.

Table 8.5 List of marketed TDP

S. No.	Product	Drug	Indication	Company
1	Alora	Estradiol	Post menstrual syndrome	Thera-Tech and Gamble, USA
2	Catapres-TTS	Clonidine	Hypogonadism	Alza, California
3	Deponit	Nitroglycerin	Angina	Schwarz Pharma, Germany
4	Duragesic	Fentanyl	Pain	Alza, California

Table 8.5 *Contd...*

S. No.	Product	Drug	Indication	Company
5	Estraderm	Estradiol	Post menstrual syndrome	Novartis, Australia
6	Habitraol	Nicotine	Smoking cessation	Parke Davis, Michigan
7	Nicoderm	Nicotine	Smoking cessation	GSK, United Kingdom
8	Ortho-Eva	Estradiol	Birth control	Ortho-McNeil Pharmaceuticals, United States

8.12 Current Limitations of TDDS

Presently the existing TDDS is suffering from various limitations and challenges, thus there is a need of modification in current TDDS or replacement by some other delivery system. Multifarious limitations of current TDDS are listed below (Kulkarni, 2010):

- Current TDDS is restricted to only a small population of drug candidates.
- There is no guarantee that the proposed TDDS can deliver the 100% of drug to systemic circulation *via* skin.
- Current TDDS is not able to alleviate the "inter and intra" subject variability and thus leads to fluctuations in results.
- Current TDDS is not able to compete with the defense strength of SC. It needs a better modification at some stages, like permeation enhancement or skin ablation.
- The performance of transdermal patches is totally adhesive dependent. They adhere to skin subjected to the effectiveness of adhesive which if not sufficient can lead to removal of patch with consequent termination of the therapy.
- Small damage to drug reservoir can lead to complete dose dumping.
- There may be chances that drug after crossing the skin may either precipitates due to pH of skin or may metabolizes by enzymes present.

8.13 Advancements in TDDS

The above mentioned limitation leads to the development of some newer and effective techniques which can bridge the existing shortfalls and provide better therapeutic results. Following section gives an insight into various latest advancements in TDDS (Fig. 8.19).

8.13.1 Iontophoresis

This technique utilizes the small amount of current (approx. 0.5 mA/cm^2) in order to deliver the charged molecule across the skin. Iontophoresis is not new to the pharmaceutical field, its origin was witnessed in around 1700's, but the first and well documented experimental evidence was carried out by Ludec in twentieth century where two polar drugs i.e., strychnine and cyanide were administered to rabbits.

It mainly works on the principle of "Like charges repel each other while opposite charges attract each other". This principle leads to the development of two basic sets of system that is 'Anodal and Cathodal'. Positively charged drugs are delivered by anodal end as they are repel by it and at the same time a fair attractive force is created in the vicinity of skin by cathodal system. In order to maintain the electro-neutrality of skin the plasma anion move towards cathode. Hence, whole system acts in a *"closed loop manner"* and finally the drug is delivered *via* skin. The possible mechanisms of drug transport by iontophoresis include electrical repulsion, electroosmosis, and alteration of skin permeability (Dhote *et al.*, 2012).

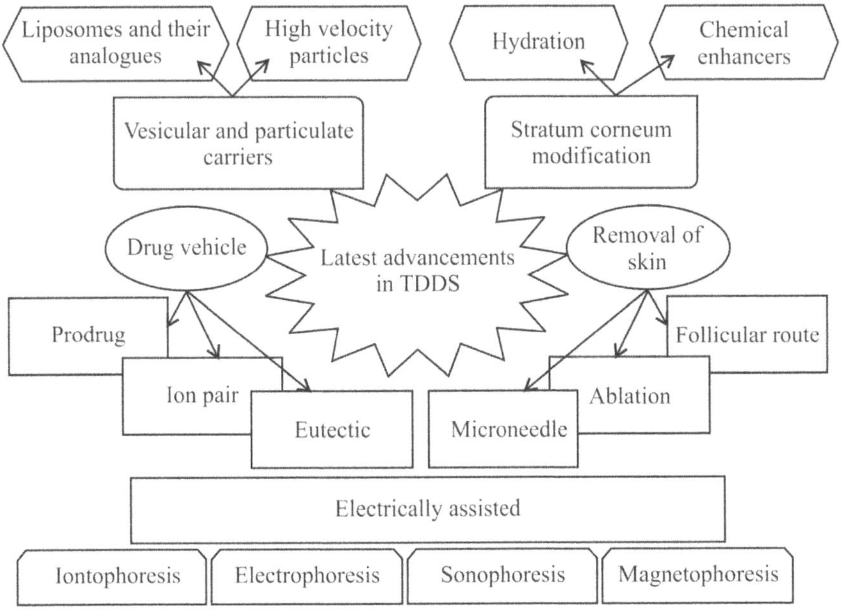

Fig. 8.19 Latest advancements in TDDS.

The list of drugs which have been administered by iontophoresis include apomorphine, rotigotine, 5-fluorouracil, 5-aminolevulinic acid, fentanyl, piroxicam, buspirone HCl, insulin, vasopressin, calcitonin, parathyroid hormone and luteinizing hormone releasing hormone. Now a day's; iontophoresis is successfully commercialized and few systems like *IONSYS*® (fentanyl iontophoresis transdermal system, Ortho-McNeil) Inc., *Hybresis*® and *GlucoWatch* ®*G2* for monitoring of glucose level have launched into market (Banga and Chien, 1988). The hypothetical drug transport *via* iontophoresis can be presented as depicted in Fig. 8.20.

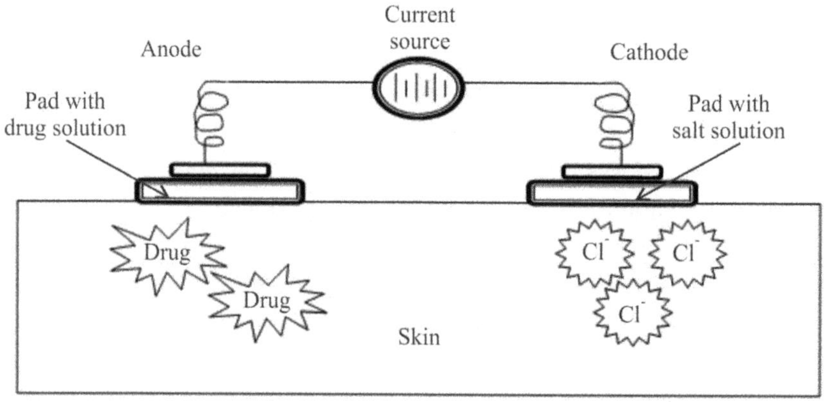

Fig. 8.20 The hypothetical drug transport *via* iontophoresis.

8.13.2 Sonophoresis or Phonophoresis

It can be defined as *"a technique which utilizes the ultrasonic sound energy for the delivery of drug via skin"*. The novel idea of using ultrasonic sound to enhance TDD *via* sonophoresis was drawn from the fact that around 1960's physiotherapist uses ultrasonic sound for the delivery of steroid in gels and creams during massage. Ultrasonic sound is a form of sound wave which is of 0.02 MHz frequency and is not audible to humans. These are mainly produced by transducer which converts electricity to sound energy *via* piezoelectric crystals. It basically works on cavitation phenomena; i.e., disturb the lipid arrangement of skin and facilitate the drug transport. Sono-prep® is the instrument which is used to facilitate drug delivery with the help of sonophoresis (Bommannan *et al.,* 1992). Some of the drugs which have been delivered using sonophoresis include insulin, interferon and erythropoietin. The representation of using sonophoresis in achieving enhanced delivery across skin is shown in Fig. 8.21.

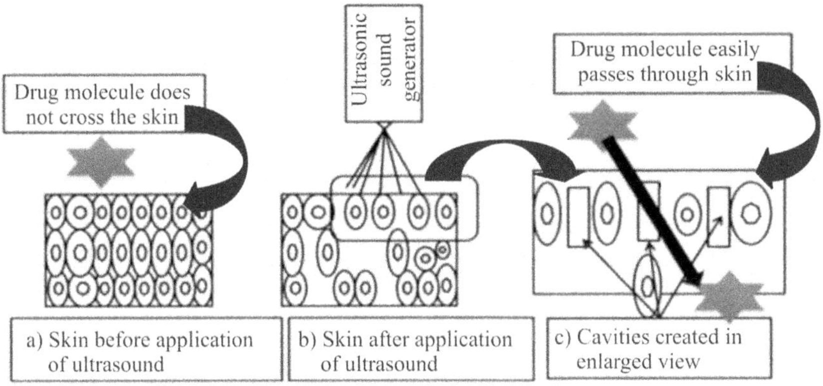

Fig. 8.21 Showing sequential steps (a, b, and c) of cavity creation by ultrasonic sound.

8.13.3 Electrophoresis

The hypothetical TDD *via* electrophoresis can be shown as in Fig. 8.22. In this method a high voltage is applied across the skin which generates the pores, ultimately facilitates the drug transport across the skin. It is proposed that it works on either one of the three principles i.e., passive diffusion, electrophoretic force of molecule, or electrosmotic effect. The drugs which are delivered by electrophoresis are fentanyl, mannitol, tetracaine, methotrexate, ascorbic acid, timolol and catechins. Electrophoresis is also reported to be capable of DNA delivery in mice (Vanbever *et al.,* 1998).

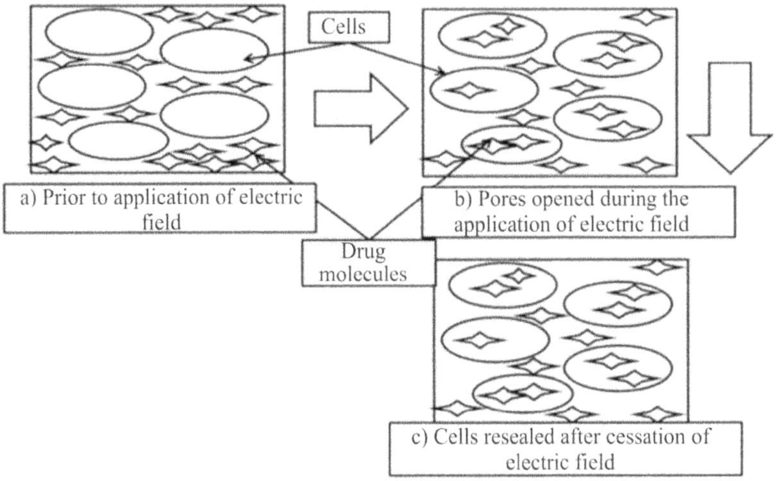

Fig. 8.22 Drug delivery *via* electrophoresis across the skin; with sequential a, b, and c steps.

8.13.4 Skin Ablation

Skin ablation fundamentally means removal of upper skin surface either with the help of surgery, laser, and vacuum suction or thermal induction. By applying any one of the techniques, pores are created which assist in facilitating drug permeation. The technique is not commonly used due to the associated pain involved in using it. The drugs which are reported to have enhanced permeation using skin ablation comprise 5-fluorouracil, hydrocortisone, indomethacin, and diclofenac (Lee *et al.,* 2001). The scheme of using this technique in achieving improved transdermal delivery is illustrated in Fig. 8.23.

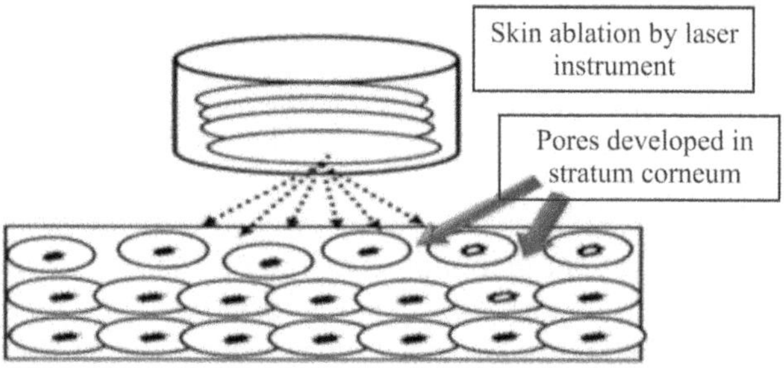

Fig. 8.23 Transdermal drug delivery by skin ablation (LASER assisted method).

8.13.5 Microneedle Technique (MN)

Transdermal drug delivery using MN was first carried out during 1990's. Finally the concept was floored up and successively patented by ALZA Corporation. Microneedles are approximately 100 to 2000 μm long structures which are provided with drug reservoir and act as a tool to increase the drug permeation across skin. They can be fabricated from variety of materials covering glass, silicon, titanium or any other biodegradable polymers. They are mainly prepared by *Etching technique.* The drugs which are primarily reported to be administered by MN are Anthrax vaccine, methyl nicotinate, ovalbumin, plasmid DNA, and bovine serum albumin (Kim *et al.,* 2012; Li *et al.,* 2009). Pictorial representation of drug delivery by MN is shown in Fig. 8.24.

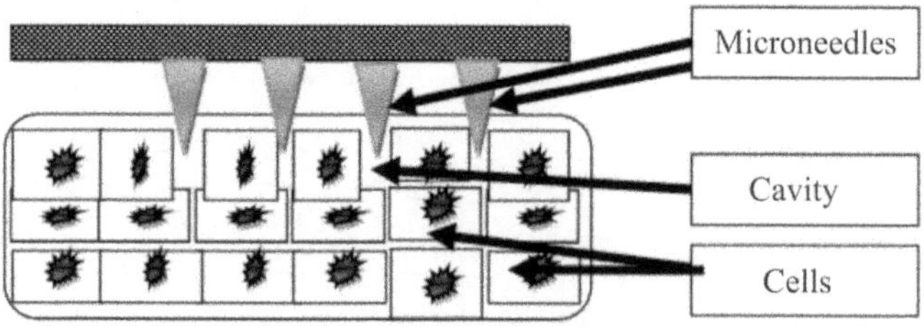

Fig. 8.24 TDD *via* microneedle technique.

8.13.6 Prodrug Method

They are basically used to alter the physiochemical properties of drug (solubility, lipophilicity and permeation etc.) in order to favour transdermal delivery. Generally the formation of prodrug enhances the lipophilicity of drug which is a major driving force assisting in permeation of drug across (shown in Fig. 8.25 in part A). Later in the biological system the prodrug is cleaved resulting in generation of parent drug that elicits desired therapeutic response (Friend *et al.*, 1988) (shown in Fig. 8.25 in part B). The drug delivery *via* prodrug method is summarized in a pictorial way in Fig. 8.25.

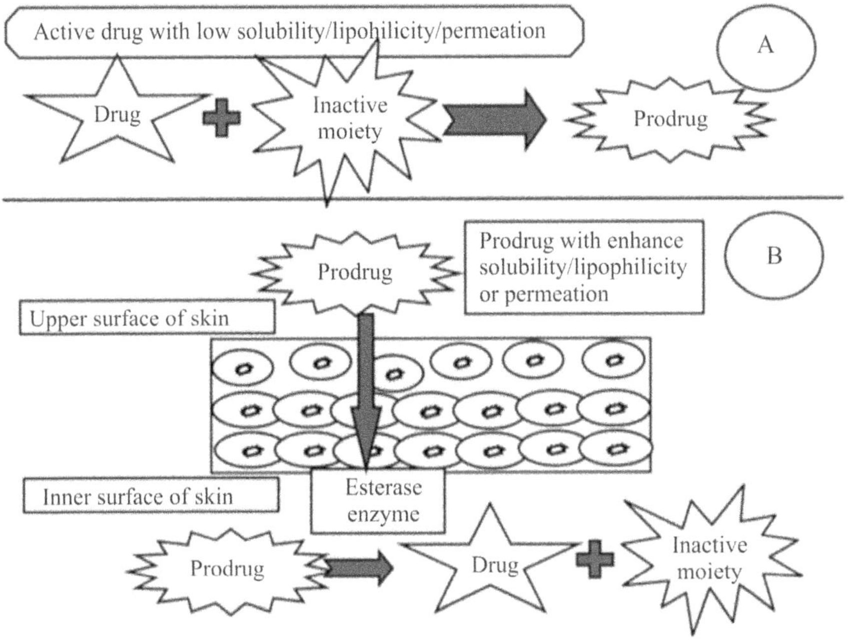

Fig. 8.25 Drug delivery across skin by prodrug technique.

8.13.7 Ion Pair Method

For an effective transdermal drug delivery the drug should be neutral, amorphous and lipophilic. This technique is most suitable for the delivery of ionic drugs across the skin as they are poorly permeable. In principle they are conjugated with an oppositely charged species so as to neutralize the charge and simultaneously become lipophilic (shown in Fig. 8.26 in part A). This endowed lipophilic nature provides easy access through the skin barrier. Finally in the dermis they are dissociated into constitute elements with the help of enzyme (shown in Fig. 8.26 in part B). The whole ion pair method is shown in an understandable way in Fig. 8.26. Lidocaine hydrochloride was conjugated with lauric acid permeation was assessed across rat ear skin (Valenta *et al.,* 2000). Approximate 20 fold of increment in permeation of propranolol was observed after conjugation with fatty acid.

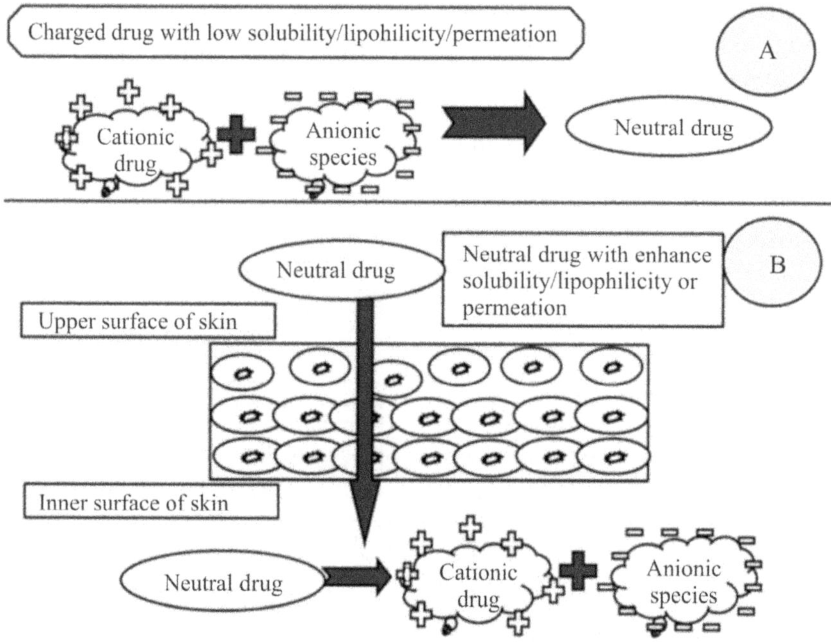

Fig. 8.26 TDD *via* ion-pair (IP) method.

8.13.8 Vesicular Systems

Lipids are integral part of skin and are present in considerable amount. The idea of using lipid based systems to increase the transdermal permeability of drugs can be of considerable importance. Delivery systems fabricated from lipids are biocompatible and biodegradable thus alleviating the concerns of safety. Vesicular systems like liposomes have wide acceptability including commercial viability on large scale. Liposomes have been tried and tested in order to increase the transdermal permeability of drugs. However liposomes have limitations in terms of depth of penetration through the skin. They cannot penetrate into deeper layers of skin, rather confined to the superficial area. Apart from liposomes two novel vesicular systems "*transfersomes and ethosomes*" have been able to gather greater attention and interest from both industrial and academic researchers. These vesicular systems consist of some favorable characteristic properties such as biodegradability, biocompatibility, and versatility of encapsulating both hydrophilic and lipophilic drugs, prolongation of duration of drug action, site specific targeting and enhanced patient compliance.

8.13.8.1 Transfersomes (TFS)

They are lipid vesicles of nanometric size range (200-300 nm) composed of drug, lipid and surfactant. They are highly elastic structure which can be used for transdermal delivery *via* into the skin or through the skin. They contain a centrally located water cavity which is suitable for encapsulation of both hydrophilic and lipophilic drugs. They are synonymously known as 'Ultra-deformable vesicles', because of their exemplary capacity that they can passes through skin. The skin penetrating ability is unbeatable work of *"edge activators"*, which get accumulated and hence cause a sudden reduction in energy required for permeation. Another key aspect of the better permeation is due to the driving force which is generated because of *'Local hydration gradient'*, between SC and deeper dermis tissue (Jain *et al.*, 2003).

8.13.8.1.1 Iconic perspectives of TFS

Various figurative features of TFS which provides an extra lead over existing vesicular system are summarized below:

- TFS consist of central cavity capable of encapsulating hydrophilic and hydrophobic drugs.
- Ultra-deformable capacity which endow properties to squeeze itself from a narrow aperture of size about 5-10 smaller than its original diameter.
- It can act as a suitable carrier for both high and low molecular weight drugs.
- They can be made from materials conforming to pharmaceutical standards making the systems biocompatible and biodegradable.
- Minimum chance of provoking immunogenic reaction.
- They can act as depot forming tool, thus can maximize the duration of drug release.
- Can be easily geared up to industrial floor.

In spite of such extraordinary features; the discussed vesicular system has some limitations. The overall processing of formulation requires lots of expenditure making it expensive in comparison to conventional systems like gels, creams or ointments. Another issue which limits wide applicability of TFS is compromised stability under normal conditions that necessitates special conditions to manufacture, transport and distribute the formulation.

8.13.8.1.2 Methods of preparation of TFS

It is prepared by thin film hydration method (Gupta *et al.,* 2005) schematically shown in Fig. 8.27.

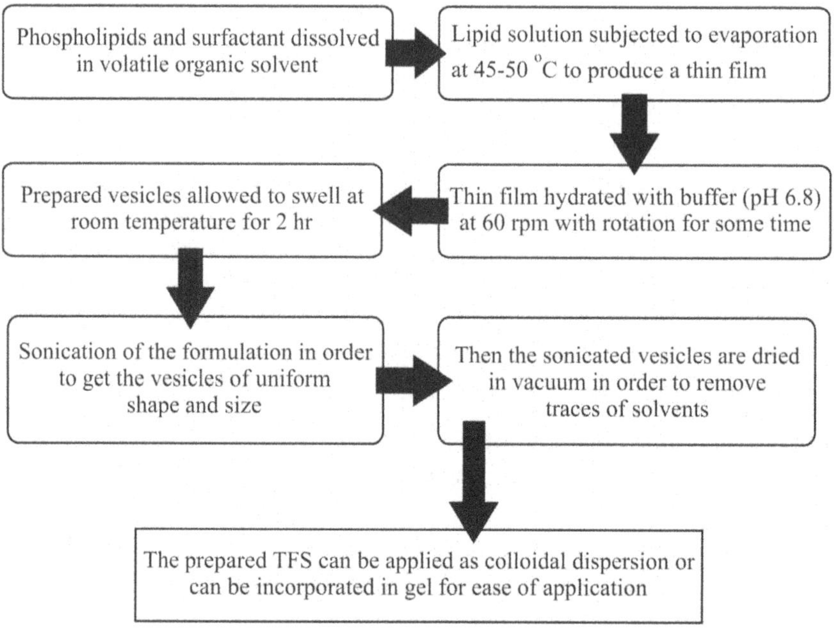

Fig. 8.27 Scheme of formulation of TFS using thin film hydration method.

8.13.8.1.3 Mechanism of drug delivery of TFS *via* skin

The drug delivery across the skin by TFS usually depends upon either the pore size of skin or its capacity to deform itself. When applied topically, they fairly interact with skin and finally squeeze themselves through pores of skin to cross the major barrier presented by SC. The overall sequence can be hypothetically illustrated as shown in Fig. 8.28. The drugs which are reported to be administered exploiting TFS are oestradiol, norgestrol, interferon, insulin, human serum albumin, methotrexate and ketoprofen.

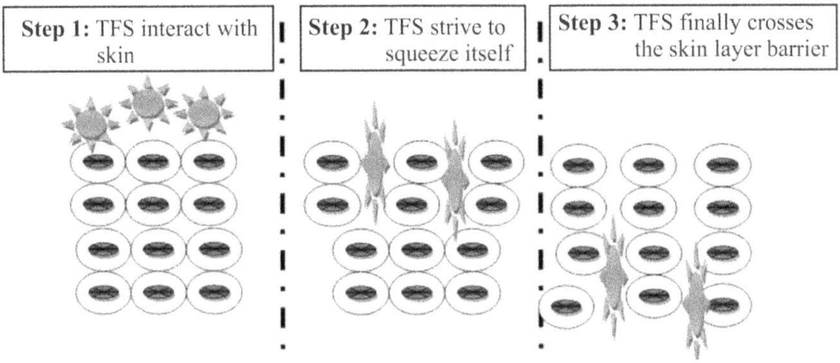

Fig. 8.28 TFS interaction and passage across the skin.

8.13.8.2 Ethosomes (ES)

Ethosomes are interesting lipid vesicles have shown potential to deliver wide variety of drugs efficiently through skin. They have lipid bi layers resembling liposomes, however principally differ in composition. Liposomes are chiefly composed of phosphatidyl choline and cholesterol, whereas in ethosomes cholesterol is replaced with large quantity of ethanol ranging from 25-40%. The ethanolic vesicles can be used for the delivery of hydrophilic, lipophilic, and amphiphilic drugs. The variation in concentration of both lipid and ethanol has prominent effect on formulation of ethosomes especially on size of vesicle. Generally a multi lamellar ethosomal vesicle shows better entrapment efficiency of drug (Touitou *et al.,* 2000).

8.13.8.2.1 Salient features of ES

- Ethosomes provide a mode for passive non-invasive delivery.
- These carriers are suitable for hydrophilic, lipophilic molecules, peptides and other macromolecules.
- They can act as a carrier for low as well as high molecular weight substances e.g., analgesics, corticosteroids, sex hormone and insulin.
- They are biocompatible and biodegradable.
- Entrapment efficiency is high due to presence of high amount of ethanol.
- They possess high cell transfection efficiency.
- They may act as depot formulation hence sustained release is achievable.
- They can be applicable for topical as well as systemic delivery.

8.13.8.2.2 Mechanism of drug delivery by ES

Several studies are reported in literature demonstrating the capability of lipid based systems in increasing the transdermal permeability of drugs. Vesicular systems act as carrier of drugs and can cross the SC carrying the entrapped drug molecule. Secondly vesicular systems act as penetration enhancers by interacting with the SC lipids leading to alteration of permeability of SC and penetration of drug molecule. Increased penetration of drug with ethosomal formulations could be due to combined effect of ethanol and lipid vesicles. Skin has densely packed structure where lipids are arranged in a systematic fashion. Alcohol being a known penetration enhancer might interact and disturb the configuration of skin lipids. Taking advantage of increased fluidity of the skin lipids, ethosomal vesicles intermingles with the skin lipids and penetrates through the SC. Fig. 8.29 is showing the penetration of ethosomal vesicles across skin. Drugs like minoxidil, testosterone, zidovudine, lamivudine, acyclovir, insulin and ketoprofen have been investigated for ability to penetrate through the skin using ethosomal vesicles.

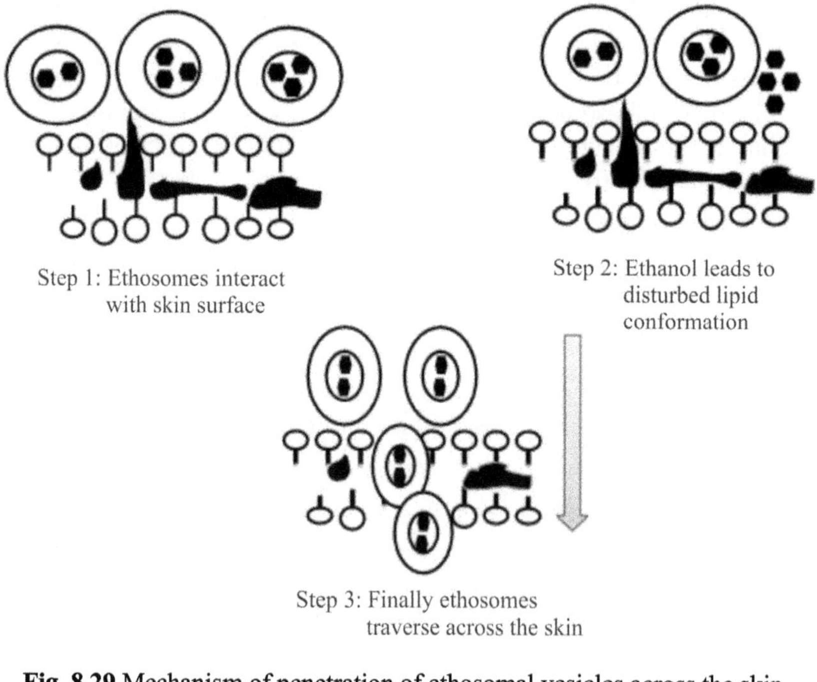
Step 1: Ethosomes interact with skin surface
Step 2: Ethanol leads to disturbed lipid conformation
Step 3: Finally ethosomes traverse across the skin

Fig. 8.29 Mechanism of penetration of ethosomal vesicles across the skin.

8.13.8.3 Evaluation of TFS and ES

Some common parameters which can be discussed for the evaluation of both TFS and ES are as follows:

- **Shape and surface morphology:** Shape and morphology of the vesicles is investigated using transmission electron microscopy and scanning electron microscopy.
- **Size distribution:** The mean size and size distribution of colloidal vesicular suspension is analyzed by dynamic light scattering technique using Zetasizer. The sample is placed in quartz cuvette and a size measurement is performed at a scattering angle of 90°.
- **Entrapment efficiency**: For determination of entrapment efficiency the vesicles are separated from the unentrapped or free drug by either Sephadex mini column centrifugation method or by ultracentrifugation. Known amount of formulation free from unentrapped drug is lysed using Triton X-100 and the amount of drug in the solution is estimated using appropriate analytical method e.g., UV Spectrophotometric/HPLC.
- **Tubidity:** The turbidity can be measured by subjecting the sample to nephelo-turbidity meter.
- **Surface charge:** Surface charge play an important role in the stability of the colloidal dispersion. It can be determined with the help of Zetasizer.
- ***In-vitro* permeation study:** *In vitro* permeation is determined using either Franz diffusion cell or flow through diffusion cell system. Epidermis (either human cadaver/animal) is mounted between the donor and receptor compartments of the flow through diffusion cell. Appropriate buffer solution is filled in the reservoir bottle. Receptor solution is thoroughly degassed to prevent the formation of bubbles beneath the epidermis. Formulation (approximately 1 ml) is placed in the donor compartment and ambient temperature of the cells is maintained at 37 ± 2 °C by circulating water bath. The receptor solution is pumped by peristaltic pump continuously through the receptor compartment. Samples are collected at various time intervals and analyzed for amount of drug using appropriate analytical technique. Value of transdermal flux is calculated with the help of graph plotted between cumulative amounts of drug permeated versus time (Chourasia *et al.*, 2011).

8.14 Future Prospects of TDDS

During last few decades, oral drug delivery systems have registered a remarkable up gradation. Multifarious oral dosage forms are available for the treatment of wide variety of diseases, but they are practically suffering from some limitations. Thus, in this case skin emerges as a preferred choice for the delivery of drug. Skin as a largest organ of body represents a unique portal for the administration of both hydrophilic and hydrophobic drugs for both systemic and local effects.

Now a days, TDDS is achieved not only with conventional formulations (creams, pastes, gels, and ointments); but with some novel approaches like transdermal films, transdermal patches, liposomes, ethosomes, transfersomes, solid lipid nanoparticles and nanoemulsion. Extensive study on transdermal delivery shows that there are various hidden shades that are still to be explored and can be used for the benefits of patients. In present scenario, the techniques like iontophoresis, sonophoresis, electrophoresis, magnetophoresis, microneedle, penetration enhancers and ion pair method can be used for effective and prolonged release of drug with minimum fluctuations in blood spike levels. Among all the systems transfersomes and ethosomes are looking promising as they can provide excellent transdermal permeability of entrapped molecules.

References

Banga A.K, and Chien Y.W (1988). Iontophoretic delivery of drugs: Fundamentals, developments and biomedical applications. *Journal of Controlled Release* **7:** 1-24.

Barry B.W (2001). Novel mechanisms and devices to enable successful transdermal drug delivery. *European Journal of Pharmaceutical Sciences : Official Journal of the European Federation for Pharmaceutical Sciences* **14:** 101-114.

Bommannan D, Menon G.K, Okuyama H, Elias P.M, and Guy R.H (1992). Sonophoresis. II. Examination of the mechanism(s) of ultrasound-enhanced transdermal drug delivery. *Pharmaceutical Research* **9:** 1043-1047.

Brown M.B, Martin G.P, Jones S.A, and Akomeah F.K (2006). Dermal and transdermal drug delivery systems: current and future prospects. *Drug Delivery* **13:** 175-187.

Chien Y.W (2003). Transdermal drug delivery, Vol 50 (NY, Marcel Dekker Inc.).

Chourasia M.K, Kang L, and Chan S.Y (2011). Nanosized ethosomes bearing ketoprofen for improved transdermal delivery. *Results in Pharma Sciences* **1:** 60-67.

Dhote V, Bhatnagar P, Mishra P.K, Mahajan S.C, and Mishra D.K (2012). Iontophoresis: a potential emergence of a transdermal drug delivery system. *Scientia Pharmaceutica* **80:** 1-28.

Elias P.M (1983). Epidermal lipids, barrier function, and desquamation. *Journal of Investigative Dermatology* **80:** 44s-49s.

Friend D, Catz P, Heller J, Reid J, and Baker R (1988). Transdermal delivery of levonorgestel II: Effect of prodrug structure on skin permeability *in vitro*. *Journal of Controlled Release* **7:** 251-261.

Gupta P.N, Mishra V, Rawat A, Dubey P, Mahor S, Jain S, Chatterji D.P, and Vyas S.P (2005). Non-invasive vaccine delivery in transfersomes, niosomes and liposomes: a comparative study. *Int J Pharm* **293:** 73-82.

Hadgraft J (2004). Skin deep. *European Journal of Pharmaceutics and Biopharmaceutics* **58:** 291-299.

Hori M, Satoh S, and Maibach H.I (1990). Classification of percutaneous penetration enhancers: a conceptional diagram. *The Journal of Pharmacy and Pharmacology* **42:** 71-72.

Jain S, Jain P, Umamaheshwari R.B, and Jain N.K (2003). Transfersomes - a novel vesicular carrier for enhanced transdermal delivery: development, characterization, and performance evaluation. *Drug Development and Industrial Pharmacy* **29:** 1013-1026.

Kim Y.C, Park J.H, and Prausnitz M.R (2012). Microneedles for drug and vaccine delivery. *Adv Drug Deliv Rev* **64:** 1547-1568.

Kulkarni V.S (2010). Handbook of noninvasive drug delivery system, First edn (NY, Elsevier Inc.).

Lee W.R, Shen S.C, Lai H.H, Hu C.H, and Fang J.Y (2001). Transdermal drug delivery enhanced and controlled by erbium:YAG laser: a comparative study of lipophilic and hydrophilic drugs. *Journal of Controlled Release : Official Journal of the Controlled Release Society* **75:** 155-166.

Li G, Badkar A, Nema S, Kolli C.S, and Banga A.K (2009). *In vitro* transdermal delivery of therapeutic antibodies using maltose microneedles. *Int J Pharm* **368:** 109-115.

Menon G.K (2002). New insights into skin structure: scratching the surface. *Adv Drug Deliv Rev* **54 Suppl 1**: S3-17.

Osborne D.W (2008). TOPICAL DRUGS-Review of Changes in Topical Drug Product Classification-This article summarizes the classification systems for topical liquid and semisolid dosage forms used for dermatological application. *Pharmaceutical Technology* **32:** 66.

Pathak Y, and Thassu D (2009). Drug delivery nanoparticles formulation and characterization, First edition edn (NY, Informa healthcare Inc.).

Prausnitz M.R, and Langer R (2008). Transdermal drug delivery. *Nature Biotechnology* **26:** 1261-1268.

Thomas B.J, and Finnin B.C (2004). The transdermal revolution. *Drug Discovery Today* **9:** 697-703.

Touitou E, Dayan N, Bergelson L, Godin B, and Eliaz M (2000). Ethosomes - novel vesicular carriers for enhanced delivery: characterization and skin penetration properties. *Journal of Controlled Release : Official Journal of the Controlled Release Society* **65:** 403-418.

Valenta C, Siman U, Kratzel M, and Hadgraft J (2000). The dermal delivery of lignocaine: influence of ion pairing. *Int J Pharm* **197:** 77-85.

Vanbever R, Leroy M.A, and Preat V (1998). Transdermal permeation of neutral molecules by skin electroporation. *Journal of Controlled Release : Official Journal of the Controlled Release Society* **54:** 243-250.

9

Nanosized Materials used in Diagnosis

Y. Singh and Manish K. Chourasia
[1]Pharmaceutics Division, CSIR-Central Drug Research Institute, Lucknow-226031, India

9.1 Introduction

Current health care system has drifted aimlessly towards symptomatic treatment protocols. Diseases are generally not diagnosed until pathological indicators become extremely overt forcing patients to seek aid of physicians, who generally adapt most trivial strategies in prescribing a treatment regimen which is general and non-specific ignoring root cause analysis. It has been due to these unscrupulous prescription practices that genuine broad spectrum antibiotics, for instance tetracyclines have lost their clinical utility. Moreover hesitancy in adapting a prompt course of action due to either patient and/or physician's casual attitude often burdens the patient with economic constraints born out of prolonged therapies necessary to overcome the mistakes committed in the first step of patient care: 'Diagnosis'. Early diagnosis of a suspected disease is thus of critical value in healthcare and medicine. Diagnosis should be fast, reliable, specific, accurate, and free of risks such as 'false positives'.

Current diagnostic modalities are tedious requiring expert execution, and riddled with invasive sampling of bodily fluids. Often samples of body fluids and/or tissues are taken to laboratories, for analysis, the results of which take several days and can still be inconclusive if the disease is at an early stage. Consequently, many diseases remain undiagnosed until long after taking root in the body and hence remain untreated too.

All this calls for a revolution in diagnostics yielding the floor for point-of-care testing (POC), or bed-side testing, which is diagnostic testing conducted at or near the site of patient care or his/her convenience like bed side or bathroom, etc., providing accurate results immediately. Tests used in medical examinations, urine test strips, simple imaging with a portable ultrasound device, regular observations such as ECG's, heart rate monitors are all amenable to POC. POC diagnostic devices should be suited to use for not only in lab but also in remote areas. Miniaturization of diagnostic devices can be a modification which paves the way for successful realization of POC principles. Small diagnostic devices require expectantly lower analyte volume and can be easily transported making marriage of diagnostics and nanotechnology inevitable. As human body is constituted by variety of building blocks (cells, organelles, signalling molecules, DNA, etc.) whose dimensions lie in the nanometric scale, it is sensible only to employ investigative methods functioning in the same size domain. Nanotechnology, applied in diagnosis at molecular level takes form of nanodiagnostics. It can be an essential tool towards development of personalized medicine. Nanodiagnostic aids have at least one dimension of their functional component in nanometres (10^{-9} m), though collectively they may form a larger composite structure on which the actual test is carried out. Owing to the unique physicochemical properties e.g., optical [surface plasmon resonance (SPR), fluorescence resonance energy transfer (FRET), surface enhanced raman scattering (SERS)] and thermal properties exhibited by size of analytical entities present on nanodiagnostic tools, they offer rapid, improved and refined diagnosis in comparison to conventional techniques. Nanoscale particles when, used as tags, labels or templates for attachment of pathogen cognizant units such as selective antibodies, membrane components, complementary DNA sequences, oligopeptides, aptamers, oligonucleotides, etc., offer massively raised surface area to volume ratios, increasing probability of pathogen recognition/and or estimation of disease markers (liver enzymes etc.), at very low levels. This increased sensitivity also facilitates analysis of relatively small sample volumes.

The current chapter dwells upon the advances made in diagnostic aids by utilizing nanotechnology and tries to furnish reader with sound knowledge of the types of materials which are being used to fabricate these intricate yet resoundingly effective aids. Simplistic schemes elaborating the mechanism of analyte detection/quantification have also been plotted. The content is interspersed with detailed examples expounding the width of clinical conditions in which nanodiagnostic tools have found relevance. We conclude with a brief foray into the toxicity issues related with these aids along with their future prospects.

9.2 Nanosized Materials used for Clinical Laboratory Diagnosis

9.2.1 Nanoparticles

Nanoparticles are a comprehensive group of colloidal sized independent (with respect to properties) objects which can be classified into numerous subtypes, viz. polymeric, lipidic, metallic (gold, silver, zinc, silver, iron-oxide), inorganic (calcium phosphate, silica), quantum dots, magnetic, dendrimers, etc. Due to several favourable and unique features attached with nanotechnology, these are being increasingly used as diagnostic tools.

9.2.1.1 Gold Nanoparticles

Gold nanoparticles (AuNPs) are the most stable nanoparticles produced so far. They are produced as suspension of submicron-sized particles by simplistic reduction of gold (III) chloride using $NaBH_4$ as reducing agent. Cetyl trimethyl ammonium bromide is concurrently used as a stabilizer in the reduction mixture to prevent aggregation of AuNPs. The generic methods for AuNPs production, like the one stated above, are thus usually very simple and result in highly reproducible size statistics with narrow distribution. Despite being a noble metal, small size of AuNPs raises the surface energy substantially, lending the surface to functionalization by variety of agents either by physisorption or chemisorption. If steric permutations permit a single AuNPs may end up being draped with over 100 functional appendages. Incubating colloidal gold with thiol terminated functional group is often adequate for decorating surface of AuNPs.

Another feature of AuNPs is their capability to exhibit differentiable optical properties with respect to subtle variations in size and shape. The suspension containing AuNPs less than 100 nm is coloured dark red whereas it has bluish to purple appearance for larger particles (Daniel and Astruc, 2004). This property is due to an optiphysical phenomenon known as Surface Plasmon Resonance (SPR). Any process which causes particulate aggregation leading to size growth will result in a distinct colorometric response easily observable by conventional light microscope. In conjunction to SPR, AuNPs also demonstrate substantial

Rayleigh Scattering, fluorescing potential and a unique phenomenon Surface Enhanced Raman Scattering making it detectible by a variety of techniques. AuNPs have promising application in detection of DNA sequencing. One such spin off for DNA detection has found its place in diagnosis of tuberculosis (TB).

Currently potential cases of TB are detected by microscopic methods of stained smears (Ziehl-Neelsen stain) and solid cultures. Smear method is extremely rapid but suffers from lack of accuracy whereas the all conclusive solid culture method takes 6-8 weeks for confirmatory growth of mycobacterium. Automation of culture method has reduced detection times by 2 weeks at least, yet the period is too long and can be the difference between early diagnosis leading to appropriate treatment initiation or development of disease to malignant stages where the bacteria enters the patients' blood circulation. The contemporary methods thus fall short of expectant standards.

Polymerase chain reaction (PCR) based assays have come up recently (Palomino, 2009). A brief outline of how these work has been plotted in the Fig. 9.1. Their execution requires special skill set and economic set up. The economic constraints posed by such tests often are beyond the reach of people residing in lower strata of society, consequently leaving them especially susceptible towards contracting TB.

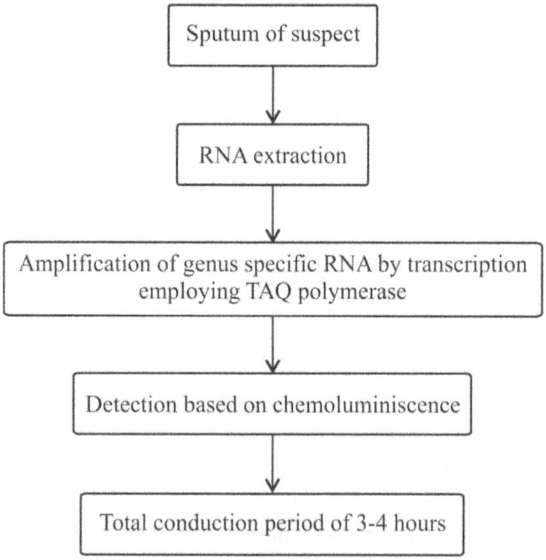

Fig. 9.1 Flow chart of sequence of steps adopted in testing for TB using PCR technique.

AuNPs based detection of TB circumvents the above shortcomings by combining rapidity with accuracy, ease of detection and cost effectiveness (Hussain *et al.,* 2013). Firstly single stranded DNA (SS DNA) sequences are produced with the aid of biotechnology. Oligo-nucleotide sequences complementary to the pathogenic DNA are cut from the prefabricated SS DNA. During actual testing the sputum of suspect is collected and treated to extract the pathogenic DNA and is incubated with SS DNA in hybridization media. This media is diluted by a small titre of red coloured AuNPs (100 nm and below) suspension. If pathogenic DNA is present in the sample it hybridizes with the SS DNA. AuNPs immediately aggregate undergoing particle size growth due to presence of salts in the hybridization media. This size growth is accompanied by SPR causing red to blue shift creating immediate visual evidence. Utilization of complementary DNA (cDNA) sequences in such probing techniques makes this experimental procedure full proof. In absence of pathogenic DNA, the SS oligo targeters very conveniently get adsorbed on surface of AuNPs and prevent aggregation retaining original red colour of the suspension ruling out potential of false positives. The above stated test has been adapted to high throughput methods (Fig. 9.2) by coating AuNPs on a 96 well plate. Using a microplate absorbance collector large numbers of samples can be screened simultaneously. AuNPs can be used to detect other microorganisms like pathogenic *E. coli, S. Aureus* and therefore can be used as replacement tool for PCR and fluorescent tags used currently.

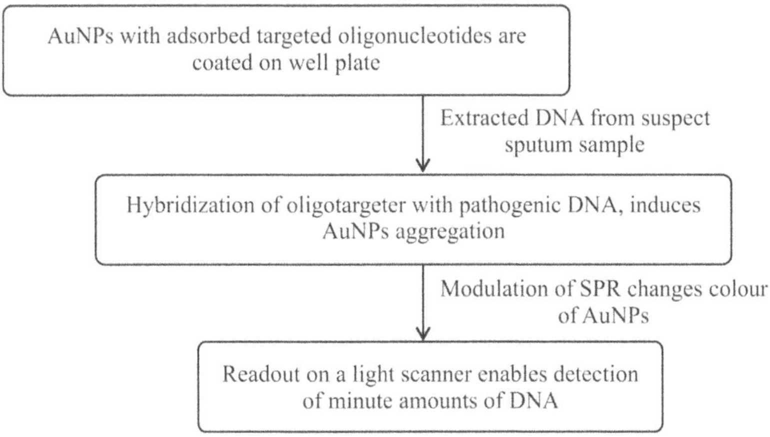

Fig. 9.2 Schematic representation of AuNPs based DNA sequence analyzing technique.

AuNPs are also used to locate cancer cells and confirm tumor (El-Sayed *et al.,* 2005). Epidermal growth factor decorated gold nanorod kit has recently made clinical inroads and is being increasingly employed to qualify patients for individualized chemotherapy. Epidermal growth factor receptor (EGFR) is overexpressed on membrane surface of variety of tumors, including colorectal adenocarcinoma, non-small cell lung carcinoma. Many targeted anticancer approaches are aimed at inhibition of EGFR, and therefore recognizing a EGFR positive tumor becomes extremely important. EGFR decorated Au nanorods in such cases accumulate selectively around the tumoral tissue, creating clear tumoral outlines when scanned under confocal laser scanning microscope. In cases where tumor is absent, the EGFR labelled nanorods are dispersed randomly throughout the body and consequently do not create any specialized fluorescent image.

9.2.1.2 Quantum Dots

Quantum Dots (QDs) are bilayered fluorescent nanocrystals made up of semiconducting material like zinc sulphide (ZnS) and cadmium selenide (CdSe). Minutely sized even with respect to nanoparticles, they can be as tiny as 2 nm with upper limits lying in 20 nm region. Upon excitation with suitable light source they fluoresce, often brilliantly, in all directions. Structurally they are constituted by a core and outer shell, both of which are often semi-conducting.

There are several methods for generating QDs tailored to varying applications. Simple QDs such as CdSe are usually synthesized by injecting coordination precursors of both Cd and Se in a hot organic solvent (hexadecylamine). The outer semiconductor shell, ZnS, is then grown around the core. Once the basic structure of a QD is built, its outer surface can be functionalized with oligonucleotides, peptides, streptavidin, oligonucleotides or aptamers to provide targeting properties. The functionalization is done in a layer by layer manner utilizing electrostatic attraction, covalent bonding, physisorption, and mercaptol exchange as attachment strategies.

QDs have several outstanding physical features (Cheki *et al.,* 2013), mainly pertaining to their quality as an inorganic fluorophore, elevating their status towards elite grade of nanodiagnostic probes. Firstly QDs absorb over a wide range of wavelengths from UV-visible to near infra-red regions thereby precluding requirement of laser based excitation sources. Secondly, QDs display substantial fluorescence lifetimes. Thirdly akin to AuNPs their optical properties are size dependent. This implies emission spectra of QDs vary with respect to their size: 2 nm (blue coloured), 3 nm (green), 4 nm (orange) and 7 nm (red). Fourthly, QDs are highly resistant to photobleaching, a phenomenon, by which a fluorescent dye loses its emission intensity against the background matrix. They also exhibit narrow emission spectra, often situated at considerable distance from the excitation zone, in so, giving rise to large Stoke's shift.

QDs sometimes sub serve as specialized donor molecules in fluorescence resonance energy transfer (FRET) systems, transferring the excitation energy to closely situated acceptor molecules. Working like this QDs can exponentially increase the fluorescent intensity of weakly luminescent probes (Zhang *et al.,* 2005). An example has been plotted in Fig. 9.3 where a hybridized sandwich of reporter cDNA, pathogenic DNA and biotinylated cDNA produces rather weak irrelevant emission spectra. Introducing a streptavidin coated QD in the diagnostic assembly dramatically alters the weak signal. Multiple biotinylated sandwich conjugate with streptavidin on QDs and create a resonance hybrid . When excited with an appropriate excitation source, QDs transfer their emission frequency to the attached sandwich due to its proximity and create an exponentially amplified emission signal.

QDs have a wide range of applications for molecular diagnostics and genotyping.

- *In vitro* imaging mainly includes three types of fluorescent QDs imaging:
  - Bio-molecular tracking in cells
  - Cellular imaging
  - Tissue staining
- *In vivo* imaging mainly covers four types of QDs imaging :
  - Bio-distribution
  - Vascular imaging
  - QDs assisted cell tracking
  - Tumour imaging
  - QDs can be used in multicolour optical marker for distinctive responses in biological assays.

Cancer diagnosis: Luminescent and stable bio-conjugates of QDs enable visualization of live cancer cells in living animals. QDs can be complemented with fluorescence microscopy to trace cells at high magnification in living animals. QDs endcapped with anti-herceptin antibody appended to polyacrylate moeity has been used for immunofluorescent labeling of breast cancer marker Her2. Elsewhere carbohydrate-encapsulated QDs with measureable fluorescent properties have also been used for cancer diagnostics.

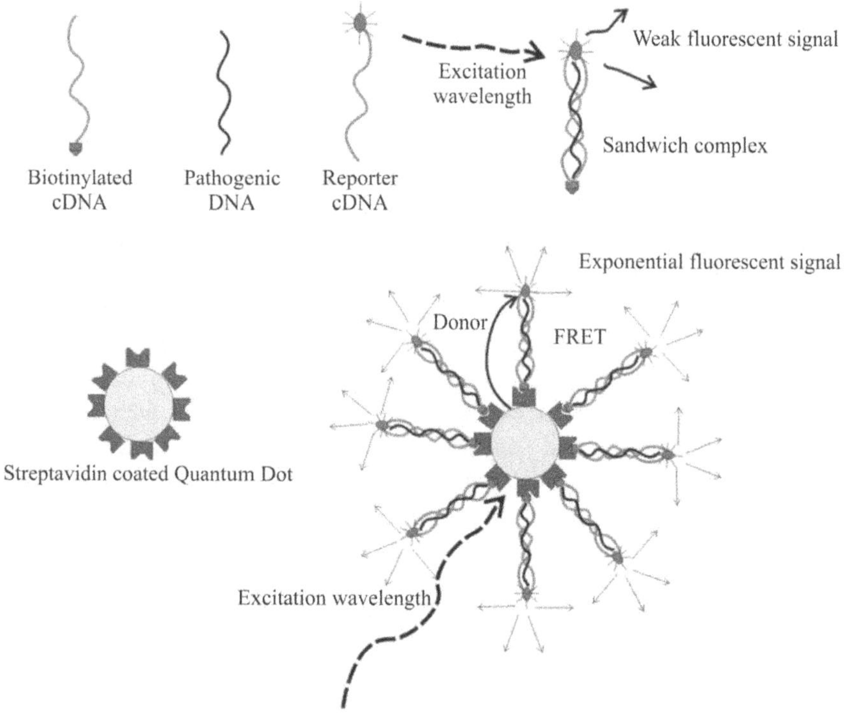

Fig. 9.3 Biotinylated SS DNA and reporter cDNA recognise and form a hybrid sandwich with pathogenic DNA (target DNA). The fluorescence intensity generated is oftentimes weak and subject to photobleaching. Introduction of streptavidin coated QD, causes close attachment of multiple sandwiched complexes, and creates an ideal set up for FRET based fluorescence enhancement.

9.2.1.3 Dendrimers

Dendrimers are distinguished nano-architectures having a core from which exponential numbers of distinct dendritic branches (analogous to dendrons protruding out of axon in a neuron) diverge out. They have well defined tree-like structure and low polydispersity due to narrow mass. Their distinctive structure furnishes a spherical shape even after production of several layers of branches with each synthesized branch being called a generation. Surfaces of dendrimers are conformable to variety of chemical alterations and its interior possess significant amount of solvent filled voids which ultimately aid host-guest interaction. Several methods such as divergent synthesis, convergent synthesis, self-assembling synthesis, lego chemistry and click chemistry have been utilized to develop dendrimers. Historically, divergent synthesis was the first method used to discover a dendrimer family termed as poly-amidoamine. This dendrimer family is unique due to availability of tree like branches in its architecture which arises from an instigator core. The size of poly-amidoamine dendrimer increases approximately 1 nm/generation and their size enhanced almost from 1 to 12 nm when they grow from first generation to tenth generation. Several times dendrimers have been employed as nano-diagnostic or MRI contrasting agents due to incomparable physical (accurate nano-scale size and morphology) and chemical properties (chemically amendable surfaces). Fluorescence tagging can be easily performed on dendrimers due to availability of highly reactive surfaces. Furthermore, unique structure of dendrimers offers several advantages over other nanostructures (polymeric nanoparticles and liposomes) such as quick cellular uptake, diminished uptake *via* reticuloendothelial system and smooth passage through biological barriers *via* transcytosis. Various disease states have been extensively evaluated using dendrimers as contrast/imaging agent (Table 9.1). In an MRI setup body is exposed to a high intensity magnetic field, followed by application of a short radiofrequency pulse causing alterations in nuclear spin precession of investigated molecule. The time taken by the nuclear spins to revert to their original states is termed as relaxation time, and during this relaxation period they emit energy which is detected by the scanner and is fourier transformed into an image. Due to their complex architecture, Dendrimers are especially adept in prolonging the transverse spin relaxation times of the ligated resonance contrast agents, improving their overall efficacy for MRI. In an illustrative publication a fourth generation dendrimer which had approximately 30 SS DNA specific to water borne pathogen *Cryptosporodium parvum* was fixated onto a quartz crystal microbalance. The microbalance serves as a mass sensitive signal transducer, converting the weight measurement into appropriate signal. Upon sample introduction, the Cryptosporodium target DNA accesses the complementary sites on SS DNA immobilized dendrimer, undergoes 3D hybridization and producing a magnified resonant frequency response. Another dendrimer of high clinical relevance is Gadomer-17. It is a

24 generation polylysine dendrimer containing a rare earth element gadolinium. The dendrimer structure is significantly larger than the constituent metal and consequently accentuates the MRI signal. Gadomer-27 is used in lymphography and angiography (Menjoge *et al.*, 2010).

Table 9.1 Applications of dendrimers for diagnosis of various diseases.

Disease state	Dendrimer	Contrast/imaging agent	Model
Breast cancer	G6-PAMAM-Cystamine	GD-DO3A MRI	Mice
Coronary artery disease	PAMAM	SH L 643A, Gadomer-17	Humans
Ovarian tumors	G2-PAMAM-Cystamine	Gd(III)-1B4M-DTPA & Rhodamine green	Nude mice
Angiography	G4-PAMAM	Gd(III))-1B4M-DTPA	Mice
Intratumoral vasculature	PAMAM	(1B4M-Gd)192 G6	Nude mice
Liver micrometastasis	(1B4M-Gd)64	DAB-Am64 (G6) DAB-Am64 (G4)	Nude mice
Blood pool	G3-6PAMAM	(1B4M-Gd)x	Nude mice

9.2.1.4 Magnetic Nanoparticles

As the name suggests magnetic nanoparticles are aligned and attracted towards magnetic source and can be willingly manipulated under the influence of external magnetic field. These are synthesized from magnetoactive compounds like iron oxides or ferrites (Fe_3O_4 and γ-Fe_2O_3), isolated metals such as iron and cobalt, spinel-type ferromagnets such as $MgFe_2O_4$, $MnFe_2O_4$, and $CoFe_2O_4$ as well as alloys $CoPt_3$ and FePt. They are extremely useful to label specific molecules, structures, or microorganisms. Magnetic nanoparticles have generated tremendous interest worldwide and researchers investigating fluid mechanics, catalysis chemistry, medicine, MRI, have been actively studying magnetic nanoparticles (Lu *et al.*, 2007).

Attaching a functional antibody to target organs or disease-causing organism is the basis of several diagnostic tests. These techniques have been broadly labelled as magnetic immunoassays. In these tests, antibodies labelled with magnetic nanoparticles give magnetic signals when exposed to a substantial magnetic field upon interacting with target antigens overexpressed in cases of specific pathological conditions. Antibodies bound to targets can thus be identified while unbound antibodies are dispersed randomly and consequently do not produce any reactionary magnetic signal. The magnetic field modulation created by the magnetically labelled targets is detected directly with a sensitive magnetometer.

Magnetic nanoparticles have shown genuine potential in estimating cancer markers such as telomerase activity. Telomeres are unique DNA structures that contain noncoding repetitive sequences. Telomerase is a ribonucleoprotein functioning as an enzyme which adds DNA repeats ("TTAGGG") to the 3' end of DNA strands in the telomere areas. As a result only 100 nucleotides are lost with each cell division cycle avoiding any harm to the organism. Telomerase levels are elevated in many malignancies making the malignant cells genomic structure conserved forever. Detector based on magnetic nanoparticles has been developed for rapid detection of telomerase activity in suspected biological samples. Magnetic nanoparticles have been appended with oligonucleotide sequences complementary to telomerase associated repeats (TTAGGG), which upon annealing produce intelligent fluctuation in focussed magnetic field. High-throughput adaptation has been implemented to accelerate sample processing (Grimm *et al.,* 2004).

Often magnetic nanoparticles are directed and concentrated within the target tissue by means of an external magnetic field. This property is exploited for detecting the specially disguised circulating cancer cells. Ferrite based magnetic nanoparticles are being used to study gene expression and angiogenesis, the primary markers of cancer.

9.2.1.5 Polymeric Nanoparticles

The exclusive purpose of biomedical analysis is to get accurate results desirably in a faster and easier way. Utilization of small amount of sample (reagent) and low limit of detection are the added features that make a biomedical diagnostic tool more reliable. Polymeric nanoparticles have gained wide acclaim because they are being used to develop diagnostic aids which comply with the above features. Polymeric nanoparticles have been employed in analysis of biomarker, diagnosis of cancer, diagnostic imaging, as well as various immunoassays. The crucial problem in the biomedical analysis is to detect the low level of target molecules/analytes which can be achieved by producing a sufficiently measurable/ quantifiable signal. Usually enzymes or dyes are employed for this purpose, which give colour or fluorescence as end point. Magnetic, thermal and pH responsive properties of the polymeric nanoparticles are also employed for the nano-diagnostic purposes. Polymeric nanoparticle for biomedical applications are prepared by (i) polymerization of monomers or (ii) processing of preformed polymers and the most commonly employed techniques are emulsion and free radical polymerization. The prepared polymeric nanoparticles are used as nanowires, nanofilms which are further attached with the bio-recognition systems. As these nanocomposites (nanowires, nanofilms) come in contact with the biological analyte, they interact leading to the change in the electrical properties of the nanocomposite, which can be detected by suitable means. Apart from the investigation of electrical properties, the bio-analysis can also be done by measuring the photochemical reaction(s) as optical output. Majorly generation and/or modulation of fluorescence emission, as well as FRET processes are employed for such purposes. Table 9.2 represents some of the reported polymeric systems for various biomedical applications.

The nanodiagnostics have application in tumour detection owing to the specific micro-environment of tumour with low pH. Lactic acid overproduction, hypoxic environment and fast metabolic rates of tumour cells are the chief reasons for weakly acidic pH (6-7) around tumour tissues. A biomimetic nano-particulate formulation based on oligopeptide self-assembly has been reported for tumour detection. This novel system shifts rapidly from self assembled into disassembeled form under the influence of subtle pH variations specific to tumor microenvironment, whilst remaining unaffected in other *in vivo* locations. Two groups of oligopeptide molecules are separately attached with fluorescent dye and quencher which are processed to form the self-assembled nanostructure. At low pH (6.8), this assembly dissociates and releases the oligopeptides. The oligopeptides attached with dye is detected by fluorescence microscopy paving the way for efficient tumour detection. These oligopeptides nanostructures are different from normal pH responsive nanoformulations in that the latter respond more slowly. Fast response makes the oligopeptides nanostructures most appropriate for biomedical diagnostic applications. Fig. 9.4 gives a diagrammatic presentation of the above mentioned phenomena.

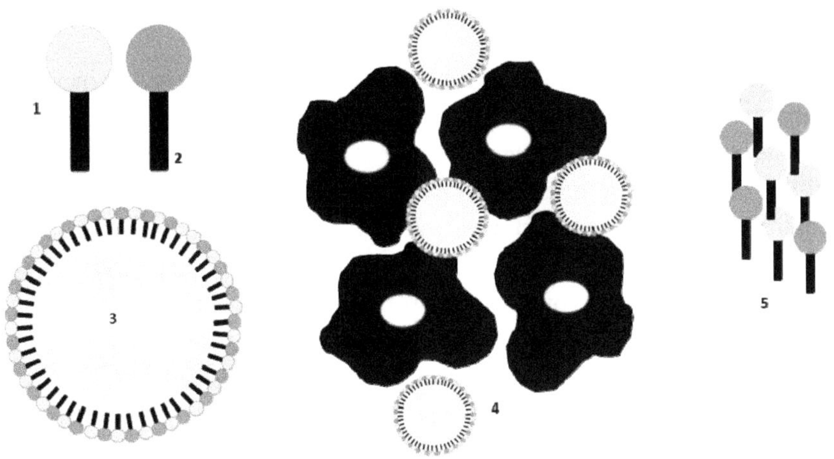

Fig. 9.4 Diagrammatic representation of tumour detection by oligopeptides nanostructures. (1) oligopeptide attached to fluorescent dye, (2) oligonucleotide attached to quencher, (3) self-assembled oligopeptides nanostructures, (4) oligopeptides nanostructures at tumour micro-environment (acidic pH; 6-7), (5) disassembled oligopeptides for detection of fluorescence.

Table 9.2 A brief account of polymeric nano-sized materials for biomedical application (Shinde *et al.*, 2012)

Polymeric nanosized materials	Application
Bio-functionalized electroactive polyaniline	Immuno-magnetic separation (biosensor). *E. coli* at a lowest limit of 7 cfu could be detected by this biosensor
Polypyrrole nanowires	Chemiresistive biosensor *B. globigii* could be detected at 1-100 cfu/mL.
Rhodamine B based fluorogenic polymeric micelles	Hg^{2+} detection (ring-opening reaction of Rhodamine B moieties occurs after the addition of Hg^{2+} ions, producing highly intense emission of fluorescence)
PEG-based thermo-responsive diblock copolymer containing coumarin	Detection of fluoride
Polymeric micelles based on Europium (EU III) complexes and fluorescein isothiocyanate (FITC)	Detection of Hg^{2+} ions inside living cells with a limit of detection of 10 nM
Polystyrene nanoparticles loaded with EU III β-diketone chelates	Detection of anthrax protective agent

9.2.1.6 Hybrid Particles

In recent years considerable work is done on hybrid particles in which inorganic nanoparticles (iron oxide, zinc oxide, gold, silver, and quantum dots) are heterogeneously incorporated in a polymeric matrix. Rationale behind development of such hybrid particles is to utilize the specific features of nano-range particles and polymeric materials in enhancing therapeutic/diagnostic potential of inorganic compounds. The physicochemical and biological properties of the nanoparticles are explored and added effects are incurred by the utilization of the polymeric systems, which in turn make these particles more efficient in performing their intended action. The basic application of hybrid particles are associated with many *in vitro* analysis where these are used as solid phase supports for biomolecules, especially in nucleic acid capture, immunoassay as well as cell sorting. Studies have also been performed on the *in vivo* applications such as drug targeting and *in vivo* imaging and successful results were observed (Shinde *et al.,* 2012). Because of opposite nature, the inorganic nanoparticles and the organic polymers show some incompatibility as well as immiscibility. In order to facilitate the formulation of hybrid particles, the inorganic nanoparticles are first functionalized by the aid of surfactants, linkers, or spacer arms. Another approach involves chemical modification of the inorganic nanoparticles, although physical approaches are comparatively easier and feasible. The functionalized nanoparticles are encapsulated in the polymeric matrix by various approaches viz. (but not limited to) physical encapsulation, emulsion polymerization, layer-by-layer encapsulation and double emulsion method. Table 9.3 enlists some of the examples of inorganic nanoparticles encapsulated in polymeric matrix. Fig. 9.5 gives a diagrammatic representation of fabrication of polymeric matrix incorporated with inorganic nanoparticles. Superparamagnetic iron oxide is one of the most widely explored inorganic candidates for development of hybrid nanoparticles. These have been investigated for many *in vitro* diagnostic applications like contrast agent, biomolecule carriers, targeted drug delivery and hyperthermia. The detection methods of the hybrid particles are similar to the polymeric particles as mentioned in previous section.

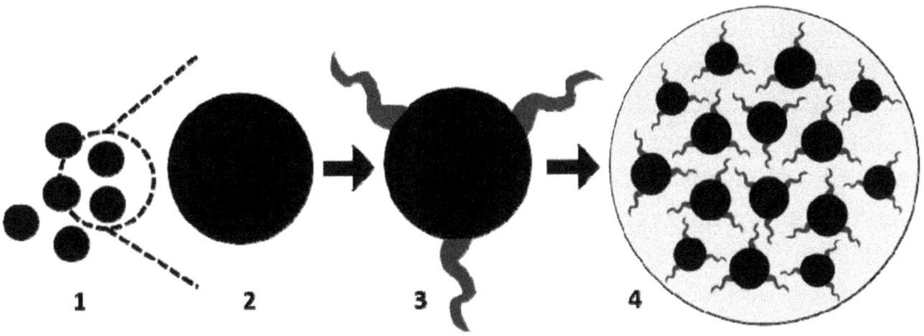

Fig. 9.5 Diagrammatic representation of functionalization and encapsulation of inorganic nanoparticles in polymeric matrix. (1) inorganic nanoparticles, (2) magnified plain nanoparticle, (3) surface functionalized nanoparticles, (4) functionalized nanoparticle dispersed in polymeric matrix.

Table 9.3 A brief account of inorganic nanoparticles encapsulated in polymeric matrix used for biomedical applications (Eissa *et al.*, 2013; Hussain *et al.*, 2005; Lutz *et al.*, 2006)

Inorganic nanoparticles	Polymeric matrix	Application
Iron oxide	Poly(divinylbenzene-co-glycidylmethacrylate)	Immunoassay
Gold	Poly(amidoamine)	Tumor cell bio-imaging
Gold and cobalt	Alkyl thioether end-functionalized poly (methacrylic acid)	Drug delivery, imaging and various biomedical applications
Maghemite	Poly(amino acid)	*In vivo* imaging
Iron oxide	poly[2-(methacryloyloxy)ethyl phosphorylcholine]-block-(glycerol monomethacrylate)	MRI, drug delivery
Iron oxide	poly-(oligo(ethylene glycol) methacrylate-co-methacrylic acid)	Imaging

9.3 Carbon Nanotubes

The biological phenomena occurring in living system involve interactions of various components at nano-meter scale. The nano-machineries of cells are therefore susceptible to alteration at their function in presence of any xenobiotic of nano-meter size. These occurrences are biologically proved by various research groups working on nanoparticle formulations. Among the several nanoparticles, carbon nanotubes (CNTs) are of considerable importance especially in the field of biomedical analysis owing to their specific features viz. high aspect ratio, biocompatibility, flexibility in functionalization, capacity to carry dyes/quenchers/drugs/ enzymes. CNTs are composed of sp^2-hybridized carbon atoms arranged in a hexagonal orientation and belong to Fullerenes. These nanostructures are formed by rolling single or multiple layers of graphene sheets into seamless cylinders. CNTs are manufactured by electric-arc discharge, catalytic chemical vapour deposition, and laser ablation methods. Purification is the next process which facilitates removal of impurities left during manufacturing process. For making CNTs suitable for biomedical applications, these are subjected to functionalization which changes physicochemical properties, and also provides ability to link molecules/ligands/enzymes/dyes/antibodies. When the analyte comes in contact with CNTs, it changes the dielectric environment, charge, conductivity and optical properties which can be analysed by suitable analytical tools. Fig. 9.6 enumerates description of the discussed phenomena.

CNTs have been explored for the bio-sensing of glucose as well as cancer biomarkers. For the bio-sensing purpose implantable/disposable devices and microfluidic techniques/immune-sensing devices are employed. An outline of *in vivo* glucose monitoring is shown in Fig. 9.7. Researchers have developed CNTs which can be implanted as miniaturized electrodes to act as biosensor, however toxicity caused by such devices are yet to be addressed.

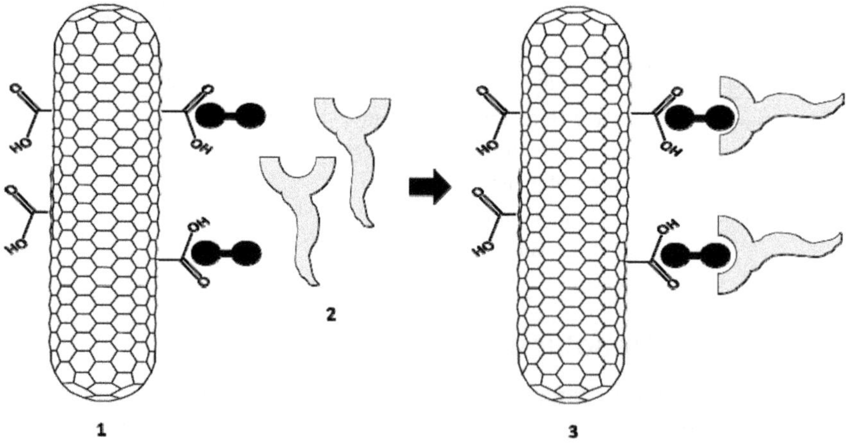

Fig. 9.6 Diagrammatic representation of the interaction of functionalized CNTs with analyte. (1) functionalized CNTs with carboxylic group and ligand, (2) analyte (antibody), (3) interaction of the functionalized CNTs with the antibody leading to change in the physicochemical characteristics (optical or electrical properties/charge) of CNTs.

CNTs functionalized with fluorescent compounds have been considered for use as a radio-opaque substance and is employed for *in vivo* imaging of the organs and tissues. Similarly CNTs labelled with radioactive isotopes are for nuclear imaging applications. A novel device viz. "piezoelectric pressure sensor" has been reported which works by employing pressure sensing capacity of CNTs. Advancements in biomedical sciences have employed CNT-based nano-biosensors in detection of DNA sequences, especially those related to cancer, and human autoimmune diseases. Functionalized CNTs are explored for the detection of DNA. Single nucleotide polymorphism, which is a mutation observed very often in DNA can be traced by the application of DNA functionalized-CNTs. The mechanism involved in this phenomenon is hybridization kinetics of DNA functionalized-CNTs and complementary sequence in the analyte solution. Apart from these applications, CNTs are also employed for small molecule detection, analysis of reactive oxygen species, tracing of biomarkers and proteins. Table 9.4 exhibits some of the important applications of CNTs in biomedical field.

Table 9.4 Examples of carbon nanotubes employed for biomedical analysis (Ji *et al.,* 2010; Kruss *et al.,* 2013).

CNTs	Application
Antibody-functionalized single walled CNTs field-effect transistor	For fast and accurate detection of Lyme disease antigen.
Multi walled CNTs-polystyrene based electrochemical transducer attached to chimeric fibrin-filaggrin peptide	Detection of anti-citrullinated peptide antibodies found in serum of rheumatoid arthritis.
Multi walled CNTs placed on the tip of glass pipette	Nanotube based endoscopy for interrogating cells at single organelle level. It can also transport fluid, perform optical and electrochemical diagnostic tests.
Vertically aligned multi walled CNTs as biosensor	Detection of cancer metastasis at single-cell level by cell membrane electrical signals.
Galactose bio-functionalized single walled CNTs	Detection of pathogenic *E. coli* by galactose binding surface proteins.
Single walled CNTs based potentiometric aptamer biosensor	Detection of living bacteria at concentration 6-26 cfu/mL in apple juice.

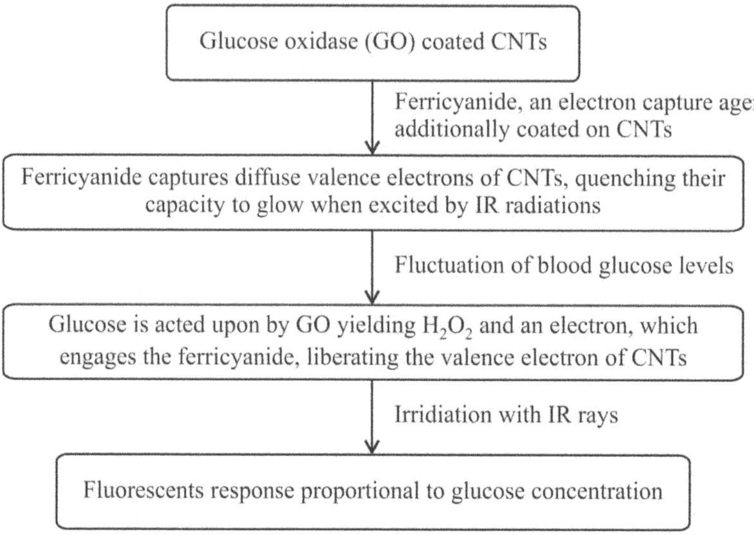

Fig. 9.7 Schematic representation of single walled CNT based *in vivo* glucose monitoring optical sensor.

9.4 NANO-BIOCHIP [LAB-ON-CHIP (LOC) Technique]

LOC concept is integration of as many analytical steps as possible on one single assembly, i.e., from sample collection to co conduction of diagnostic test followed by obtainment and quantification of results. Nano-biochips come under miniaturised *in vitro* diagnostic devices which transpire to follow the LOC principle. These are small but highly integrated devices fabricated using microelectronic techniques and are made up of microfluidic systems which are chambers interconnected by narrow channels, pumps, valves and nano-sized electrodes. These are solid phase assays in which one of the reactive species interacting with the analyte to elicit a quantifiable response is present in solid state. Due to the miniscule dimensions of the nanobiochip relatively small sample volume is expended, which remains undiluted, causing fast diffusion movements, increasing the reaction rates and the associated sensitivity. This technique tenders various advantages including high accuracy, high sensitivity, fast and economic way, minimum sample extraction and waste production.

9.5 Toxicity Aspects of Nano-Diagnostics

Any nano-sized formulation is always associated with risk of toxicity due to their ultra-small size. It is recognized that the biological phenomena at cellular levels occur at nanometre range, so there are substantial possibilities of interaction of the nanostructures with the nano-machinery of cells. Due to intentional surface modification of nanostructures for therapeutic effect, it is difficult for the defence cells of body to counteract these materials. As a consequence these nano-materials get more opportunity to interact with normal cells of body, leading to toxicity. Researchers have found that CNTs successfully bind and interfere with the normal behaviour of multi-protein intracellular assemblies. Other cellular components like voltage dependent ion channels of mitochondria, DNA and RNA interact with CNTs leading to conformational changes and altered function of these components. The nanomaterials also cause adverse action at the organ level e.g., these items affect eye, liver, kidney and lung by causing aggregation of the nanoparticles (Azzazy *et al.*, 2006; Lam *et al.*, 2004). Similarly potential toxic effects of other nanosized materials are reported in literature. Inorganic nanoparticles are often found to be deposited in various sites inside the body and their delayed clearance cause severe inflammatory and hypersensitive reactions. However, rigours work is going on in order to improve the safety profile of these nanomaterials so that these can be successfully employed for healthcare of human beings.

9.6 Future Outlook

Therapeutic intervention of diseases solely depends on the early and accurate detection of the pathophysiologic symptoms, hence advancement in the biomedical analysis techniques has been forever a challenging and demanding segment in healthcare. Nanodiagnostics are gradually spreading their wings in almost all segment of biomedical analysis. The rapid advancement in electronics technology and biomedical engineering together is a positive sign in the development of nanodiagnostics. It has been noticed that due to their specific features the nanomaterial has got immense potential in molecular diagnosis of various disease conditions. Nanodiagnostics, viz. polymeric nanoparticles, hybrid particles, CNTs, dendrimers, magnetic particles, quantum dots or inorganic (silver, gold, iron oxide) particles are to be understood in terms of biocompatibility, toxicity, and risk/benefit ratio for successful clinical application. A number of nanotechnology based diagnostics devises/tools are available in market and many more are patented by researchers which are expected to accomplish commercialization opportunity in near future. A variety of novel nanodiagnostics viz. nanowires, nanoprobes, nanobarcodes, cantilever array, nanochip, nanosensors are yet to find clinical approval. Apart from the day-to-day diagnostic tests, these nanosized materials are projected to be employed for various applications such as DNA mapping, viral RNA detection, multiplexed diagnostics, advanced and more sensitive immune assay as well as genotyping. Development of safe, effective and stable nanodiagnostics with added features like automated, portability, cost-effectiveness should be the prime future prospects in this field of research which needs a multidisciplinary approach.

References

Azzazy H.M, Mansour M.M, and Kazmierczak S.C (2006). Nanodiagnostics: a new frontier for clinical laboratory medicine. *Clinical Chemistry* **52:** 1238-1246.

Cheki M, Moslehi M, and Assadi M (2013). Marvelous applications of quantum dots. *European Review for Medical and Pharmacological Sciences* **17:** 1141-1148.

Daniel M.C, and Astruc D (2004). Gold nanoparticles: assembly, supramolecular chemistry, quantum-size-related properties, and applications toward biology, catalysis, and nanotechnology. *Chemical Reviews* **104:** 293-346.

Eissa M.M, Rahman M, Zine N, Jaffrezic N, Errachid A, Fessi H, and Elaissari A (2013). Reactive magnetic poly (divinylbenzene-co-glycidyl methacrylate) colloidal particles for specific antigen detection using microcontact printing technique. *Acta Biomaterialia* **9:** 5573-5582.

El-Sayed I.H, Huang X, and El-Sayed M.A (2005). Surface plasmon resonance scattering and absorption of anti-EGFR antibody conjugated gold nanoparticles in cancer diagnostics: applications in oral cancer. *Nano Letters* **5:** 829-834.

Grimm J, Perez J.M, Josephson L, and Weissleder R (2004). Novel Nanosensors for Rapid Analysis of Telomerase Activity. *Cancer Research* **64:** 639-643.

Hussain I, Graham S, Wang Z, Tan B, Sherrington D.C, Rannard S.P, Cooper A.I, and Brust M (2005). Size-controlled synthesis of near-monodisperse gold nanoparticles in the 1-4 nm range using polymeric stabilizers. *Journal of the American Chemical Society* **127:** 16398-16399.

Hussain M.M, Samir T.M, and Azzazy H.M (2013). Unmodified gold nanoparticles for direct and rapid detection of Mycobacterium tuberculosis complex. *Clinical Biochemistry* **46:** 633-637.

Indira T.K, and Lakshmi P.K (2010). Magnetic Nanoparticles - A Review. *International Journal of Pharmaceutical Sciences and Nanotechnology* **3:** 1035-1042.

Ji S.R, Liu C, Zhang B, Yang F, Xu J, Long J, Jin C, Fu D.L, Ni Q.X, and Yu X.J (2010). Carbon nanotubes in cancer diagnosis and therapy. *Biochimica et Biophysica Acta (BBA)-Reviews on Cancer* **1806:** 29-35.

Kruss S, Hilmer A.J, Zhang J, Reuel N.F, Mu B, and Strano M.S (2013). Carbon nanotubes as optical biomedical sensors. *Advanced Drug Delivery Reviews* **65:** 1933-1950.

Lam C.W, James J.T, McCluskey R, and Hunter R.L (2004). Pulmonary toxicity of single-wall carbon nanotubes in mice 7 and 90 days after intratracheal instillation. *Toxicological Sciences* **77:** 126-134.

Lu A.H, Salabas E.L, and Schuth F (2007). Magnetic nanoparticles: synthesis, protection, functionalization, and application. *Angewandte Chemie (International ed in English)* **46:** 1222-1244.

Lutz J.F, Stiller S, Hoth A, Kaufner L, Pison U, and Cartier R (2006). One-pot synthesis of pegylated ultrasmall iron-oxide nanoparticles and their *in vivo* evaluation as magnetic resonance imaging contrast agents. *Biomacromolecules* **7:** 3132-3138.

Menjoge A.R, Kannan R.M, and Tomalia D.A (2010). Dendrimer-based drug and imaging conjugates: design considerations for nanomedical applications. *Drug Discovery Today* **15:** 171-185.

Palomino J.C (2009). Molecular detection, identification and drug resistance detection in Mycobacterium tuberculosis. *FEMS Immunology and Medical Microbiology* **56:** 103-111.

Shinde S.B, Fernandes C.B, and Patravale V.B (2012). Recent trends in *in-vitro* nanodiagnostics for detection of pathogens. *Journal of Controlled Release* **159:** 164-180.

Zhang C.Y, Yeh H.C, Kuroki M.T, and Wang T.H (2005). Single-quantum-dot-based DNA nanosensor. *Nature Materials* **4:** 826-831.

10

Solid Lipid Nanoparticles: A Promising Colloidal Carrier

D. Mishra[1], V. Dhote[2] and P.K. Mishra[3]

[1]College of Pharmacy, IPS Academy, Indore-452012, India.

[2]Truba Institute of Pharmacy, Karond - Gandhi Nagar By Pass Road, Bhopal-462038, India.

[3]Translational Research Lab, School of Biological Sciences, Dr. H S Gour Central University, Sagar- 470003, India.

10.1 Introduction

In the last few decades, pharmaceutical field has registered most outstanding landmarks in the field of medicines and drug delivery. Reminiscing the pharmaceutical dosage form development starting from conventional powders to till date more sophisticated and reliable nano technological strategies equipped drug delivery systems, we have treaded a long way. Nanotechnology has not only created a deep impression on medicinal field, but also massively expanded its area in diagnosis, treatment, cure and patient monitoring. The effective use of nanotechnology in drug delivery leads to the development of a new branch of pharmacy i.e., "Nanomedicine". Various categories of nanomedicines including liposomes, niosomes, transfersomes, dendrimers, nanoshells, nanocapsules, nanowires and solid lipid nanoparticles are available in market and all are gaining vital importance in comparison to conventional drug carriers (Acosta, 2009), (Ahlin Grabnar, 1998), (Aji Alex *et al.,* 2011), (Almeida and Souto, 2007).

Amongst the various nanocarriers, solid lipid nanoparticles (SLN) have gained a tremendous attention from both industrial and academic perspective. They can be simply epitomize as new epoch of colloidal carriers of submicron size where liquid lipid of emulsion is replaced by solid lipid; which ultimately provide smaller size, larger surface area, high drug loading capacity and controlled drug release profile. SLN not only enjoys the combine benefits of conventional colloidal carriers (e.g., like liposomes, niosomes, nanoparticles) but at the same time it has the capacity to attenuate or obliterate the adversities associated with them (Alvarez-Roman *et al.,* 2004), (Benita *et al.,* 1986). It can be competently used for the delivery of copious amounts of drugs *via* various possible drug delivery routes. The roles and classification of various colloidal carriers can be summarized in Table 10.1 and Fig. 10.1 carriers (Aji Alex *et al.,* 2011), (Chakraborty *et al.,* 2009), (Diepold *et al.,* 1989), (Eldem *et al.,* 1991).

Table 10.1 Roles of various colloidal carriers

S. No.	Colloidal carriers	Materials used	Applications
1.	Nanosuspension and Nanocrystal	Drug powder is dispersed in surfactant solution	Stable system for controlled delivery of poorly water soluble drug
2.	Solid Lipid Nanoparticles (SLN)	Melted lipid is dispersed in aqueous surfactant	Least toxic and most stable system carrier system as alternative system to polymer
3.	Polymeric nanoparticles	Biodegradable polymers	Controlled and targeted drug delivery
4.	Polymeric micelles	Amphiphilic block co-polymers	Controlled and systemic delivery of water insoluble drugs
5.	Magnetic Nanoparticles	Magnetite Fe_2O_3 coated with dextran	Drug diagnostic tool kit
6.	Carbon Nanotubes	Metals, semiconductor or carbon	Controlled delivery of gene and DNA
7.	Liposomes	Phospholipid vesicles	Controlled and targeted drug delivery
8.	Nanoshells	Dielectric core and metal shell	Tumor targeting
9.	Ceramic Nanoparticles	Silica, aluminum and titanium	Drug and biomolecule delivery
10.	Nanopores	Aerogels, which is cell gel based chemistry	Controlled release of drug carries
11.	Nanowires	Silicon, copper, gold and cobalt	Transport electron in nanoelectronics

Table 10.1 *Contd...*

S. No.	Colloidal carriers	Materials used	Applications
12.	Quantom dots (QD's)	Cadmium selenide and sulphide	Imaging and diagnostic agent
13.	Nanofilms	Polypeptide	Systemic and local delivery
14.	Ferrofluids	Iron oxide NP's encapsulated in polymers	For capturing cells and other drug target

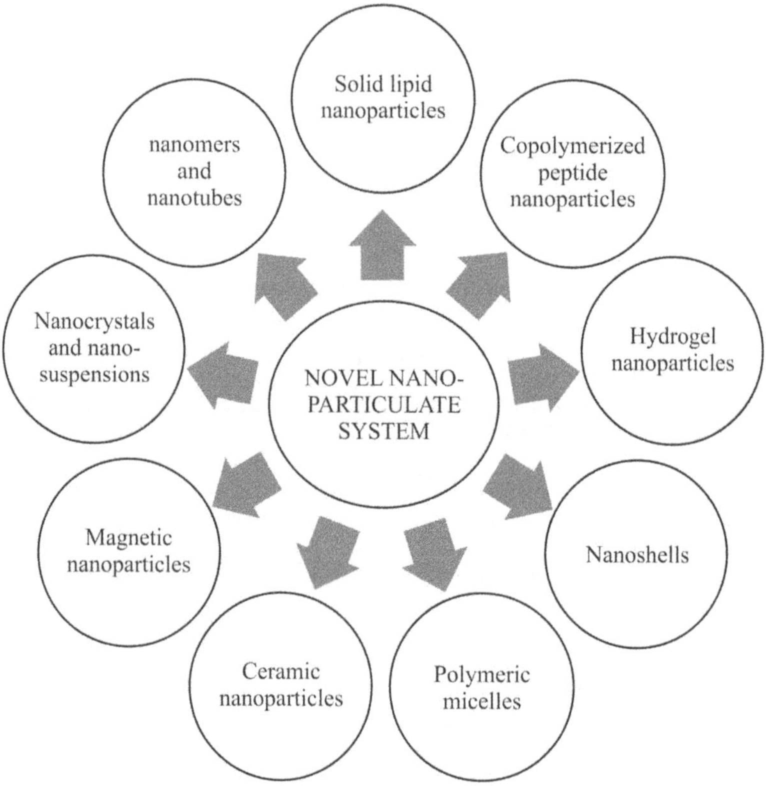

Fig. 10.1 Nanomedicines used for drug delivery.

Solid lipids have been used for long to obtain a sustained or controlled release drug profile. But in earlier 1980 it was Speiser and its co-workers who have proficiently developed solid lipid micro-particles and lipid pellets (Mucosolvan®) for drug delivery (Fang *et al.*, 2008). They have claimed that this novel carriers possessed voluminous capacity for drug delivery which can be seen in comparative way in Table 10.2 (Kaur *et al.*, 2008), (Ye *et al.*, 2008), (Tabatt *et al.*, 2004).

Table 10.2 Comparative aspects of colloidal carriers

S. No.	Parameters	SLN	Lipid emulsion	Liposomes	Polymeric nanoparticles
1	Systemic toxicity	Low	Low	Low	> SLN
2	Cytotoxicity	Low	Low	Low	> SLN
3	Organic solvent residue	No	No	—	Yes
4	Sterilization by autoclaving	Yes	Yes	No	No
5	Sustained release	Yes	No	Yes	Yes
6	Avoidance of RES	Yes	Yes	Yes	Yes
7	Large scale production	Yes	Yes	Yes	No

As it is clear from the Table 10.2, that SLN possess an extra-edge advantage over other colloidal carriers and can be effectively employed as promising drug delivery tool (Westesen and Siekmann, 1997).

10.2 Solid Lipid Nanoparticles (SLN)

SLNs are nano-sized colloidal carriers (50-1000 nm), which are composed of lipid, surfactants, and drugs in appropriate ratios. The small size and lipid core provide some unbeatable properties to SLN which make it superior over other existing carriers (Lippacher *et al.,* 2001), (Magenheim *et al.,* 1993), (zur Muhlen *et al.,* 1996). Its small size offers several advantages like larger surface, high drug loading capacity, interaction with target site up to molecular level and may enhance bioavailability of drug. Whereas the lipid core facilitates the incorporation wide variety of drugs (Eldem *et al.,* 1991) which get dissolved, dispersed, or entrapped in it. SLN may be used to deliver lipophilic drugs, macromolecules, proteins, peptides, genes, antigens, food molecules, hydrophilic drugs and diagnostics molecules (zur Muhlen *et al.,* 1998), (Schwarz and Mehnert, 1999), (Muller *et al.,* 2000). A cross sectional view of SLN delineate that the drug moiety is embedded in phospholipid layer (Fig. 10.2). The beneficial aspect of solid lipid core is that, it reduces the "*drug mobility*" and hence reduces the chances of its degradation (Muller *et al.,* 2008).

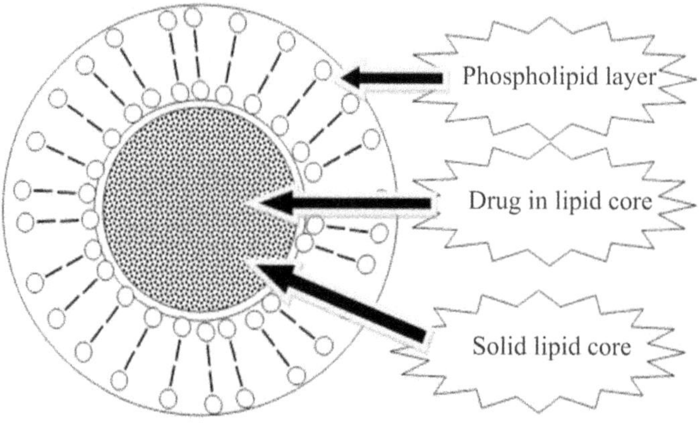

Fig. 10.2 Cross sectional view of SLN.

10.2.1 Mechanism of Preparation of SLN

SLN is usually prepared from oil-in-water type of emulsion. The liquid lipid faces the shortfall of drug mobility and hence is more prone to drug degradation. On the contrary, solid lipid of SLN reduces the drug mobility and subsequently improve the stability of formulation (Muller, 1998). The solidified lipid matrix (Fig. 10.3) is achieved by

- Use of surfactants (Tween-80, sodium dodecyl sulphate (SDS), lecithin etc.)
- Using *stearic stabilizer* (poloxmer-180)
- Using some *viscosity enhancers* (ethyl cellulose solution, PEG600, Miglyol 812) for drug distribution (Cavalli *et al.,* 2002).

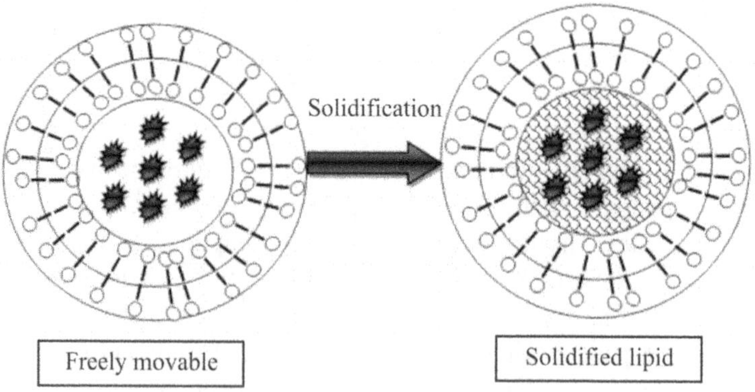

Fig. 10.3 Mechanism of SLN preparation.

10.2.2 Advantages of SLN

SLNs are of tremendous advantages. Some of the prominent ones have been enlisted below (Kaur *et al.,* 2008), (del Pozo-Rodriguez *et al.,* 2009), (Runge *et al.,* 1996):

- Controlled and/or targeted drug release
- Enhanced bioavailability
- Excellent biocompatibility
- Very high long-term stability
- Easy scale up
- Application versatility
- Avoidance of organic solvents
- No toxic metabolites are produced
- Surface modification can be done
- Can be lyophilized as well as spray dried
- Protection of incorporated drug against chemical degradation
- Possible sterilization by autoclaving and gamma irradiation
- Small size and relatively narrow size distribution provide biological opportunities for site specific drug delivery

10.2.3 Disadvantages of SLN (del Pozo-Rodriguez *et al.,* 2009)

- Drug expulsion
- Particle growth
- Unpredictable gelation tendency
- Co-existence of several colloidal species
- High pressure induced drug degradation

10.2.4 Aims of SLN Preparation

SLN are selected because they are well tolerated by body and are able to reduce fluctuations in blood spike at target site with reduced toxicity. It has been suggested that SLN possess numerous advantages over existing colloidal carriers with minimum loopholes (Runge *et al.,* 1996), (Scheffel *et al.,* 1972), (Serpe *et al.,* 2010). Unique features which gave a breakthrough to SLN are as follows:

- Impart stability to carrier and encapsulated drug
- Drug release profile can be tailored per need

- Voluminous capacity of delivering and encapsulating both hydrophilic and lipophilic drugs
- High drug loading capacity
- Can be made of polymers which impart minimal or no immunogenicity
- Can be easily floor up to commercial scale of production

10.2.5 Components of SLN

The basic components of SLN are phospholipids, and surfactants which provide excellent acceptable features. Various constitute elements of SLN are effectively summarized in Table 10.3 (Souto and Muller, 2006), (Uner, 2006).

Table 10.3 List of various lipids and excipients used for the preparation of SLN

S. No.	Lipids	Surfactant
1	***Triacylglycerols*** Tricaprin Trilaurin Trimyristin Tripalmitin Tristearin	***Phospholipids*** Soy lecithin Egg lecithin Phosphatidylcholine
2	*Acylglycerols* Glycerol monostearate Glycerol behenate Glycerol Palmitostearate	**Ethylene oxide/propylene oxide copolymers** Poloxamer 188 Poloxamer 182 Poloxamer 407 Poloxamine 908
3	***Fatty acids*** Stearic acid Palmitic acid Decanoic acid Behenic acid	***Sorbitan ethylene oxide/propylene oxide copolymers*** Polysorbate 20 Polysorbate 60 Polysorbate 80
4	***Waxes*** Cetylpalmitate	***Alkylaryl polyether alcohol polymers*** Tyloxapol
5	***Cyclic complexes*** Cyclodextrin	**Bile salts** Sodium cholate Sodium glycocholate Sodium taurocholate Sodium taurodeoxycholate
6	***Hard fat types*** Witepsol W 35 Witepsol H 35	***Alcohol*** Ethanol Butanol

10.3 Formulation of SLN

SLN can be prepared by various methods, but some of the important and commercially scale-able techniques are summarized in Fig. 10.4. Out of various methods high pressure homogenization (HPH) play a vital role in manufacturing of SLN but other methods like spray drying, ultrasonic homogenization, microemulsion, double emulsion and supercritical methods are also popularly used (Westesen and Siekmann, 1997) (Jenning *et al.,* 2000), (Mehnert and Mader, 2001), (Kuo and Chen, 2009).

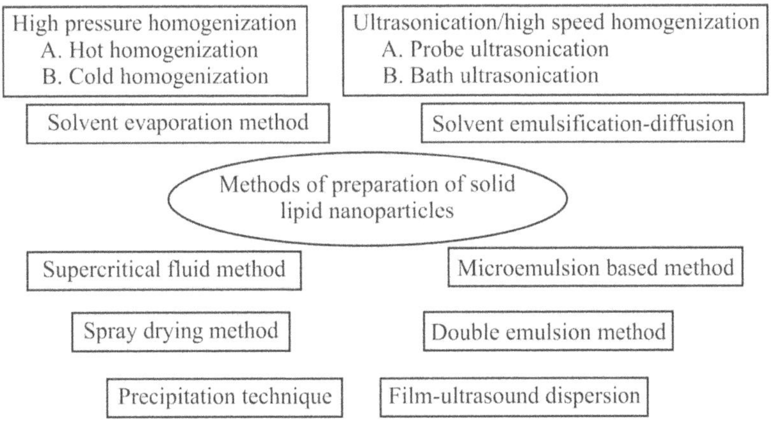

Fig. 10.4 Methods of SLN preparation.

10.3.1 High Pressure Homogenization (HPH)

In this method a high pressure is applied to molten drug-lipid solution, so as to reduce the particles size up to nano range and also promote its homogenization in solution. HPH can be carried out in either conditions i.e., hot or cold HPH.

10.3.1.1 Hot HPH

In this method the lipid is heated over 5-10 °C above its melting point followed by addition of drug which is allowed to dissolve/disperse throughout the molten lipid. Subsequently, molten drug-lipid solution and emulsifier is subjected to high shear mixing in order to form a pre-emulsion. Finally, the prepared pre-emulsion is subjected to high pressure homogenization (approx 5-10 cycles at 500 bars). Finally the formulation is rapidly cooled down to room temperature to get SLN. A schematic representation of formulation of SLN by hot HPH is shown in Fig. 10.5 A.

10.3.1.2 Cold HPH

The preliminary step of preparation of SLN is somewhat similar to hot HPH. The drug is either dispersed or dissolved in molten lipid to prepare a solution which is allowed to cool for solidification. Afterwards, the solidified masses are crushed down to yield microparticles. The prepared microparticles are suspended in cool aqueous surfactant solution in order to get a pre-suspension. Finally, the pre-suspension is passed through HPH (5-10 cycles at 500 bars) to get the desired SLN (Kang *et al.,* 2010). The process is schematically depicted in Fig. 10.5 B.

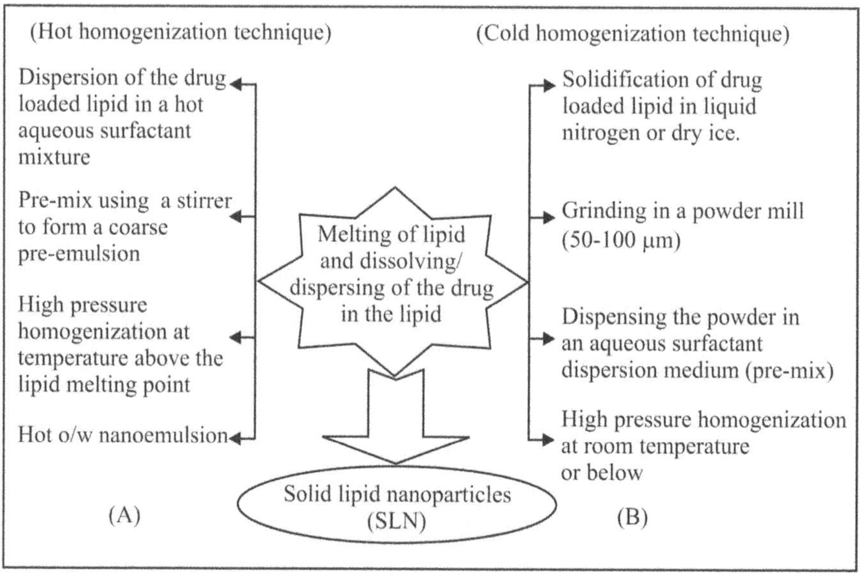

Fig. 10.5 (a) Hot homogenization technique
(b) Cold homogenization technique.

10.3.2 Ultrasonic Homogenization

The basic process is carried out by dissolving drug in molten lipid, which is initially maintained at approx. 5-10 °C above its melting point. After that the prepared drug-lipid solution is added to aqueous surfactant solution, with high shear homogenization (8000 rpm for 15 min) (Cavalli *et al.,* 2002), (Runge *et al.,* 1996) (Scheffel *et al.,* 1972). Subsequently, the prepared emulsion is subjected to sonication in a probe sonicator, which finally reduces the size and produce cavities for better entrapment of drug molecules. Finally, the sonicated emulsion is poured in vial and rapidly cools down to get SLN. The process can be envisioned as shown in Fig. 10.6 (Gasco, 1993).

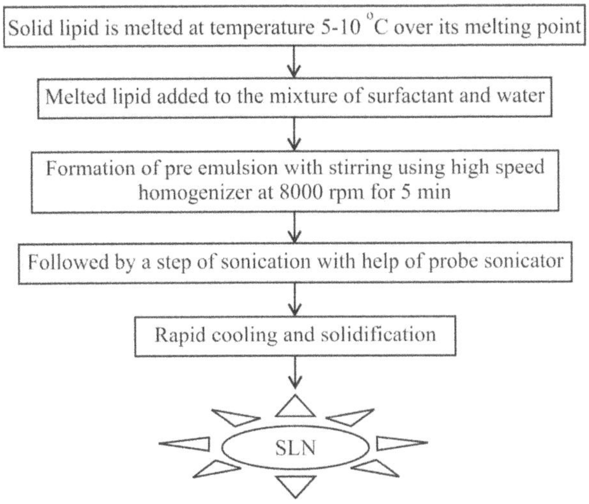

Fig. 10.6 Flow diagram of Ultra-sonic homogenization.

10.3.3 Micro-emulsion based Method

This method involves preparation of a microemulsion (ME) of drug, emulsifier, co-emulsifier, low melting point lipid and water. The prepared ME is almost optically transparent in nature and prepared at high temperatures (65-75 °C). In next step the ME is dispersed in cold water maintained at 2-3 °C with stirring. At the end the prepared SLN is collected by ultracentrifugation. The process can be summarized as shown in Fig. 10.7.

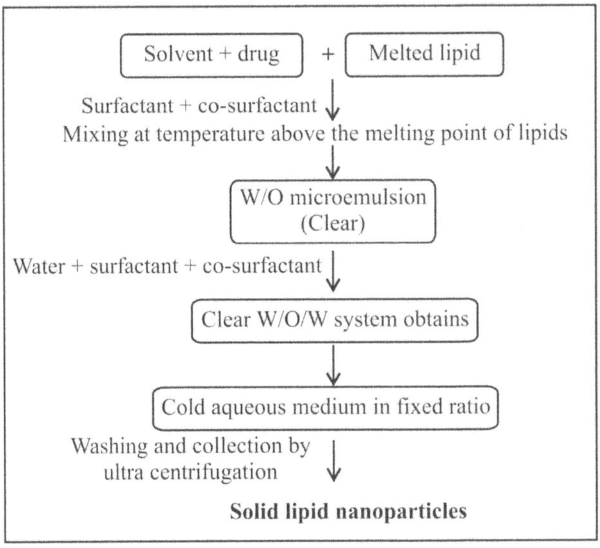

Fig. 10.7 Flow diagram of microemulsion based method.

10.3.4 Spray Drying Technique

It is a closed system process which consists of four basic steps i.e., atomization, drying, evaporation, and separation. It is most suitable for lipids with somewhat high melting point i.e., above 70 °C. The molten drug-lipid solution is sprayed in a drying vessel (Gasco, 1993). This vessel is maintained at a specific temperature and pressure conditions, which also facilitates the rapid drying of nanodroplets leaving behind nanosized SLN (Gasco, 1993), (Kaur *et al.,* 2008). The basic scheme is summarized in Fig. 10.8.

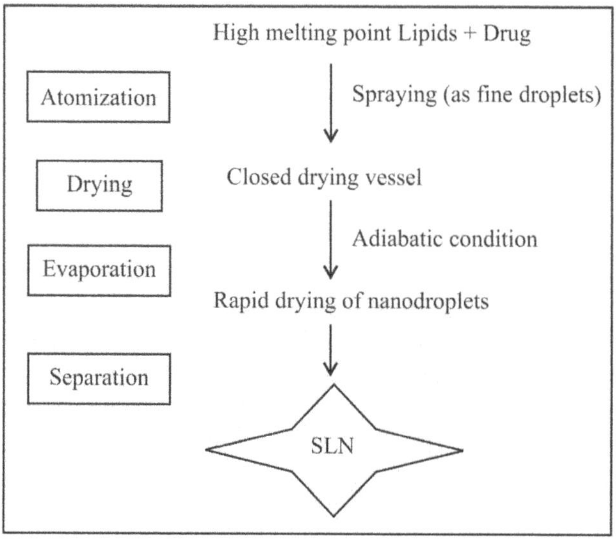

Fig. 10.8 Flow diagram of Spray drying technique.

10.3.5 Supercritical Fluid (SCF) Method

This method is also a closed system process and thus eliminate the chances of drug contamination and all process variables can be checked efficiently (Kaur *et al.,* 2008), (Ye *et al.,* 2008). In this method, lipid and drug is dissolved in supercritical fluids like CO_2, nitrous oxide, methane, propane, ammonia etc., subsequently the medicated fluid is subjected to homogenization in a vessel which is maintained at specific temperature and pressure (Runge *et al.,* 1996). The homogenized fluid is allowed to spray through atomizer in expansion vessel, where the fluid is rapidly evaporated from the surface of droplets. Finally, SLNs are prepared and further filtered in order to get a narrow sized product (Scheffel *et al.,* 1972). The process can be summarized as represented in Fig. 10.9.

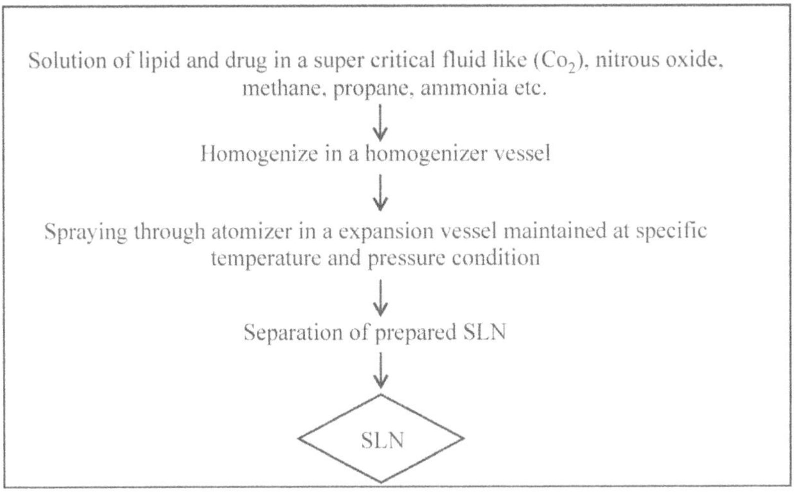

Fig. 10.9 Flow chart of SCF method for SLN preparation.

10.4 Ancillary Processing of SLN

SLN can be successfully prepared either by one of the above mentioned methods but they appear to be in non-deliverable form. It requires some extra efforts or auxiliary process like sterilization, drying, lyophillization, etc., to put them into the market or in dispensable form (Kang *et al.,* 2010). Sterilization is one of the most crucial steps involved in manufacturing of SLN. It can be achieved by steam sterilization, γ-sterilization, chemical sterilization or filtration. Steam sterilization is the preferred technique. However, upon exposure to steam, SLN sometimes re-melt and appear as O/W emulsion of larger particles size and leads to

(a) recrystallization of lipid
(b) chances of drug and lipid degradation
(c) production of some by-products.

In such case, sterilization by filtration is preferable option but it is not viable for the SLN of more than 0.2 μm size range because it may lead to the blockage of the filter. Sterilization by γ-radiation can also be used which doesn't not causes particle size enlargement, however may lead to the production of free radicals which can interfere with performance and stability of SLN. Extensive research shows that each sterilization process is striving with its own shortcomings but can be efficiently used by keeping proper process variable under check. An ideal sterilization process should be such that it should not interfere with the performance, stability and *in-vivo* fate of drug.

10.5 Exsiccation of SLN

The SLN has to pass through the stage of drying after sterilization. Usually the prepared SLN is in dispersed form which is thermodynamically unstable. Also the drug and lipid incorporated in manufacturing of SLN is also prone to oxidation, hydrolysis, racemization and transformation reaction. Therefore, it is essential to ensure that the SLN should sustain for longer period of time and may be administrated as reconstituted powder form (Tabatt *et al.,* 2004), (Westesen and Siekmann, 1997), (Lippacher *et al.,* 2001), (Magenheim *et al.,* 1993).

The mentioned task can be achieved by the proper drying of SLN using one of the techniques like lyophilization, drying in nitrogen stream or by spray drying. In lyophilization, the SLN is dried in vacuum at freezing conditions and all the water is removed from its bulk and surface (Diepold *et al.,* 1989), (Eldem *et al.,* 1991). Though, lyophilization is better technique but it has some practical limitations like probable re-solubilization of SLN, re-aggregation and particle size enlargement, induced drastic changes in osmolarity and pH of SLN. In order to alleviate such problems there is need to add some cryoprotectants like sucrose, trehalose, maltose, mannitol, glycerol and PEG 3350.

Spray drying can also be used for eradicating excess of water. It is a closed system process, in which SLN is sprayed in an expansion vessel where rapid drying is achieved but the practical impediment is that there are some chances of lipid degradation and particle aggregation which ultimately reduce the shelf- life of SLN (Chakraborty *et al.,* 2009).

10.6 Characterization of SLN

The prepared SLN has to be characterized for some basic physico-chemical parameters *(in-vitro)* which will ensure the correct *in-vivo* performance of this novel colloidal carrier after administration in patients for specific disease conditions (Alvarez-Roman *et al.,* 2004). It can be characterized on parameters shown in Fig. 10.10.

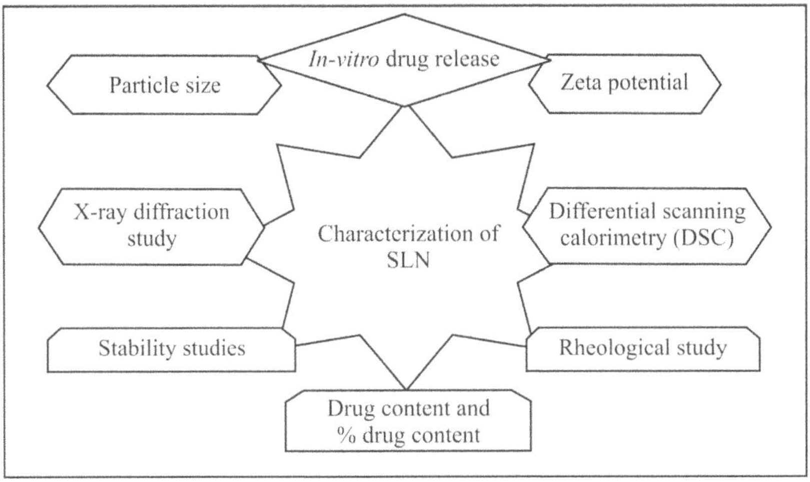

Fig. 10.10 Characterization parameters of SLN.

10.6.1 Particle Size

Particle size is a crucial factor for determining the possible *in-vivo* fate and stability aspect of SLN. It can be effectively determined by employing one of the techniques like photon correlation spectroscopy (PCS), laser diffraction (LD), coulter counter method, electron microscopy and phase-sensitive-intensity-difference (PSID) technique. Out of the mentioned techniques PCS and LD are most commonly employed techniques for particles size measurement. They mainly measure the scatter light rather than actual size of particles. PCS can measure from few micrometres upto approximately 3 μm scale but not able to detect larger particles, (R, 1993) (Kuo and Chen, 2009). In contrast LD can measure from μm to few mm range. Nowadays greater emphasis is posed on Field flow fraction technique (FFF) that usually separates the SLN on the basis of size, density or charge. The basic advantage of FFF technique is that the separated particle can be further characterized by some other techniques (Muller, 1998).

10.6.2 Zeta Potential

Zeta potential is the electric potential difference across the ionic layer around a charged colloid ion. The charge on the surface of SLN plays an important role not only in determining the stability of prepared SLN but also define its impact over bioavailability. The surface charge can be trimmed so that the particle repels each other in a dispersed system. This enhances the shelf-life of product and can be used to modify the uptake from reticuloendothelial system. It is usually determined by zetasizer and the observed potential is termed as zeta potential (Tabatt *et al.,* 2004).

10.6.3 Drug Content Estimation

The amount of drug incorporated can be determined by this technique. In this formulated SLN are digested with suitable surfactant solution so as to separate the drug from lipid. Actual separation is confirmed by the use of ultracentrifugation/gel permeation chromatography (Fang *et al.,* 2008). After ultra-centrifugation the dense lipid settles down and drug containing supernatant fluid is filtered out. The drug content in the supernatant after suitable dilution is estimated using appropriate analytical technique i.e., UV spectrophotometry or HPLC.

10.6.4 Differential Scanning Calorimetry (DSC)

This technique is employed for ensuring the compatibility and stability of drug and lipid involved. The prepared SLN is taken in aluminium pan and exposed to a temperature range from 20-200 °C which is elevated at definite rate in an inert atmosphere of nitrogen. The temperature at which the lipid or drug will melt is recorded and reported in form of thermograms. The corresponding endothermic peaks will determine the stability and purity of SLN.

10.6.5 Fourier Transform Infrared Spectroscopy (FTIR)

It is used to determine the lipid or drug modification during the formulating period or shelf life. It mainly measures the characteristic peak shift of functional groups. Prior to test, the SLN is lyophilized, a pellet is made with potassium bromide and is allowed to scan from 4000 to 400 cm^{-1} range and corresponding absorbance is reported and interpreted from graph.

10.6.6 X-ray Diffraction

By means of X-ray scattering it is possible to assess the length of the long and short spacing of the lipid lattice. The recommendation to measure the SLN dispersion themselves is reported in literature because solvent removal can lead to structural modification. Sensitivity problems and long measurement times of conventional X-ray sources might be overcome by synchrotron irradiation (Lippacher *et al.,* 2001).

10.6.7 *In vitro* Drug Release

It is usually determined by diffusion through a dialysis tube. For the experiment, a definite volume of the SLN formulation is placed in the cellophane membrane dialysis tubing, both the ends of which are sealed and suspended in a dissolution vessel/beaker having definite volume of dissolution media at 37 ± 1 °C. The medium is stirred with the help of a stirrer at 50-100 rpm and samples are collected at predetermined time intervals. The collected volume is replaced with equal quantity of fresh dissolution media and analyzed for the amount of drug released using either UV spectrophotometry or HPLC (Acosta, 2009), (Ahlin Grabnar, 1998), (Aji Alex *et al.,* 2011).

10.6.8 Stability Studies

Stability studies are conducted as per ICH guidelines. The study is carried out in stability chamber which can provide varying temperature and relative humidity. Accelerated stability studies are conducted by keeping the samples for six months. At predetermined time interval samples are collected and analysed for amount of the drug present in the formulation.

10.7 Route of SLN Administration

A suitable route to deliver the formulated SLN is a prerequisite to obtain the desired drug release profile in order to provide the effective therapeutic benefits to patient population. The projected routes which can be used for the administration of SLN are as follows (Fig. 10.11).

10.7.1 Oral Route

This route is always preferred over other routes for drug administration. SLN can be given by this route in aqueous dispersion or in other solid oral dosage form like tablets, pellets or can be filled in the capsules. They can be used either at the place of granulating fluid to prepare the granules. They can be either spray dried or dried with the help of SCF technique in the form of powder and can be mixed with tablet powders to be compressed as tablets (Westesen and Siekmann, 1997). It can also be dispensed as soft gelatin capsules (SGC) or hard gelatin capsules (HGC) (zur Muhlen *et al.,* 1998). For SGC the SLN has to be poured in liquid PEG 600 and filled in soft capsules. Likewise it can be filled in powder form to formulate HGC. Oral route shows better therapeutic activity and enhancement in bioavailability of poorly water soluble drug for e.g., camptothecin loaded SLN shows remarkable enhancement in bioavailability when given orally (zur Muhlen *et al.*, 1996).

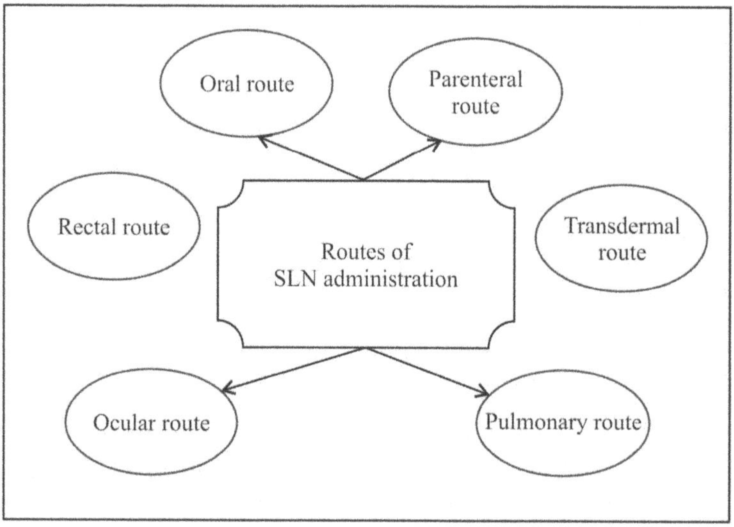

Fig. 10.11 Routes of SLN administration.

10.7.2 Topical Route

SLN has also been employed in transdermal drug delivery system (TDDS). They are mainly given *via* skin portal system and usually applied as pharmaceutical or cosmaceuticals preparations (Lippacher *et al.,* 2001). They have some unique features like ability to firmly adhere to skin in order to produce film, prevent drug from degradation and ability to modulate drug release because of which they are utilized. Apart from that the key benefit is that it can be easily registered for production and marketing aspects (Almeida and Souto, 2007).

Various drugs like retinol, coenzyme Q10, vitamin E and its derivatives are applied on skin using SLN as a carrier by various researchers. They have found a marked increase in their serum level and also demonstrated that the formulation is able to prolong the drug release. Mimicking the concept some researchers have put-forward the concept of *"Intelligent SLN" (ISLN)*, which are able to trim the drug release profile (Ahlin Grabnar, 1998).

10.7.3 Parenteral Route

SLN can also be administered *via* parenteral route. Studies have carried on stealth and non-stealth SLN for the delivery of paclitaxel on cultured macrophages (Fang *et al.*, 2008). Data revealed some surprising positive facts, that both the macrophages of liver and spleen showed slower uptake of SLN which ultimately indicate that the SLN has capacity to prolong the drug release. This particular property is useful for the delivery of anticancer drugs which needs prolonged circulation of carriers in blood in order to increase the possibility of entrapped drug reaching target site. Similarly, they have been given by intra-articular route and found that they are capable of releasing the drug inside macrophages and are able to reduce inflammation (del Pozo-Rodriguez *et al.*, 2009).

10.7.4 Pulmonary Administration

Pulmonary administration is one of the alternative routes for drug administration. SLN can be administered either in the form of aqueous suspension or in dry powder by using nebulizer. This route is mainly used for prolonged release of drug and they also ensured that after achieving therapeutic breakthrough it will degrade and dispose the by-products (Uner, 2006).

10.8 Pharmaceutical Applications of SLN

SLN have rapidly gained an indispensible position in drug delivery system. They are widely accepted and adopted by all allied field of medicines (Cavalli *et al.*, 2002). Multifarious applications of SLN can be summarized as shown in Fig 10.12.

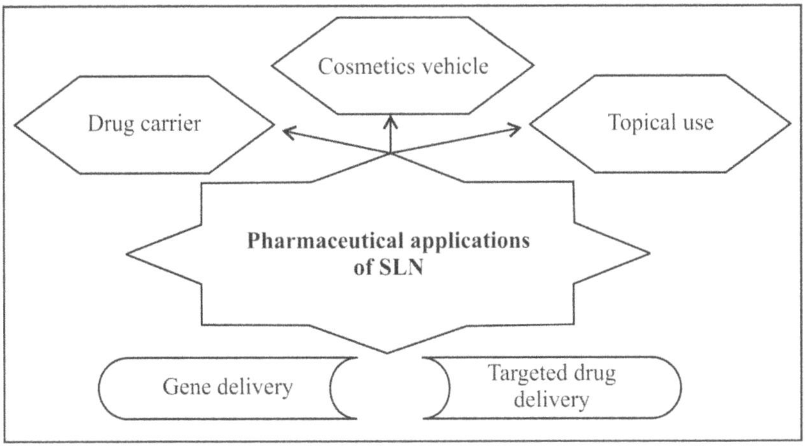

Fig. 10.12 Pharmaceutical applications of SLN.

10.8.1 Cosmetics Vehicle

SLN has appeared as a choice of preference for the delivery of not only the drug but for the application of cosmetics to skin. They are considered to be safe and efficient in crossing the stratum corneum barrier. After application of SLN dispersion the water evaporates from the surface of skin leaving behind a thin film of SLN layer which is "*occlusive*" in nature. This occlusive layer increases transdermal hydration which in turn facilitates drug permeation and also reduces drug crystallization (Alvarez-Roman *et al.,* 2004).

10.8.2 Drug Carrier

They are mainly used as drug delivery tool for various hydrophilic and hydrophobic drugs (Eldem *et al.,* 1991). They are able to deliver the drug at controlled rate and in the vicinity of target organ in order to achieve better therapeutic benefits. They have been successfully used for the delivery of various drugs including paclitaxel, methotrexate, doxorubicin and many more.

10.8.3 Gene Delivery

They can be used for the delivery of proteins, peptides or genes and DNA at cellular level. Nowadays they are assisted with acoustic i.e., ultrasonic sound in order to release the drug. By combining the two techniques much better results can be obtained (Westesen and Siekmann, 1997). SLN has capacity to deal upto molecular level and reaches inside the cancerous cells. Finally with the help of ultrasonic sound SLN release the drug and therapeutic action is achieved (Chakraborty *et al.,* 2009).

10.8.4 Targeted Delivery

SLNs are also used for the targeted drug delivery in various cases like cancer, HIV, malaria, tuberculosis and brain targeting. In general either their surface are modified or activated with some polymers so as to reach to target sites or bind to specific receptors so as to provide effect (Muller *et al.,* 2008). Generally adjuvants are used in vaccines to improve the immune response. One of the new developments in the adjuvant sector is SLN that slowly degrades to ensure prolonged exposure to the immune system. The extremely small size of SLN is beneficial for drug targeting. They have the capability to penetrate the blood- brain barrier for treating central nervous system disorders. These nanoparticles are evaluated for lymphatic uptake upon intra-duodenal administration to rats. They have also been proved to be successful in encapsulating anti tubercular drugs in tuberculosis chemotherapy (Diepold *et al.,* 1989).

Delivery of drugs to the specific organs or sites is the biggest challenge in pharmaceutical sciences. However, with the use of colloidal delivery systems like SLN, improved and precise drug delivery can be achieved. Recent studies have suggested that SLN when incorporated with essential oil from Artemisia arborescens L can be used as a convenient carrier for safe pesticides. In addition, cationic SLN are being formulated for gene transfer with the help of cationic lipids that control the *in vitro* transfection performance (Mehnert and Mader, 2001), (Jenning *et al.,* 2000).

References

Acosta E (2009). Bioavailability of nanoparticles in nutrient and nutraceutical delivery. *Current Opinion in Colloid & Interface Science* **14:** 3-15.

Ahlin Grabnar P.K.J.S.m.-K.J (1998). Optimization of procedure parameters and physical stability of solid lipid nanoparticles in dispersions. *Acta Pharmaceutica* **48:** 259-267.

Aji Alex M.R, Chacko A.J, Jose S, and Souto E.B (2011). Lopinavir loaded solid lipid nanoparticles (SLN) for intestinal lymphatic targeting. *European Journal of Pharmaceutical Sciences : Official Journal of the European Federation for Pharmaceutical Sciences* **42:** 11-18.

Almeida A.J, and Souto E (2007). Solid lipid nanoparticles as a drug delivery system for peptides and proteins. *Advanced Drug Delivery Reviews* **59:** 478-490.

Alvarez-Roman R, Naik A, Kalia Y.N, Guy R.H, and Fessi H (2004). Skin penetration and distribution of polymeric nanoparticles. *Journal of Controlled Release : Official Journal of the Controlled Release Society* **99:** 53-62.

Benita S, Friedman D, and Weinstock M (1986). Physostigmine emulsion: a new injectable controlled release delivery system. *International Journal of Pharmaceutics* **30:** 47-55.

Cavalli R, Gasco M.R, Chetoni P, Burgalassi S, and Saettone M.F (2002). Solid lipid nanoparticles (SLN) as ocular delivery system for tobramycin. *Int J Pharm* **238:** 241-245.

Chakraborty S, Shukla D, Mishra B, and Singh S (2009). Lipid-an emerging platform for oral delivery of drugs with poor bioavailability. *European Journal of Pharmaceutics and Biopharmaceutics : Official Journal of Arbeitsgemeinschaft fur Pharmazeutische Verfahrenstechnik eV* **73:** 1-15.

Del Pozo-Rodriguez A, Solinis M.A, Gascon A.R, and Pedraz J.L (2009). Short- and long-term stability study of lyophilized solid lipid nanoparticles for gene therapy. *European Journal of Pharmaceutics and Biopharmaceutics : Official Journal of Arbeitsgemeinschaft fur Pharmazeutische Verfahren-stechnik eV* **71:** 181-189.

Diepold R, Kreuter J, Guggenbuhl P, and Robinson J.R (1989). Distribution of poly-hexyl-2-cyano-[3-14C]acrylate nano-particles in healthy and chronically inflamed rabbit eyes. *International Journal of Pharmaceutics* **54:** 149-153.

Eldem T, Speiser P, and Hincal A (1991). Optimization of spray-dried and -congealed lipid micropellets and characterization of their surface morphology by scanning electron microscopy. *Pharmaceutical Research* **8:** 47-54.

Fang J.Y, Fang C.L, Liu C.H, and Su Y.H (2008). Lipid nanoparticles as vehicles for topical psoralen delivery: solid lipid nanoparticles (SLN) versus nanostructured lipid carriers (NLC). *European Journal of Pharmaceutics and Biopharmaceutics: Official Journal of Arbeitsgemeinschaft fur Pharmazeutische Verfahrenstechnik eV* **70:** 633-640.

Gasco M.R (1993). Method for producing solid lipid microspheres having a narrow size distribution (Google Patents).

Jenning V, Mader K, and Gohla S.H (2000). Solid lipid nanoparticles (SLN) based on binary mixtures of liquid and solid lipids: a (1)H-NMR study. *Int J Pharm* **205:** 15-21.

Kang K.W, Chun M.K, Kim O, Subedi R.K, Ahn S.G, Yoon J.H, and Choi H.K (2010). Doxorubicin-loaded solid lipid nanoparticles to overcome multidrug resistance in cancer therapy. *Nanomedicine : Nanotechnology, Biology, and Medicine* **6:** 210-213.

Kaur I.P, Bhandari R, Bhandari S, and Kakkar V (2008). Potential of solid lipid nanoparticles in brain targeting. *Journal of Controlled Release : Official Journal of the Controlled Release Society* **127:** 97-109.

Kuo Y.C, and Chen H.H (2009). Entrapment and release of saquinavir using novel cationic solid lipid nanoparticles. *Int J Pharm* **365:** 206-213.

Lippacher A, Muller R.H, and Mader K (2001). Preparation of semisolid drug carriers for topical application based on solid lipid nanoparticles. *Int J Pharm* **214:** 9-12.

Magenheim B, Levy M.Y, and Benita S (1993). A new *in vitro* technique for the evaluation of drug release profile from colloidal carriers - ultrafiltration technique at low pressure. *International Journal of Pharmaceutics* **94:** 115-123.

Mehnert W, and Mader K (2001). Solid lipid nanoparticles: production, characterization and applications. *Advanced Drug Delivery Reviews* **47:** 165-196.

Muller R.H, Mader K, and Gohla S (2000). Solid lipid nanoparticles (SLN) for controlled drug delivery - a review of the state of the art. *European Journal of Pharmaceutics and Biopharmaceutics : Official Journal of Arbeitsgemeinschaft fur Pharmazeutische Verfahrenstechnik eV* **50:** 161-177.

Muller R.H, Runge S.A, Ravelli V, Thunemann A.F, Mehnert W, and Souto E.B (2008). Cyclosporine-loaded solid lipid nanoparticles (SLN): drug-lipid physicochemical interactions and characterization of drug incorporation. *European Journal of Pharmaceutics and Biopharmaceutics : Official Journal of Arbeitsgemeinschaft fur Pharmazeutische Verfahrenstechnik eV* **68:** 535-544.

Muller R.R, S (1998). Solid lipid nanoparticles (SLN) for controlled drug delivery. (Amsterdam: Harwood Academic Publishers.).

R G.M (1993). Method for producing solid lipid microspheres having a narrow size distribution, U.s. patent, ed. (US: Gasco Maria R).

Runge S, Mehnert W, and Muller R.H (1996). SLN (Solid Lipid Nanoparticles), A Novel Formulation for the oral administration of drugs. *European Journal of Pharmaceutical Sciences* **4:** 132-132.

Scheffel U, Rhodes B.A, Natarajan T.K, and Wagner H.N, Jr. (1972). Albumin microspheres for study of the reticuloendothelial system. *Journal of Nuclear Medicine : Official Publication, Society of Nuclear Medicine* **13:** 498-503.

Schwarz C, and Mehnert W (1999). Solid lipid nanoparticles (SLN) for controlled drug delivery. II. Drug incorporation and physicochemical characterization. *Journal of Microencapsulation* **16:** 205-213.

Serpe L, Canaparo R, Daperno M, Sostegni R, Martinasso G, Muntoni E, Ippolito L, Vivenza N, Pera A, Eandi M, *et al.,* (2010). Solid lipid nanoparticles as anti-inflammatory drug delivery system in a human inflammatory bowel disease whole-blood model. *European Journal of Pharmaceutical Sciences : Official Journal of the European Federation for Pharmaceutical Sciences* **39:** 428-436.

Souto E.B, and Muller R.H (2006). The use of SLN and NLC as topical particulate carriers for imidazole antifungal agents. *Die Pharmazie* **61:** 431-437.

Tabatt K, Kneuer C, Sameti M, Olbrich C, Muller R.H, Lehr C.M, and Bakowsky U (2004). Transfection with different colloidal systems: comparison of solid lipid nanoparticles and liposomes. *Journal of Controlled release : Official Journal of the Controlled Release Society* **97:** 321-332.

Uner M (2006). Preparation, characterization and physico-chemical properties of solid lipid nanoparticles (SLN) and nanostructured lipid carriers (NLC): their benefits as colloidal drug carrier systems. *Die Pharmazie* **61:** 375-386.

Westesen K, and Siekmann B (1997). Investigation of the gel formation of phospholipid-stabilized solid lipid nanoparticles. *International Journal of Pharmaceutics* **151:** 35-45.

Ye J, Wang Q, Zhou X, and Zhang N (2008). Injectable actarit-loaded solid lipid nanoparticles as passive targeting therapeutic agents for rheumatoid arthritis. *Int J Pharm* **352:** 273-279.

zur Muhlen A, Schwarz C, and Mehnert W (1998). Solid lipid nanoparticles (SLN) for controlled drug delivery-drug release and release mechanism. *European Journal of Pharmaceutics and Biopharmaceutics : Official Journal of Arbeitsgemeinschaft fur Pharmazeutische Verfahrenstechnik eV* **45:** 149-155.

zur Muhlen A, zur Muhlen E, Niehus H, and Mehnert W (1996). Atomic force microscopy studies of solid lipid nanoparticles. *Pharmaceutical Research* **13:** 1411-1416.

11

Niosomes Mediated Drug Delivery

J.G. Meher[1], M. Chaurasia[2] and Manish K. Chourasia[1]

[1]Pharmaceutics Division, CSIR-Central Drug Research Institute, Lucknow-226031, India.

[2]Amity Institute of Pharmacy, Amity University, Lucknow-226028, India.

11.1 Introduction

Vesicular drug delivery systems are among the effective tools in delivering therapeutically active drug molecules. As evident from literature, liposomes are very much efficient in transporting both lipophilic as well as hydrophilic drugs. The lipophilic bilayers and the aqueous core are responsible in holding as well as transporting active ingredients (almost all BCS-class) to the target site (Elsayed *et al.,* 2007). Presently several therapeutic agents like amphotericin B (Lambin, AmBisome), daunorubicin (DaunoXome), vincristine (Marqibo), doxorubicin (Doxil, Caelyx) are used clinically in liposomal form. Natural and/or synthetic phospholipids are the major constituents for formulation of liposomes, but the limitations are their high cost and poor stability. From pharmaceutical and regulatory point of concern stability is an important issue, whereas cost-effectiveness is the need of manufacturing industries. Hydrolysis (ester bonds in phospholipids) and oxidation (unsaturated double bonds in phospholipids) are the foremost cause of liposomal instability and often seen due to improper storage. Fusion, sedimentation or alterations in the bilayer structure adversely affect the liposome formulations while chemical changes associated with the phospholipids (deacylation) are also chief reasons of failure in lipid based vesicular formulations. Apart from these technical problems the high cost of phospholipids has encouraged research for alternative methods/tools in vesicular drug delivery.

In 1970s researcher started investigating substitutes to liposomes which can address both the stability and economic matters. Vanlerberghe and group in 1972 for the first time reported an alternative to liposomes as a non-ionic vesicular system (niosomes) for cosmetic use (Vanlerberghe *et al.,* 1972). Later, niosomes for skin moisturizing and tanning products were reported in *International journal of cosmetics* by Handjani-Vila *et al.,* as an useful tool for delivery of active substances to the skin (Handjani-Vila *et al.,* 1979). Better penetration into stratum corneum and lower toxicity further encouraged to explore niosomes in drug delivery research. Since then niosomes have considerably attracted researchers over the globe and a large number of scientific texts are generated in last few decades. Niosomes are concentric bilayers of non-ionic amphiphilic substances (surfactants) in aqueous medium. In order to be in the most stable form, the amphiphiles arrange themselves as the concentric bilayers in aqueous environment, which is also termed as self-assembly of surfactants. The hydrophobic tails face each other, whereas the hydrophilic heads remain in contact with the water, consequently developing a bilayer. The development of bilayers is a spontaneous process (sometimes need input of energy), where amphiphiles attempt to decrease high energy hydrophobic-hydrophilic interactions (hydrophobic tail of amphiphiles and water) and increase low energy hydrophilic-hydrophilic (hydrophilic head of amphiphiles and water) interactions. Figure 11.1 exhibits the diagrammatic representation of niosomes and building block of niosomes; an amphiphile molecule (sorbitan ester).

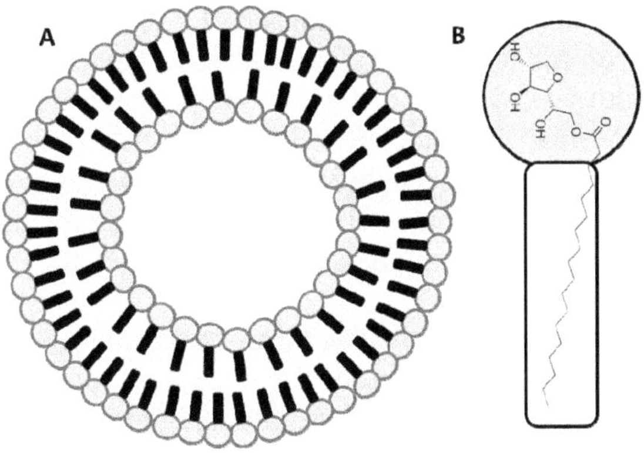

Fig. 11.1 Diagrammatic representation of niosomes.

A. Concentric bilayer of niosomes in aqueous environment; hydrophobic tails shielded away from aqueous phase and hydrophilic head oriented towards aqueous phase.
B. Building block of niosomes; an amphiphile (sorbitan ester) with hydrophilic head (dark color) and hydrophobic tail (light color).

The basic components of niosomes are non-ionic surfactants, cholesterol, drug molecules and other charged molecules. The size of niosomes varies in a wide range measuring few nanometers to several micrometers and shape may be of different types. Conventional niosomes are spherical in nature because of the spatial orientation of amphiphiles in aqueous media, but by varying the amphiphiles composition, vesicles of different shapes (disc, polyhedral) can also be developed. The shape of niosomes not only depends on the amphiphiles, but additives, method of formulation and physicochemical properties of drug molecules to be entrapped also play an important role. Vesicular aggregations are seen very often with niosomes and molecules such as the cholesteryl poly(oxyethyleneether)-Solulan or the ionic molecule dicetyl phosphate is used to achieve steric and electrostatic stabilization. Many drug delivery complications related to bioavailability, solubility, stability, targetability, spatial and temporal control of drug and much such kind of huddles can be resolved through niosomal drug delivery systems.

In the further sections of this chapter reader will come across a brief description of route of niosomal administration. As the use of non-ionic surfactants is abundant in pharmaceutical and food industries, there is no dilemma in administration of niosomes by oral or topical route. In topical route it may either be transdermal or ocular. As niosomes are homologous to liposomes, the formulation and characterization are to some extent similar. Some of the popular methods of preparation, characterization are discussed in details. Several factors such as effect of non-ionic surfactant structure, cholesterol, temperature, membrane additives, pH of the hydration medium, surfactant and lipid amount, encapsulated drug as well as method of preparation are highlighted in context of niosomal formulations. The competence of niosomes to manage the supply of entrapped moiety within the body for drug delivery, diagnostic imaging and vaccine delivery has also been narrated in details.

11.1.1 Classification

There are no strict criteria for classifying niosomes but many kinds of niosomes are reported in literature viz. elastic niosomes, proniosomes, discomes, aspasomes, surfactant ethosomes and bola niosomes (Manosroi *et al.,* 2013). A brief description of different niosomes is discussed below.

11.1.1.1 Elastic Niosomes

Niosomes are elastic in nature due to the inherent nature of surfactant molecules but elastic niosomes as the name explains, exhibit additional elastic properties. These are composed of non-ionic surfactant, water and ethanol. These vesicles are capable of passing through pores of diameter less than (up to 10 times) the vesicle size. Because of this specific characteristic, elastic niosomes are capable of passing the intact skin through stratum corneum. The first detergent-based elastic or deformable niosomes are prepared by using surfactant L-595 (sucrose laurate ester) and the micelle forming surfactant PEG-8-L (octaoxyethylene laurate ester). The mechanism of transportation of elastic niosomes are believed to be concentration independent and driven by transepidermal hydration (Chen *et al.,* 2013).

11.1.1.2 Proniosomes

The physical stability issues of niosomes are resolved by the conceptualization of proniosomes. These are dry form of niosomes and usually reconstituted to give a fine dispersion immediately before use. It is composed of non-ionic surfactant, carrier and drug molecules. Vesicular aggregation, fusion, alteration of vesicular shape which are frequently observed in conventional niosomes are overcome by proniosomes (Sankar *et al.,* 2010). Topically applied proniosomes, under occlusive conditions gets converted to niosomes due to hydration by water in the skin itself. Many drug molecules viz. ketoprofen and estradiol have been therapeutically found to be effective upon niosomal drug delivery.

11.1.1.3 Discomes

Discomes are also known as polyhedral or giant vesicles (Uchegbu *et al.,* 1992). These are morphologically disc shaped and larger vesicles up to 25-100 μm in size. Discomes were reported by Uchegbu *et al.,* that the addition of Solulan C24 to hexadecyl diglycerol ether niosomes resulted in the development of mixed micelles. Solulan C24 at 20-40 mole percent concentrations tends to develop giant vesicles (discomes). These giant polyhedral vesicles are capable to entrap water soluble solutes.

11.1.1.4 Aspasomes

Aspasomes are composed of acorbyl palmitate, cholesterol and highly charged lipid diacetyl phosphate. These vesicles are hydrated with aqueous solution and then sonicated to get the niosomes. Aspasomes can be used to increase the transdermal permeation of drugs. It has inherent antioxidant property.

11.1.1.5 Surfactant Ethosomes

Ethosomes are the lipoidal vesicular systems containing high quantity of ethanol. Surfactant ethosomes are the vesicular systems containing non-ionic surfactants, water and high quantity of ethanol or isopropyl alcohol. Surfactant ethosomes exhibit deeper penetration into the skin through pores of stratum corneum. The mechanism of enhanced permeation is hypothesized to be due to the increase in trans-epidermal hydration by high concentration of alcohol.

11.1.1.6 Bola Surfactant Niosomes

Omega-hexadecyl-bis-(1-aza-18 crown-6) are known as Bola surfactants. Niosomes composed of Omega-hexadecyl-bis-(1-aza-18 crown-6) and span-80/cholesterol in 2 : 3 : 1 molar ratio are known as Bola surfactants niosomes. These are efficient in crossing the lipoidal barrier of skin. Both hydrophilic and hydrophobic drugs can be accommodated in these niosomes.

11.1.2 Advantages and Disadvantages

Every drug delivery system has its own advantages and disadvantages. Advantages in-term of scientific subject is of prime concern for successful delivery as well as stability, at the same time optimization must be accomplished with respect to several other factors related to trade and economy (industrial prospects). Table 11.1 enlists an account of advantages and disadvantages of niosomal drug delivery systems.

Table 11.1 An account of advantages and disadvantages of niosomal drug delivery systems.

S. No.	Advantages	Disadvantages*
1.	Ability to incorporate both hydrophilic and hydrophobic drug molecules	Aggregation/coalescence of surfactants
2.	Sustained, controlled and targeted drug delivery can be achieved	Sedimentation or fusion of vesicles
3.	Biocompatible, biodegradable and non-immunogenic to body	Phase separation upon any change in temperature or pH
4.	Comparatively cheaper than other vesicular drug delivery systems (liposomes, phyto-somes) as non-ionic surfactants are less costlier than phospholipids	Hydrolysis of entrapped drug molecule
5.	Better stability (comparatively less chances of hydrolysis and oxidation)	
6.	Reduced toxicity of potent drugs	
7.	Enhanced penetration of poorly soluble/bio-available drug molecules	

*These disadvantages are observed in aqueous suspension of niosomes

11.1.3 Root of Administration

For any drug delivery, the route of administration is forever being a point of apprehension. As the route of drug administration directly governs the patient compliance, stability (protection against enzymatic, acidic degradation) as well as efficacy of drug delivery systems, utmost emphasis is paid on this area of research. Niosomes as a vesicular drug delivery can be administered through oral, intravenous and topical routes. In oral and intravenous route it might be given as either oral suspension or emulsion formulations. Topically, niosomes may be administered as gels, creams, emulsions, suspensions, films/patches through ocular and transdermal routes.

11.1.3.1 Oral

Oral route is the most preferred one in delivery of drugs due to many advantages primarily patient compliance. Many niosomes formulations have been administered through this route and found to be therapeutically more effective than conventional formulations. Niosomes containing griseofulvin, rifampicin, acyclovir and methotrexate exhibit increase in oral bioavailability than conventional dosage forms. Proficient delivery of mannosylated nonionic surfactant containing plasmid DNA encoding small subunit proteins of hepatitis B virus have been developed for oral immunization. Sustained delivery of drug can be achieved through the niosomes as these vesicles act as drug reservoir. Enzymatic/acidic degradations and fist pass metabolisms are the major limitations in oral route of administration of niosomes.

11.1.3.2 Transdermal

Lipoidal architecture of skin is the main barrier for transdermal delivery of drugs. Preferably penetration enhancers are used for the effective administration of drugs through any transdermal drug delivery device. Niosomes by their inherent amphiphilic characteristics can easily pass through the phospholipid bilayers of skin. Under occlusive conditions, topically applied proniosomes get converted to niosomes due to hydration by water in the skin itself. The mechanism of enhanced permeation is supposed to be due to the increase in transepidermal hydration. Aceclofenac, meloxicam, estradiol and cyclosporine showed increased permeation through transdermal route in the niosomal formulations. Hydrophobic as well as amphiphilic drugs can be successfully administered through transdermal route. Figure 11.2 diagrammatically represents the interaction of phospholipid bilayers of skin and the niosomes. As clearly depicted in Figure 11.2, niosomes which are composed of non-ionic surfactant (sorbitan ester) and cholesterol interact with each other by hydrogen bonding to frame the structural block (bilayers) of niosomes. Further it is attempted to show the interaction of the phospholipid bilayer with the cholesterol molecule of niosomes facilitating the deeper penetration of the niosomes to skin (phospholipids).

11.1.3.3 Ocular

Sustained release (zero order kinetic) delivery is achieved by drug delivery systems based on niosomes. In the treatment of eye diseases/infection like glaucoma, keratitis such delivery is useful. Prolonged period of drug release at the corneal surface also prevents the unwanted enzymatic metabolism of the drug molecules. Many drugs viz. timolol, ofloxacin, brimonidine, acetazolamide, gentamicin, acyclovir are therapeutically more effective in niosomal than conventional formulations.

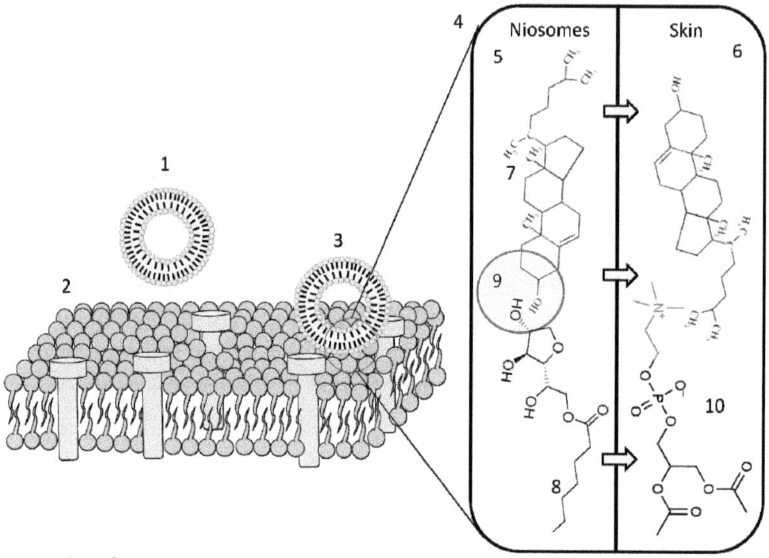

1. niosomes,
2. phospholipid bilayer of skin,
3. niosomes in contact with phospholipid bilayer of skin,
4. magnified representation of interaction between niosomes and phospholipid bilayer of skin at molecular level,
5. enlarged representation of niosomes,
6. representation of skin using amplified image,
7. cholesterol,
8. sorbitan ester,
9. interaction of cholesterol and sorbitan ester in niosomes,
10. cholesterol and phospholipid (lipid content) of skin.

Fig. 11.2 Diagrammatic representation showing interaction of niosomes and phospholipid bilayers of skin.

11.2 Materials used in Niosomes Preparation

The essential components of niosomes formulations are non-ionic surfactants, membrane additives and water. Drug molecules and their physicochemical properties are also important in the formulation and development of niosomes. In this section the readers will be receptive to the different raw materials used in niosomes formulation.

11.2.1 Non-ionic Surfactants

Non-ionic surfactants are chief component of niosomes. These ingredients are usually less irritating, less toxic and less hemolytic to cells and also uphold physiological pH in solution. Functionally they act as permeability enhancers, solubilizers, emulsifiers and wetting agents. As already mentioned non-ionic surfactants form bilayers in aqueous environment and can accommodate both hydrophilic and lipophilic drug molecules. These surfactants also have useful property in enhancing drug absorption by inhibiting action of P-glycoprotein (which transports a wide variety of substrates across extra- and intracellular membranes) because high intestinal expression of P-glycoprotein can diminish the absorption of many drug molecules leading to reduced bioavailability and poor therapeutic effect. Critical packing parameters (CPP), HLB and chain length are important parameters in the formation of niosomes.

The following formula is used for the calculation of CPP.

$$\mathrm{CPP} = \frac{\mathrm{v}}{l_c \times \mathrm{a}_o}$$

v = hydrophobic group volume, l_c = critical hydrophobic group length, a_0 = area of the hydrophilic head group.

Theoretically CPP below 0.5 favors formation of micelles, CPP between 0.5-1.0 forms spherical vesicles and inverted micelles are developed when CPP is greater than 1.0. Surfactants of higher HLB value (14-18) do not favor formation of niosomes but comparatively lower HLB (7-9) give niosomes with the maximum entrapment efficiency. As the HLB scale decreases from 8 to 1, entrapment efficiency reduces. A brief account of different non-ionic surfactants used in the formulation of niosomes is enlisted in Table 11.2.

Table 11.2 Raw materials (excipients) used in the formulation of niosomes.

Raw materials	Category	Examples	Descriptions
Non-ionic surfactants	Alkyl ethers and alkyl glyceryl ethers	Polyoxyethelene-lauryl ether, Polyoxyethylene-cetyl ethers, Polyoxyethylene stearyl ethers (BRIJ series)	These surfactants are stable, non-irritant to the skin and compatible with other surfactants. Compatibility of these surfactants with other drugs must be checked before formulation. Alkyl ethers are widely used in the formulation of niosomes.
	Sorbitan fatty acid esters	Sorbitan monooleate, sorbitan monostearate, sorbitan monolaurate etc. (SPAN series)	These surfactants are very much efficient in accommodating fixed and essential oils. In combination with cholesterol their encapsulation efficiency increases. These surfactants are preferably employed in the formulation of niosomes.
	Polyoxyethylene fatty acid esters	Polyoxyethylene sorbitan monooleate, Polyoxyethylene sorbitan monostearate, Polyoxyethylene Sorbitan monolaurate etc. (TWEEN series)	These surfactants are polysorbates, more specifically PEGylated sorbitan esterified with fatty acids. These surfactants might have incompatibility with phenolic contents/drugs. In combination with other surfactants such as SPAN/BRIJ, the encapsulation efficiency increases.
Additives	Cholesterol	Cholesterol	Cholesterol increases rigidity, encapsulation efficiency, fine dispersion and rehydration of pro-niosomes. It also checks aggregation/fusion of vesicles by the addition of other molecules that stabilize the system.

Table 11.2 *Contd...*

Raw materials	Category	Examples	Descriptions
	Charged molecules	Diacetyl phosphate, phosphatidic acid, steary-lamine, stearyl pyridinium chloride	Increase stability of niosomes by electrostatic repulsion which prevents coalescence, fusion or aggregation.
Dispersion/ Hydration medium		Phosphate buffers	Phosphate buffer at various pHs is used as dispersion or hydration medium for preparation of niosomes

11.2.2 Additives

Apart from non-ionic surfactants, other additives are also frequently used in the formulation and development of niosomes such as cholesterol and other charged molecules. Without these additives it is difficult to formulate a stable niosomes formulation. Briefly these additives are discussed below.

11.2.2.1 Cholesterol

Cholesterol is used as one of the membrane manipulating additives in niosomes. Of course it has no role to play in the development of bilayers/ self-assembly, but it can effectively interfere with the permeability, fluidity, and rigidity as well as encapsulation efficiency of niosomes. It is well known that the skin is composed of phospholipids and cholesterol contributes a small fraction of skin total lipid content. The presence of cholesterol in niosomes thus facilitates penetration into deeper skin layer. Being incorporated in the bilayers of surfactant molecules, it regulates the rigidity of niosomes. Cholesterol is also useful in inclusion of other charged molecules that enhance the overall stability of niosomes (Devaraj *et al.*, 2002).

11.2.2.2 Charged Molecules

In the advantages and disadvantages section we have seen many shortcomings of niosomes in the dispersion state. In order to avoid such situations, pro-niosomes concept was developed. After reconstitution/ hydration of pro-niosomes a fine dispersion of niosomes in the hydration medium is obtained, but the chances of fusion, aggregation or coalescence may not be avoided. In such situation it is always preferable to use any charged molecules (depending upon the niosomes formulation) so that the niosomes will be in fine dispersion state due to electrostatic repulsion. Caution must be taken in the use of these charged molecules because these might interfere in the formation of niosomes. Measurement of zeta-potential of the niosomes should be the evaluating parameters in employing the charged molecule for stability of the system. Incorporation of charged molecule takes care of stability of niosomes. A few examples are enlisted in Table 11.2.

11.2.3 Dispersion Medium

As previously discussed, pro-niosomes are now-a-days preferred than niosomes to achieve better stability. In order to disperse the pro-niosomes to form niosomes, different dispersion media are used. Buffers of different pH are used for this purpose, which depends on the solubility of the drug(s) entrapped in the niosomes. Table 11.2 enlists some of the preferred buffers used in the formulation of niosomes.

11.3 Methods of Preparation of Niosomes

For the preparation of niosomes various methods are reported. Even though some of these methods are realized in the industrial setup but these are primarily suitable for laboratory scale. Scale up is an important step from laboratory to manufacturing plant, in bringing these niosomes to the market. Some of the popular methods in formulation of niosomes are discussed below (Arunothayanun *et al.,* 1999).

11.3.1 Reverse Phase Evaporation Method

In the reverse phase evaporation method, the surfactants, lipids and organic solvent is mixed together, at the other end the aqueous solvent and drug (water soluble) is mixed separately. Both the phases are homogenized under reduced pressure to get the niosomes (Figure 11.3). This is one of the easiest methods for the formulation of niosomes. Many drug molecules can be accommodated in niosomes by this method. Reverse phase evaporation method is schematically presented below.

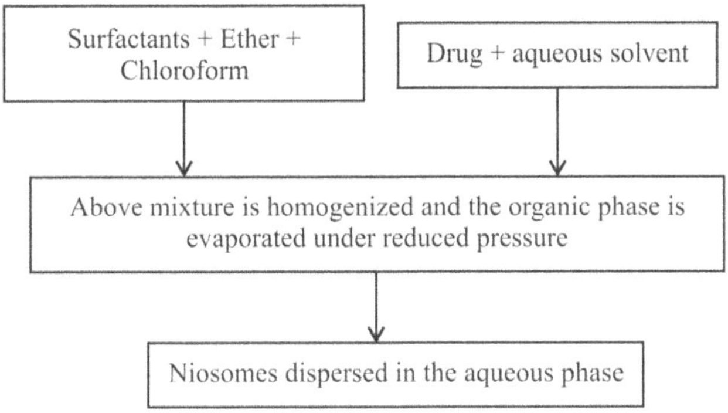

Fig. 11.3 Formulation of niosomes by reverse phase evaporation method.

11.3.2 Ether Injection Method

Ether injection method is a useful method of niosomes' formulation. As exhibited in the flowchart, aqueous phase is added to the mixture of lipid, surfactant, drug and organic solvent. The above mixture is heated above the boiling point of the organic solvent, to evaporate the same. Larger niosomes are formed in the aqueous medium, which might be subjected to size reduction (Figure 11.4).

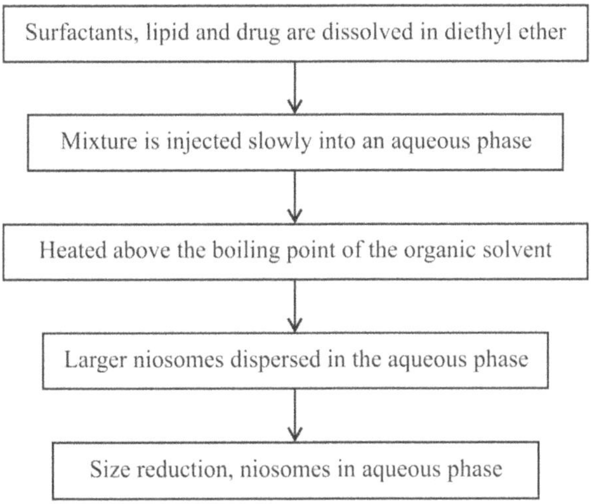

Fig. 11.4 Basic steps involved in ether injection method for preparation of niosomes

11.3.3 Trans-membrane pH Gradient Method

In this method first of all a thin film of surfactant and cholesterol is prepared by evaporation under reduced pressure condition. Then the film is hydrated with buffer. This hydrated mixture is passed through freeze-thaw cycle and finally aqueous solution of drug is added and properly mixed. For the adjustment of pH, additional buffer may be added (Figure 11.5).

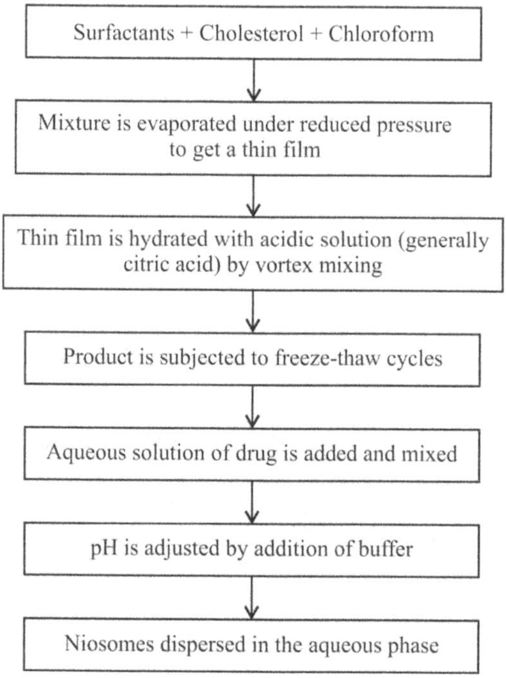

Fig. 11.5 Trans-membrane pH gradient method.

11.3.4 Sonication Method

Sonication method is one of the widely used methods for the formulation of niosomes. The dispersed surfactants and lipid is subjected to sonication for a specific period of time and niosomes are formed as uni/ multilamellar vesicles (Figure 11.6).

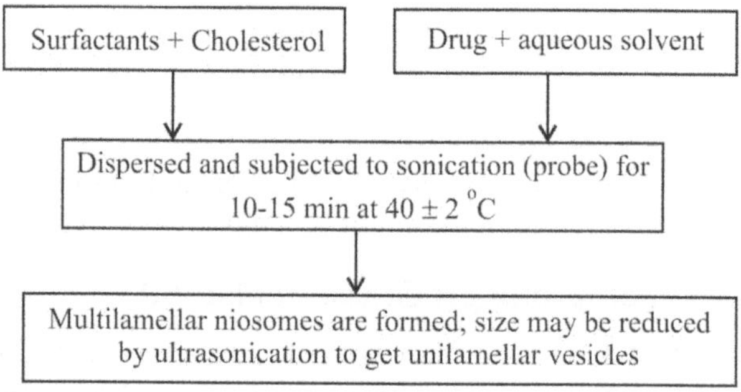

Fig 11.6 Scheme showing sonication methods for the formulation of niosomes.

11.3.5 Lipid Layer Hydration Method

Similar to the trans-membrane pH gradient method, a thin film of lipids and surfactants is formed. The aqueous solution of drug is added to the thin film and is subjected to constant agitation. Temperature above the phase transition temperature of surfactant is maintained for a specified period of time in order to get niosomes dispersed in the aqueous medium.

11.3.6 Bubbling of Nitrogen Method

In some scientific texts, bubbling of nitrogen method is reported. Initially the surfactants are homogenized for required time. Then nitrogen gas is passed through these surfactants mixture to get the large unilamellar vesicles. In-order to get the desired size, these vesicles may be subjected to size reduction using techniques such as sonication. As the method involves use of nitrogen, any reaction with either drug or other excipients must be ensured before.

11.3.7 Extrusion Method

In extrusion method, a thin film of surfactants and lipid is prepared and hydrated with buffer. After hydration the mixture is extruded through polycarbonate membrane multiple times to get uniform sized niosomes (Figure 11.7).

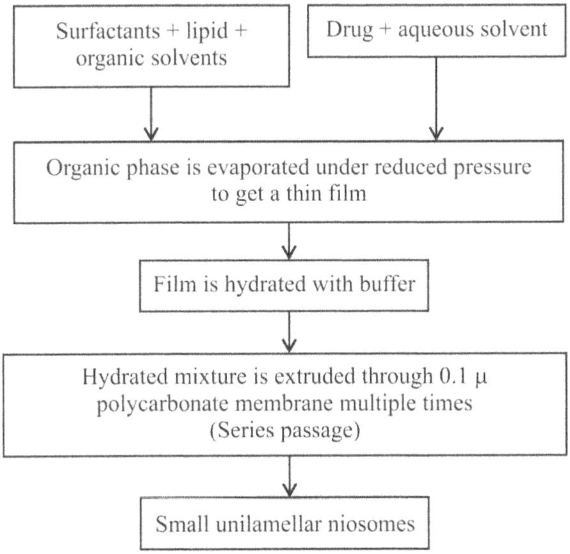

Fig. 11.7 Flowchart illustrating extrusion method for the formulation of niosomes.

11.3.8 Hand Shaking Method

This is primarily a laboratory method but not preferred now-a-days. It involves the formulation of thin lipid-surfactant layer by rotary evaporation method, which is further hydrated with buffer containing drug by continuous shaking. The vesicles are formed after adequate swelling.

11.3.9 High Pressure Homogenization

The principle of high pressure homogenization is adopted for the formulation of niosomes. Both the drug and surfactants are interacted in the fluidized state with very high velocity in the interaction chamber. The mixture is then passed through a cooling loop to reduce the heat generated during high pressure homogenization. It is again returned to the reservoir for recirculation. The process is continued until vesicles of the uniform size are produced (Figure 11.8).

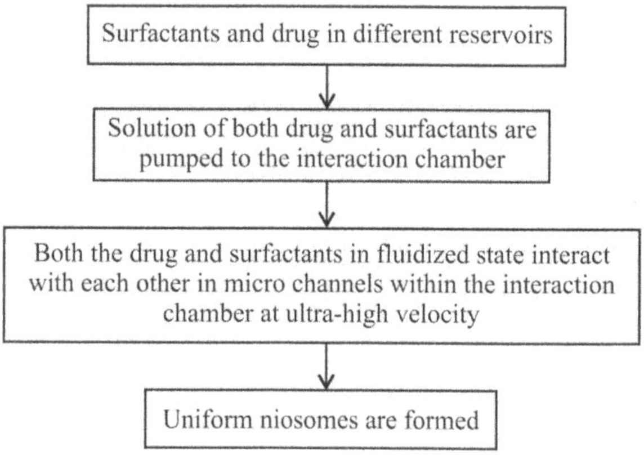

Fig. 11.8 High pressure homogenization method for the formulation of niosomes.

11.4 Characterization

Any vesicular systems (niosomes, liposomes) are characterized for their size, shape, surface characteristics and electrical potential (thermo-dynamic stability). Further from pharmaceutical aspects vesicles may be characterized for *in vitro-in vivo* drug release, toxicity, entrapment efficacy, physical stability as well as therapeutic efficacy (Pando *et al.,* 2013).

11.4.1 Size, Shape and Surface Morphology

Niosomes are in nanometer range so high magnification and resolution techniques are used to evaluate the size, shape, lamellarity and overall morphology. Advanced microscopic techniques such as optical microscopy, scanning electron (SEM) and transmission electron microscopy (TEM), atomic force microscopy (AFM), cryo-electron, fluorescence and confocal microscopy are widely used to investigate the size and shape of niosomes (Mehta and Jindal, 2013).

Size (mean diameter), size distribution and zeta potential of the niosomes are determined by particle size analyzer such as zeta/master/metasizer which are based on dynamic light scattering principles. TEM is one of the versatile techniques to determine the size, shape as well as lamellarity of niosomes. In this technique appropriately diluted sample is adsorbed onto a grid with carbon-coated formvar film. Excess sample is blotted off and the grid is covered with a small drop of staining solution (uranyl acetate/phosphotungstic acid). This staining is called as the negative staining. It is left on the grid for few minutes and excess solution is drained off. The grid is allowed to dry thoroughly in air before examined in the transmission electron microscope. SEM is another useful technique that shows the surface morphology of the niosomes. Here the sample is fixed on stubs and coated with gold palladium with the help of a gold sputter module in a high vacuum evaporator. Sample is then analyzed using secondary electron imaging. The shape and the morphological characteristics such as fracture, leaky area and improperly formed niosomes may be visualized through the highly resolute micrograph. Other techniques such as confocal microscopy and AFM are also used for these purposes. AFM facilitates to examine samples with sub-nanometer resolution in three dimensions. Intermittent contact mode AFM allows the examination of samples with least sample alteration. Phase imaging permits evaluation of information ahead of the sample's topography and force spectroscopy experiments allow understanding the intrinsic structure by recording the elastic/adhesion behavior. Readers are encouraged to grasp much information on the different microscopic analytical tools through many peer reviewed articles available in scientific text.

Confocal microscopy is one of the advanced techniques in visualizing nano and micro particulate systems. In confocal microscopy, a single diffraction-limited point at the focal plane is illuminated. Due to the optical configuration of lenses with pinholes, confocal microscopy displays improved resolution compared to other microscopy techniques.

Stage scanning, beam staining and tandem staining are the different scanning designs in confocal microscopy. Latest technologies are used in the processing of confocal images either during or after acquisition. The 3D re-construction presents a clear picture of the spatial arrangement of the vesicles. Different optical slices can be observed and different angle of view of the niosomes can be analyzed by processing the images with software.

11.4.2 Vesicle Charge

Aggregation and/or fusion are common problems encountered in formulation and development of niosomes, hence charged molecules are employed for the purpose of stabilization. The charge developed on these niosomes is measured as zeta-potential of the system. Henry's equation is applied in the determination of zeta potential.

$$\mu E = \frac{2\varepsilon z f(ka)}{\eta}$$

Where, μE = Electrophoretic mobility, ε = Dielectric constant, z = Zeta potential, $f(Ka)$ = Henry's function, η = Viscosity

The values of zeta-potential are usually preferable in the range of 30 to 50 mV (both positive and negative). Depending upon the formulations as well as drug entrapped in the niosomes, other charged molecules are used to alter zeta-potential of the niosomes. The instruments which are used to measure zeta potential include zetasizer and laser doppler micro-electrophoresis. With zetasizer, the sample is placed in a quartz cuvette and size measurement is generally performed at a scattering angle of 90°. In case of laser doppler micro-electrophoresis, an electric field is applied to a dispersion of particles (solution of molecules), which travel with a specific velocity. This velocity, which is related to the zeta-potential, is measured and further used in the calculation of electrophoretic mobility. From the electrophoretic mobility, the zeta potential of the system is calculated (Henry's equation).

11.4.3 Entrapment Efficiency (EE)

EE is one of the crucial parameters to be determined in any vesicular or particulate formulation. Entrapment of drug at high level is always desirable in formulation and development of novel drug delivery systems. EE is the actual amount of drug entrapped in the niosomes in comparison to the total amount of drug added in the formulation. It can be denoted by the following formula

$$EE = D_E / D_A \times 100$$

Where, D_E = amount of drug entrapped in niosomes

D_A = total amount of drug added

For estimation of EE, the unentrapped or free drug is separated from the niosomal formulation by sephadex mini column centrifugation or ultracentrifugation. The vesicles free from un-entrapped drug are lysed and drug content is determined using suitable analytical technique.

11.4.4 *In vitro* Drug Release

As there is no official method available in the text (pharmacopoeia, regulatory guidelines), so the *in vitro* drug release is performed by different methods reported by researchers. One of the widely used methods for this purpose is membrane dialysis method. Here dialysis membrane (commercially available in different molecular weight cut off range) is activated before conducting the test. After activation of the membrane, an accurately weighed amount of formulation is placed in the membrane and tied at both the end to give it a shape of a bag. This bag is further dipped in the buffer media (dissolution medium of the drug) and subjected to dissolution study. The dissolution study may be carried out in a locally assembled dissolution setup (magnetic stirrer with hot plate). Periodically sample is withdrawn from the dissolution media, replaced with equal quantity of fresh media and analyzed by appropriate analytical technique. Physicochemical characteristic of the drugs like heat, light sensitivity need to be considered during release study and suitable measures are to be taken to prevent drug degradation. Figure 11.9 represents a diagrammatic view of *in vitro* drug release study using niosomes.

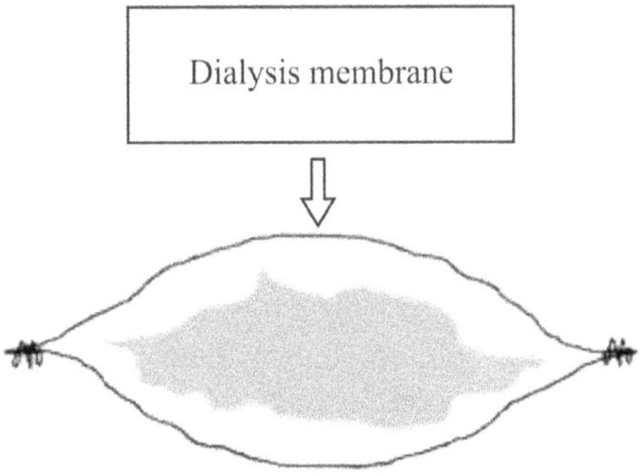

Prepared dialysis membrane bag containing niosomes

(a)

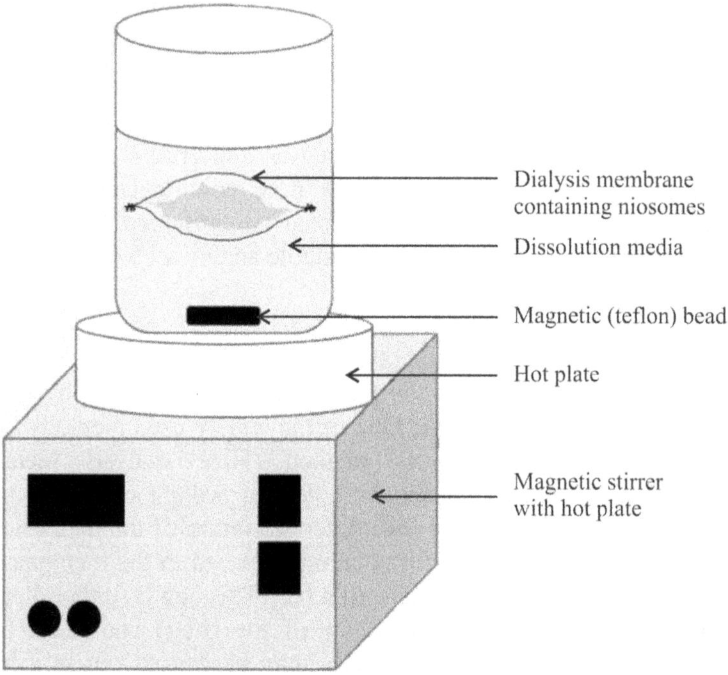

(b)

Fig. 11.9 (a) Dialysis membrane and preparation of dialysis membrane bag containing niosomes, (b) *In vitro* drug release setup for dissolution test of niosomes.

11.4.5 *In vitro* Toxicity

Before performing the *in vivo* studies for therapeutic activity as well as toxicity, *in vitro* toxicity studies are performed. This is in accordance to the animal cruelty act 1960, that any formulations cannot be directly administered in animals before ensuring *in vitro* safety. *In vitro* cell lines for both animal as well as human are available commercially, which are used for this purpose (Palozza *et al.,* 2006).

11.4.6 *In vivo* Studies

The final stage in the pre-clinical evaluation of niosomes is the *in vivo* studies of the developed formulation. Any *in vivo* studies may be for toxicity or activity evaluation of the niosomal formulation. The excipients/ingredients used in the formulation of niosomes are of Generally Recognized as Safe (GRAS) grade, but still there are chances of contamination/degradation which may cause harm to the users. In order to ensure safety, toxicity studies are conducted in animal models as per the guidelines of different recognized agencies such as institutional ethical committee, The Organization for Economic Co-operation and Development (OECD) (Martínez *et al.,* 2011) and Food and Drug Administration (FDA) (Stumpf, 2007), International Conference on Harmonization (ICH). Pharmacological and therapeutic activity of the formulation is also evaluated in the animal models as per the regulatory guidelines.

11.4.7 Stability

There have always been apprehensions over the stability of novel formulations like liposomes, niosomes and other lipids based systems. It was considered that such formulations have space and utility in laboratory only. However with the advent of liposomal formulations in the market bias has changed regarding commercial viability and utility of such systems. For the stability evaluation, niosomes are subjected to different accelerated and conventional stability testing. ICH guidelines for the stability testing are followed and certain parameters are evaluated at definite time intervals and compared with the original data. There are two types of stability evaluation viz. long term and accelerated stability testing. In long term stability testing niosomes formulations are kept at 5 ± 3 °C for 12 months. Samples are drawn at 0, 3, 6, 9 and 12th month time intervals and evaluated for stability. In the accelerated stability evaluation, formulations are kept at 30 ± 2 °C/65 ± 5% RH for 6 months and are evaluated for stability at 0, 3 and 6th months. Size, shape, morphology, charge and EE are the evaluation parameters to be checked during the stability studies. Any significant change in the above mentioned parameters are taken seriously and formulation is redeveloped (Mehta *et al.,* 2011).

11.5 Factors affecting the Preparation of Niosomes

In this section readers will come across the key factors that influence the formulation of niosomes. These factors include the method of preparation, surfactants and other excipients, pH, temperature, drug molecule and hydration medium. Variation in different evaluation parameters viz. size, shape, morphology, EE and stability is observed with the change in the above mentioned factors (Mokhtar *et al.,* 2008).

11.5.1 Method of Preparation

Many methods for the formulation of niosomes are narrated in the previous section of this chapter. These methods are different in various aspects such as ease, economy, EE, stability, size and shape. The hand shaking method is comparatively less efficient than other methods such as ether injection, high pressure homogenization and trans-membrane pH gradient methods with respect to the size and shape of niosomes. The reasons might be the specific and mechanical process utilized in the later methods whereas in hand shaking method the same is not achieved. Smaller and unilamellar niosomes are developed by high pressure homogenization technique as it is one of the sophisticated methods (Zidan *et al.,* 2011). Drug entrapment also differs with different method of niosomes formulation. The process variables involved in these methods of formulation are responsible for the variation in resulted niosomal formulations. The process variables are volume of excipient and drug, method of addition of excipients and aqueous phase, temperature and rotation speed in case of rotary evaporation method.

11.5.2 Effect of Excipients

Non-ionic surfactant, cholesterol and charged molecules are different excipients used in the formulation of niosomes. These excipients have significant effect on the development of niosomes. As already mentioned in the earlier part of this chapter, CPP, HLB and chain length are important parameters in the preparation of niosomes. CPP is very much specific to the surfactant which depends on the volume of hydrophilic and hydrophobic content, whereas each surfactant has a unique HLB which determines the development of niosomes in aqueous environment. The second important excipient used in niosomes is cholesterol. Details of this excipient have been discussed earlier in this chapter. In order to prevent the aggregation, fusion or coalescence, charged molecules are also added to the niosomes which act by the mechanism of charge repulsion and ensure stability (Devaraj *et al.,* 2002).

11.5.3 Effect of Temperature

Temperature and surfactants have an integral relation with respect to either emulsification or vesicle formation. As in case of emulsification, adequate temperature is required and beyond or below that temperature emulsification does not take place, similarly in case of niosomes formation, temperature plays an important role. The temperature should be more than the gel to liquid phase transition temperature of the system. Very high temperature negatively affects the vesicles formation. At different temperature the shape and size of niosomes also change. Usually it is observed that at low temperature polyhedral shaped niosomes are formed whereas at comparatively high temperature spherical niosomes are developed. Reason behind such changes in the size and shape may be attributed to the different energy state and arrangement of the surfactant molecules in the aqueous environment.

11.5.4 Effect of pH of the Dispersion Medium

pH of the dispersion medium is crucial in the development of niosomes. pH has got direct relation to the intactness (unionized form) of the drug. The EE of any drug molecule is directly related to its unionized form i.e., high EE is seen when the drug is in unionized form. As and when the drug gets converted to the ionized (at specific pH) form EE decreases. One of the classical examples in this case is EE of ibuprofen at acidic pH (pH 5.5) which shows a maximum encapsulation efficiency of 94.6%. With the increase in pH (towards base) of the dispersion medium the EE decreases. So the optimum encapsulation of drug to niosomes depends upon the pH of hydration/dispersion medium.

11.5.5 Effect of Encapsulated Drug

In the above section the effect of pH is discussed where the ionized and unionized form of drug plays important role in EE of niosomes. From this it is clear that drug's physicochemical properties such as dissociation constant (*pKa*), solubility, melting point, log *p*, molecular weight as well as crystalline/amorphous state influence its EE in niosomes. Specific mechanisms are involved in each of the mentioned parameters in entrapment of drug in niosomes. Quantity of drug also affects the entrapment efficiency into the niosomes. Depending upon the characteristics of drug molecules, the excipient for the formulation of niosomes is chosen. If the drug is water soluble then hydrophilic surfactant may be of interest and vice versa. However a combination /blend of surfactants is also preferred in niosomes formulation. The compatibility of the drug and excipient must be checked prior to the formulation. Any incompatibility issue may later cause degradation or instability of the developed niosomes. Compatibility of drug-excipient may be evaluated by DSC, X-Ray diffraction, NMR and FRIR analysis.

11.6 Applications

Niosomes as a novel drug delivery have wide applications. The applications may be with respect to the therapeutic efficacy by increasing targetability or by increasing the physicochemical characteristics of drug molecules. The basic aim of formulation scientists to enhance the therapeutic efficacy of drug is resolved to a major extent by the development of niosomes. It is already proved to be successful in the laboratory but yet to be realized at the commercial scale.

11.6.1 Controlled/Sustained Drug Delivery

Achievement of sustained and/or controlled drug delivery is the art of manipulating therapeutic activity of drugs. Need of such delivery arises based on the physicochemical properties (less $t_{1/2}$) or requirement of prolonged/targeted delivery of drugs. Entrapment of both hydrophilic and hydrophobic drug in the surfactant bilayers and further sustained release is possible using niosomes. The drug depending upon its partition co-efficient gets released from niosomes and becomes available to the target site for therapeutic action. Amount of surfactants and other additives such as cholesterol control the release of drug from the vesicles. Targeting of drug is also possible by niosomes because of their small size and inherent lipophilic characteristics. Small size and flexible shape facilitates the entry of these niosomes utilizing the enhanced permeability and retention (EPR) effect seen in the cancer tissue. Attachment of different ligands to the niosomes allows targeting of drugs to the specific receptor. So in a nutshell niosomes can be utilized in the sustained/controlled and targeted drug delivery of therapeutic agents (Mahale *et al.*, 2012).

11.6.2 Modulation of Physicochemical Characteristics of Drug

Many drug molecules have poor solubility or penetrability to skin or even poor oral bioavailability. By the formulation of niosomes some of these characteristics of drug molecule are improved. Because of the lipoidal nature of niosomes the penetrability of the drug loaded to niosomes increases. It has also been investigated and reported that the oral bioavailability of drugs like acyclovir, peptide, griseofulvin and ergot alkaloid increases in the niosomal drug delivery systems.

11.6.3 Transdermal Delivery

It is very difficult for many drug molecules to cross the lipid bilayers of skin. Because of the specific bilayer arrangement of phospholipid, skin prevents entry of any xenobiotics. The major barrier of the skin is the stratum corneum, the top most layer of the epidermis. Low molecular weight ($\leq$ 500 Da) and lipophilicity are desirable characteristics in transdermal drug delivery. Niosomes because of its lipoidal nature interact well with phospholipid bilayer of skin and act as a carrier of drug in to the skin (Manosroi *et al.*, 2010). The presence of cholesterol in the niosomes also facilitates the skin-niosome interaction and enhances penetration. Figure 11.2 represents the transdermal application of niosomes. Anti-inflammatory, analgesic, NSAID, antiseptic, antioxidant as well as anti-rheumatic drugs can be delivered suitably as niosomes through transdermal route. Elastic niosomes are novel vesicles and of special interest for transdermal delivery.

11.6.4 Pulmonary Delivery

Delivery of drug through the pulmonary route is being a difficult task for researchers. This route exhibits obstacles due to the hydrophilic mucosa. Niosomes prepared by the hydrophilic non-ionic surfactants has been used to enhance the therapeutic efficacy of drug. Due to the hydrophilic nature the niosomes interact well with the pulmonary mucosal layer and release drug for a sustained period of time. Niosomes of beclomethasone dipropionate is developed for the treatment of asthma. Similarly other drugs in the treatment of chronic obstructive pulmonary disease are developed as niosomal delivery system (Manosroi *et al.,* 2012).

11.6.5 Treatment of Infectious Disease

Infectious diseases such as leishmaniasis, tuberculosis, yellow fever, malaria and others are serious health problem. Drugs in the treatment of such diseases usually show unwanted adverse effects. In order to reduce the adverse effects, drug targeting approach is adopted as discussed in the previous section. Drug molecule like amphotericin B is successfully designed, developed and now clinically available as vesicular drug delivery system. The therapeutic efficacy of drugs is significantly improved by such approaches. Niosomes formulation of many drugs in the treatment of infectious disease is developed and therapeutically found to be more effective than conventional drug delivery (Mehta and Jindal, 2013).

11.6.6 Ophthalmic Delivery

Certain drugs need to be delivered through the ophthalmic route for the purpose of sustained and site specific release. Niosomes are proposed as an ocular delivery system for drugs to delay precorneal residence time and increase corneal uptake. Niosomes can be administered or instilled conveniently onto the surface of the eye as drops. Discomes, a type of non-conventional niosomes better fit in the cul-de-sac of the eye and improve ocular drug bioavailability due to slower nasolacrimal drainage. Disruption of the tight junctions of the corneal epithelium is believed to be responsible for increasing corneal uptake whereas better spreading of lipophilic niosomes on the corneal surface are other reason for better therapeutic effect (Abdelkader *et al.,* 2012).

11.6.7 Vaccine Delivery

Vaccine delivery system should be a simple and stable formulation that can be easily administered to the patient and could provide lifetime immunity against a specific pathogen. There is a number of infectious diseases viz. malaria and HIV for which no effective vaccine is available also there are example of disease such as tuberculosis, whooping cough for which existing vaccines provide insufficient immunity. Niosomes has shown promising efficacy in vaccine delivery e.g., subcutaneous vaccination of mice with purified gp63 entrapped in niosomes, induced partial resistance against *L. mexicana* infection (Badiee *et al.,* 2013).

11.6.8 Protein and Peptide Delivery

The delivery of protein, peptides to the blood circulation through oral route is obstructed by several hurdles, including proteolytic enzymes, pH gradients as well as low epithelial permeability. Niosomes are successfully developed and evaluated at the pre-clinical level for different proteins and peptides viz. bovine serum albumin, alpha-interferon, GnRH-based anti-fertility immunogen, haemagglutinin, influenza viral antigens, insulin and luteinizing hormone releasing hormone. Polyoxyethylene alkyl ether type of non-ionic surfactants can be used for preparation of insulin entrapping niosomes for better therapeutic efficacy (Pardakhty *et al.,* 2007).

11.6.9 Cancer Chemotherapy

Anticancer drugs are well known for their side effects. The prime aim is to increase the targetability of the drug to reduce side effects. In cancer tissues EPR effect is seen, which can be used to achieve site specific delivery of anticancer drugs. Because of the leaky vasculature at these area niosomes can easily get entry into the tumor tissue. More specifically grafting of ligand molecule (folic acid, antibody or other ligands) on the niosomes achieves cellular drug delivery of anticancer drugs. 5-fluorouracil, doxorubicin and many other anticancer drug molecules are successfully developed and pre-clinically evaluated for anticancer activity (Paolino *et al.,* 2008).

11.7 Future Prospects

Increasing stability and achieving scalability of vesicular as well as particulate drug delivery systems are the current needs in novel drug therapy. The story of AmBisome®, DOXIL® and other marketed formulations have witnessed the successful journey of novel drug delivery systems from laboratory to the market. Such achievements in novel drug delivery are signs of encouragement in realizing drug delivery at industrial scale. Niosomal formulations have potential to be a successful product with the added advantages of low cost and better stability. If it could be developed at the industrial scale, many pharmacokinetic issues of concerns associated with drug molecules (especially chemotherapeutic drugs) will be shorted out. The key strategies for successful niosomal formulations include employment of generally recognized as safe (GRAS) excipients (surfactants) in preparation of niosomes, use of upgradable/scalable manufacturing techniques, and compliance of regulatory guidelines as well as achieving stability as per ICH norms.

References

Abdelkader H, Ismail S, Hussein A, Wu Z, Al-Kassas R, and Alany R.G (2012). Conjunctival and corneal tolerability assessment of ocular naltrexone niosomes and their ingredients on the hen's egg chorioallantoic membrane and excised bovine cornea models. *International Journal of Pharmaceutics* **432:** 1-10.

Arunothayanun P, Uchegbu I.F, Craig D.Q.M, Turton J.A, and Florence A.T (1999). *In vitro/in vivo* characterisation of polyhedral niosomes. *International Journal of Pharmaceutics* **183:** 57-61.

Badiee A, Heravi Shargh V, Khamesipour A, and Jaafari M.R (2013). Micro/nanoparticle adjuvants for antileishmanial vaccines: Present and future trends. *Vaccine* **31:** 735-749.

Chen J, Lu W.L, Gu W, Lu S.S, Chen Z.P, and Cai B.C (2013). Skin permeation behavior of elastic liposomes: role of formulation ingredients. *Expert Opin Drug Deliv* **35(7):** 1704-16.

Devaraj G.N, Parakh S.R, Devraj R, Apte S.S, Rao B.R, and Rambhau D (2002). Release Studies on Niosomes Containing Fatty Alcohols as Bilayer Stabilizers Instead of Cholesterol. *Journal of Colloid and Interface Science* **251:** 360-365.

Elsayed M.M.A, Abdallah O.Y, Naggar V.F, and Khalafallah N.M (2007). Lipid vesicles for skin delivery of drugs: Reviewing three decades of research. *International Journal of Pharmaceutics* **332:** 1-16.

Handjani-Vila R.M, Ribier A, Rondot B, and Vanlerberghie G (1979). Dispersions of lamellar phases of non-ionic lipids in cosmetic products. *Int J Cosmet Sci* **1:** 303-314.

Mahale N.B, Thakkar P.D, Mali R.G, Walunj D.R, and Chaudhari S.R (2012). Niosomes: Novel sustained release nonionic stable vesicular systems - An overview. *Advances in Colloid and Interface Science* **183-184:** 46-54.

Manosroi A, Chankhampan C, Manosroi W, and Manosroi J (2013). Transdermal absorption enhancement of papain loaded in elastic niosomes incorporated in gel for scar treatment. *European Journal of Pharmaceutical Sciences* **48:** 474-483.

Manosroi A, Khanrin P, Lohcharoenkal W, Werner R.G, Götz F, Manosroi W, and Manosroi J (2010). Transdermal absorption enhancement through rat skin of gallidermin loaded in niosomes. *International Journal of Pharmaceutics* **392:** 304-310.

Manosroi A, Ruksiriwanich W, Abe M, Manosroi W, and Manosroi J (2012). Transfollicular enhancement of gel containing cationic niosomes loaded with unsaturated fatty acids in rice (Oryza sativa) bran semi-purified fraction. *European Journal of Pharmaceutics and Biopharmaceutics* **81:** 303-313.

Martínez C.E, Pamies D, Sogorb M.A, and Vilanova E (2011). Chapter 10 - OECD guidelines and validated methods for *in vivo* testing of reproductive toxicity. In Reproductive and Developmental Toxicology, C.G. Ramesh, ed. (San Diego, Academic Press), pp. 123-133.

Mehta S.K, and Jindal N (2013). Formulation of Tyloxapol niosomes for encapsulation, stabilization and dissolution of anti-tubercular drugs. *Colloids and Surfaces B: Biointerfaces* **101:** 434-441.

Mehta S.K, Jindal N, and Kaur G (2011). Quantitative investigation, stability and *in vitro* release studies of anti-TB drugs in Triton niosomes. *Colloids and Surfaces B: Biointerfaces* **87:** 173-179.

Mokhtar M, Sammour O.A, Hammad M.A, and Megrab N.A (2008). Effect of some formulation parameters on flurbiprofen encapsulation and release rates of niosomes prepared from proniosomes. *International Journal of Pharmaceutics* **361:** 104-111.

Palozza P, Muzzalupo R, Trombino S, Valdannini A, and Picci N (2006). Solubilization and stabilization of β-carotene in niosomes: delivery to cultured cells. *Chemistry and Physics of Lipids* **139:** 32-42.

Pando D, Gutiérrez G, Coca J, and Pazos C (2013). Preparation and characterization of niosomes containing resveratrol. *Journal of Food Engineering* **117:** 227-234.

Paolino D, Cosco D, Muzzalupo R, Trapasso E, Picci N, and Fresta M (2008). Innovative bola-surfactant niosomes as topical delivery systems of 5-fluorouracil for the treatment of skin cancer. *International Journal of Pharmaceutics* **353:** 233-242.

Pardakhty A, Varshosaz J, and Rouholamini A (2007). *In vitro* study of polyoxyethylene alkyl ether niosomes for delivery of insulin. *International Journal of Pharmaceutics* **328:** 130-141.

Sankar V, Ruckmani K, Durga S, and Jailani S (2010). Proniosomes as drug carriers. *Pak J Pharm Sci* **23:** 103-107.

Stumpf W.E (2007). Memo to the FDA and ICH: appeal for *in vivo* drug target identification and target pharmacokinetics: Recommendations for improved procedures and requirements. *Drug Discovery Today* **12:** 594-598.

Uchegbu I.F, Bouwstra J.A, and Florence A.T (1992). Large disk-shaped structures (discomes) in nonionic surfactant vesicle to micelle transitions. *The Journal of Physical Chemistry* **96:** 10548-10553.

Vanlerberghe G, Handjani-Vila R.-M, Berthelot C, and Sebag H (1972). Chemistry, physical chemistry and Anwendunggstechnik cross-active substances. In Reports from Vi International Congress for surface-active agents (Carl Hanser Verlag, Zurich).

Zidan A.S, Rahman Z, and Khan M.A (2011). Product and process understanding of a novel pediatric anti-HIV tenofovir niosomes with a high-pressure homogenizer. *European Journal of Pharmaceutical Sciences* **44:** 93-102.

12

Microparticles as Drug Delivery Systems

J.G. Meher and Manish K. Chourasia

Pharmaceutics Division, CSIR-Central Drug Research Institute, Lucknow-226031, India.

12.1 Introduction

Drug delivery science is growing at its full swing by keeping pace with first-hand expansion in multi-disciplinary sciences. Advancement in combinatorial chemistry, high throughput/content screening, biotechnology, virtual screening and genomics-proteomics, the major mainstays in drug discovery have produced a wide variety of new, potent and target specific therapeutics/new chemical entities. These new therapeutics are better than the older drugs but at the same time they exhibit many physicochemical shortcomings especially low solubility, and/or poor stability on storage (Drews, 2000; Lipinski *et al.,* 1997). Such physicochemical hitches (poor bioavailability/stability of anticancer, antileishmanial, antitubercular drugs etc.) are also encountered with many older drugs that are already existing in the market in different dosage forms (Adler-Moore and Proffitt, 2002; Pham *et al.,* 2013). Overall such complications lead to the decrease in therapeutic efficacy and increase in undesirable effects, particularly in chemotherapeutics. In such scenario augmenting therapeutic efficacy and achieving required storage stability have been the primary objectives of professionals involved in health care research. Augmentation of therapeutic action may be achieved by *Spatial* (related to position/space) and/or *temporal* (related to time) control in delivering therapeutic agents. A major success has been achieved in this regard since last couple of decades at laboratory scale as evident from a large number of research publications and patents. Vesicular (liposome, niosomes, phytosomes etc.) and particulate (nano-, micro-particles etc.) drug delivering tools are experimentally found to be over-the-hill in this endeavor (Muthu *et al.,* 2012; Owens III and Peppas, 2006).

As and when these competent delivery systems are attempted to be manufactured at industrial scale, many interfering factors come to the picture viz. regulatory requirement, scale up at bulk, and economy of the product/project. Regulatory constrain in terms of (i) use of generally recognized as safe (GRAS) excipients, (ii) the allowable quantity of excipients, (iii) avoidance of using fancy excipients (excipients not having a significant function) as well as (iv) filling the product to different regulatory authorities for approval, and many such kind of issues are mandatorily addressed for new products. Similarly, many process variables in manufacturing and packaging as well as transporting play major hindrance in development of drug delivery systems. Additionally, other important aspects that come on the way of developing the therapeutics into novel drug delivery systems is the economy of product and patient compliance. Pharmaceutical industries pay serious attention in this field and estimate the market size as well as economic viability of the product to be developed.

Overcoming these impediments, many pharmaceutical industries as well as research laboratories have come up with various novel drug delivery systems as medicine (dosage forms) and medical devises (Benita, 2005). When it comes to see the developed delivery systems and advancement in drug delivery since last few decades, *microparticles/ microencapsulation-technology* seems to hold a luminary position in comparison to other delivery systems. The market size of microspheres was estimated to be $2 billion in 2010 and projected to be $3.5 billion by 2015 (Lipovetskaya, 2010).

Spatial and *temporal* modulation of drug molecules for better therapeutic effect could be achieved at an industrial measure through microparticulate drug delivery system. Microparticles (1-1000 μm diameter) are used in drug delivery, cosmetics and personal care products, which can encapsulate a variety of drugs including small molecules (hydro-/lipo-philic), proteins, and nucleic acids etc. Biocompatibility, higher bioavailability, and proficiency of sustained release of drugs are some of the attractive features in microparticles drug delivery (Mathiowitz *et al.,* 1997). There are numerous medicines available in market in a variety of dosage form as microparticles. A brief account of these medicines are depicted in Table 12.1. Microparticles technology is a successful model both in research and trade, and this chapter brings about the fine points of microparticles comprising preformulation, formulation, characterization, scale up, route of administration, factors influencing microspheres, applications as well as the future potential.

Table 12.1 A brief account of medicines in market as microparticles (www.drugs.com).

Name of product	Drug	Ingredients/ Excipients	Indication
Lupron Depot® (lyophilized microspheres as injectable suspension)	Leuprolide acetate [gonadotropin-releasing hormone (GnRH) agonist]	Biodegradable copolymer of lactic and glycolic acids (PLGA)	Treatment of advanced prostate cancer
Nutropin Depot® (micronized particles as injectable suspension)	Somatropin (rDNA origin) [long acting dosage form of recombinant human growth hormone (rhGH)]	Biodegradable polylactide coglycolide	Long term treatment of growth failure due to lack of adequate endogenous growth hormone secretion
Tretinoin gel, USP (porous microspheres in aqueous gel)	Tretinoin (member of the retinoid family of compounds, and a metabolite of naturally occurring Vitamin A)	Methyl methacrylate/ glycol di-methacrylate cross-polymer	Topical treatment of acne vulgaris
Arestin®	Minocycline hydrochloride (Broad-spectrum tetracycline antibiotic)	Bio-resorbable polymer PLGA	As adjunct to scaling and root planning procedures for reduction of pocket depth in patients with adult periodontitis
Optison (microspheres injectable suspension)	Perflutren Protein-Type A	Human serum albumin, N-acetyltry-ptophan, Caprylic acid in 0.9% aqueous sodium chloride	Contrast agent (Making the heart easier to see during a certain diagnostic procedure)

Table 12.1 *Contd...*

Name of product	Drug	Ingredients/ Excipients	Indication
Risperdal® Consta® (extended-release microspheres for injection)	Risperidone (Atypical antipsychotic drug)	PLGA	Prescribed in schizophrenia and symptoms of bipolar disorder (manic depression)
Zoladex® (injectable implant containing microparticles)	Goserelin acetate (GnRH agonist)	D,L-lactic and glycolic acids copolymer	Management of locally confined Stage T2b-T4 carcinoma of the prostate
Trelstar LA, (lyophilized biodegradable micro-granule)	Triptorelin pamoate (GnRH agonist)	PLGA copolymer, mannitol, carboxymethylcellulose sodium, polysorbate 80	Palliative treatment of advanced prostatic cancer
Bydureon (extended-release microsphere formulation)	Exenatide (Antidiabetic drug, glucagon-like peptide-1 agonist)	PLGA copolymer, sucrose	Treatment of Type 2 diabetes
Vivitrol® (extended-release injectable microsphere suspension)	Naltraxone (opioid receptor antagonist)	PLGA copolymer, carboxymethylcellulose sodium salt, polysorbate 20, sodium chloride	Treatment of alcohol dependence, opioid dependence
Sandostatin LAR (depot injectible available as powder microspheres for suspension)	Octreotide acetate (octapeptide that mimics natural somatostatin)	PLGA, Mannitol	Treatment of acromegaly, relieve stomach or bowel symptoms associated with gastroentero-pancreatic tumors, neuroendocrine tumors located in the gut

12.1.1 A Brief History of Microparticles

Microparticles as encapsulation system was introduced by H.G. Bungenberg de Jong (Dutch chemist) in 1932 and he had used the term *coacervate* (from the Latin words acervus: mass) to describe droplets containing a colloid. Later in 1953, the first commercial product using microencapsulation technique was carbonless copy paper developed by L. Schleicher and B. Green. In 1960s, for the first time the idea of controlled release from polymers by utilizing silicone rubber and polyethylene was discussed by Folkman and Long (1964). This concept was not that much successful due to lack of degradability of polymers in these systems and surgical removal was the only way to overcome this problem. The next demand in controlled release delivery was for biodegradable polymers and in the 1970s these types of polymers were proposed as suitable drug delivery ingredients sidestepping the surgical operation in removing the non-degradable polymer (Jalil and Nixon, 1990). A step ahead in this field of research, the idea of polymer microcapsules as delivery systems was reported in the early 1960s by Chang (1964) and co-worker. First pharmaceutical application of microcapsule was patented in 1970 by W.M. Holliday and co-worker. The patented product was a sustained release formulation of acetylsalicylic acid encapsulated in a thin coating of ethyl cellulose (Holliday *et al.,* 1970). Smith (1986) had demonstrated the use of poly (lactic acid) as biodegradable delivery system in parenteral administration. Progressively a large number of research work were reported in different journals as a potential drug delivery system. These original research were also complied periodically by reviewers and readers are encouraged to study these reviews for more information on different aspects like targetability, drug loading/entrapment, disease area, immunogenicity/biocompatibility as well as bulk scale manufacture potential (Freiberg and Zhu, 2004; Jalil and Nixon, 1990; Kawaguchi, 2000; Muller *et al.,* 2001).

12.1.2 Types of Microparticles

Broadly microparticles are categorized as microcapsules and microspheres based on the structure and internal construction. Microparticles where the active pharmaceutical ingredients (API) is homogeneously dispersed in the raw polymer matrix is termed as microsphere, whereas microparticles designed with a central core of API (solid, liquid or gas) is designated as microcapsule (Campos *et al.,* 2013). Microparticles may also be categorized on the basis of any specific function. Interestingly it has been noticed that many researchers use the term microspheres synonymously with microparticles, which might be due to the over shading popularity and viability of microspheres in comparison to microcapsules. Table 12.2 enumerates a systematic classification of microparticles on the above outlines. Fig. 12.1 diagrammatically presents the structure and internal construction of microcapsules and microspheres. It is shown in the figure that polymeric microcapsule is containing Minocycline (API) in the core coated by the outer PLGA polymer (PLGA, Minocycline) and the polymeric microspheres containing homogeneously dispersed Minocycline in the matrix of PLGA polymer. The API may be incorporated as a central core or even in micro/nano capsular manner inside a microcapsule. Similarly in case of microspheres the API may be homogeneously dispersed or even incorporated as a micro/nano-capsular dispersion. Fig. 12.2 and 12.3 show the illustrative representation of microcapsules and microspheres respectively.

Table 12.2 Classification of microparticles based on structure and function.

Based on structure		
Category	**Description**	**Example**
Microcapsules	The drug material is inside the core of a polymeric coat. It is a reservoir type system.	Chitosan microcapsules containing 5-Flurouracil for anticancer activity (Yan *et al.*, 2012) PVA engineered microcapsules for targeted delivery of camptothecin to HeLa cells (Galbiati *et al.*, 2011)
Microspheres	The drug material is uniformly dispersed in the polymeric matrix.	BSA microspheres containing Taxol for anticancer activity (Grinberg *et al.*, 2007) Porous large PLGA microspheres adsorbed with palmityl-acylated exendin-4 as a long-acting inhalation system for treating diabetes (Kim *et al.*, 2011)
Based on function		
Polymeric	The microparticles are made up of biodegradable and biocompatible polymers.	Alginic acid and PLGA biodegradable microspheres for controlled delivery of paracetamol and protein at different stages from core-shell (Wang *et al.*, 2010) Erythromycin-loaded biodegradable gelatin microspheres (Wang *et al.*, 2008)
Mucoadhesive	These are the polymeric microparticles but with additional advantages of mucoadhesion.	Acyclovir-loaded mucoadhesive microspheres with ethyl-cellulose as matrix and Carbopol 974P NF as mucoadhesive polymer (Tao *et al.*, 2009) Mucoadhesive microspheres of HPMC containing gentamicin sulfate for nasal administration (Hasçiçek *et al.*, 2003)

Table 12.2 *Contd...*

Based on structure		
Category	**Description**	**Example**
Floating	These are polymeric microparticles with floating properties.	Ranitidine hydrochloride loaded floating microspheres fabricated with ethyl-cellulose and polyethylene glycol blend (Saravanan and Anupama, 2011) Floating alginate microspheres containing diltiazem hydrochloride in combination with calcium carbonate as gas-forming agent (Ma *et al.*, 2008)
Magnetic	In magnetic micro-particles, particles of magnetite (Fe_3O_4) is incorporated, which is guided by an external magnetic field after administration.	Monodispersed cross-linked superparamagnetic poly(St-AA)/Fe_3O_4 microspheres with carboxyl group for adsorption on BSA (Liu *et al.*, 2014) Magnetic polylactic acid micro-spheres containing curcumin for sustained release (Li *et al.*, 2011)
pH-responsive	These are polymeric microparticles which release drug at specific pH.	Acrylamide-modified chitin based fast responsive pH sensitive micro-spheres containing vancomycin for controlled drug release (Shang *et al.*, 2014) pH-responsive composite micro-spheres of cross-linked poly (methacrylic acid) containing doxorubicin hydrochloride for tumor targeting (Wen *et al.*, 2013)
Based on function		
Category	**Description**	**Example**
Thermo-sensitive	These are polymeric microparticles which release drug at specific temperature.	N-isopropylacrylamide grafted ther-mo-responsive gelatin microspheres loaded with diclofenac sodium as delivery systems (Curcio *et al.*, 2010) Thermo-responsive super-hydro-phobic TiO_2/poly(N-isopropyla-crylamide) microspheres as drug delivery system (Chen *et al.*, 2012)

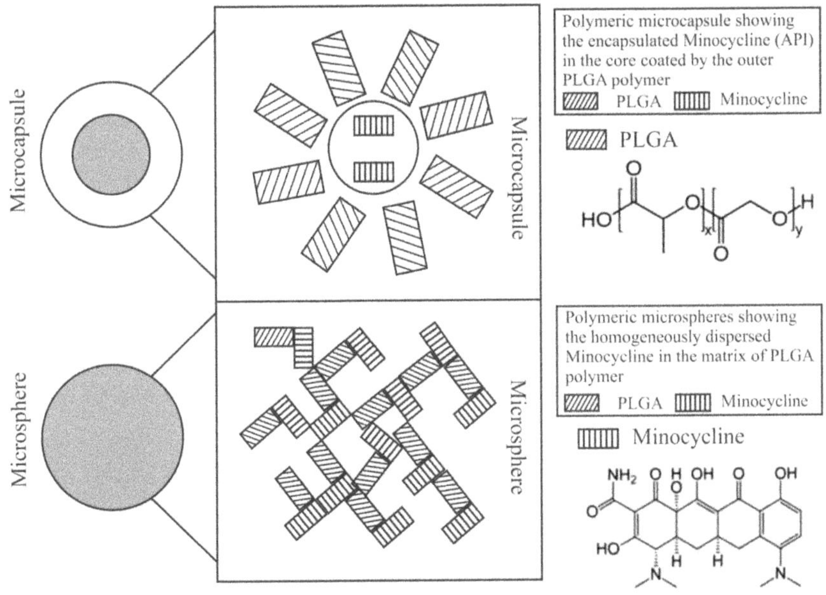

Fig. 12.1 Diagrammatic representation of microparticles and their magnified molecular orientation.

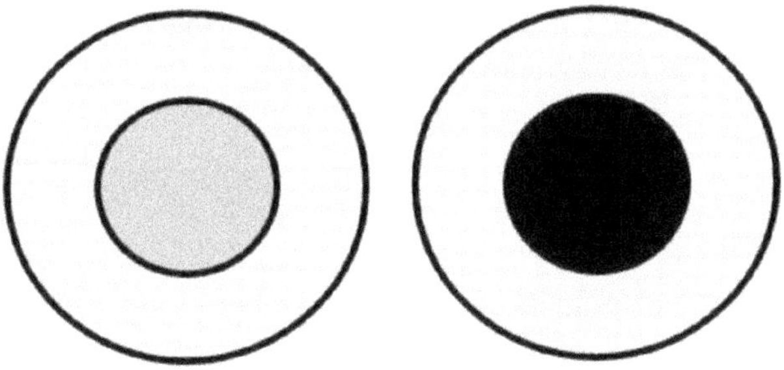

a b

Fig. 12.2 Diagrammatic representation of type of microcapsules, **a**: polymeric microcapsules containing liquid/gaseous drug as core materials, **b**: polymeric microcapsules containing solid drug as core materials.

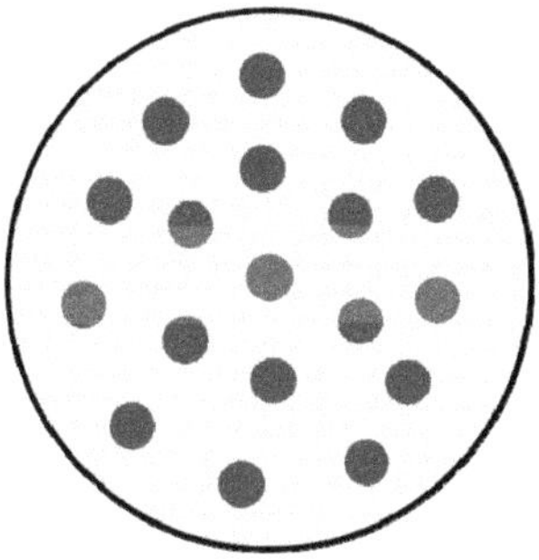

Fig. 12.3 Diagrammatic representation of polymeric microsphere having drug homogeneously dispersed in a matrix.

12.1.3 Salient Features and Drawbacks

Microparticles must comply with some of the features as per the requirement set by the formulation scientists. These features may vary in different formulation but there are some of the generalized criteria for appropriate formulation. As like other drug delivery systems microparticles also have some limitations, which must be seriously considered during the formulation and development.

Salient features

- Controlled and/or sustained release of API
- Biocompatible and biodegradable (depending on type of polymer used)
- Protection of the API from any physical/chemical degradation
- Masking of color, odour and taste of API
- Non-toxic and non-immunogenic
- Easy manufacturing and handling
- Targetability of API
- Spherical size and nearly mono-size distribution (depending on type of polymer and method of formulation)
- Adequate flowability and stability

Drawbacks

- Burst release of API
- Hindrance in coating because of larger distribution of particles
- Difficulties in removing undesired solvent/chemical used during manufacturing
- Poor syringeability in case of parenteral drug delivery
- Higher cost and special manufacturing setup

12.2 Pharmaceutical Excipients and Active Pharmaceutical Ingredients used in Microparticles

In any conventional or novel drug delivery systems, the pharmaceutical excipients contribute a lot in term of stability, manufacturing, cost, acceptance by patient as well as regulatory approval. Hence it's a very crucial step to choose the suitable excipients in the formulation and development. Many excipients exhibit inter-excipients as well as excipient-API incompatibility. In such conditions the compatibility issues must be addressed by suitable investigation before proceeding towards the formulation and development. It is always to be at the safer side by employing the GRAS excipients at their allowable quantity. Currently many text books for excipients are available which describe all these above mentioned issues (Rowe *et al.,* 2009; Wade and Weller, 1994). Information regarding the physicochemical properties, compatibility and toxicity etc., are also available with the manufacturer in their respective websites as technical/specification/toxicological/material safety data sheets. Readers are encouraged to read these books and follow these websites for more information. The following section details the pharmaceutical excipients as well as core materials used in the formulation of microspheres.

12.2.1 Polymers

Polymers are the chief excipients employed in the formulation of microspheres containing drugs. Polymers may be from natural, synthetic or semi-synthetic origin. Natural polymers are having the advantages of biodegradability and biocompatibility but also pose some limitations such as poor stability, chances of microbial growth, complex structure and sometimes variation in the physicochemical properties due to regional and/or climatic variation. On the other hand synthetic polymers are very widely available with featured physicochemical properties. There is always a race between the natural and synthetic polymers in terms of quality and applicability. Some of the semi-synthetic polymers are also available in the market, which are usually the modified/semi-synthesized polymers of natural origin. Table 12.3 gives a brief account of different polymers, used in the formulation of microparticles. As already discussed in the previous section, the drug molecule is either encapsulated or dispersed in the polymer and hence the release of drug from the polymer depends on the type of polymer used in the formulation. Depending upon the type of formulation and the characteristics of the polymers employed, the release may be either diffusion or dissolution controlled manner. Literature reveals that encapsulation efficiency and the particle size (distribution) of microspheres decreased when prepared with the polymer containing uncapped (free) carboxyl groups as compared to those formed with the polymer containing ester end groups (capped) (Mao *et al.,* 2007).

Table 12.3 A brief account of polymers used in the formulation of microparticles.

Name of polymers	Examples of the specific polymers with their structure		
	Natural polymers		
Protein	Albumin, gelatin, collagen (these polymers have complex three dimensional structure)		
Polysaccharide	Agarose 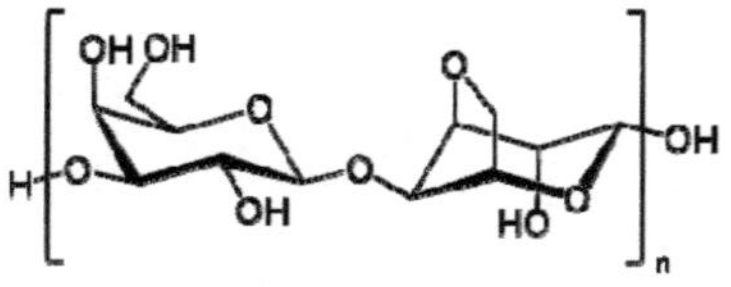	Carrageenan 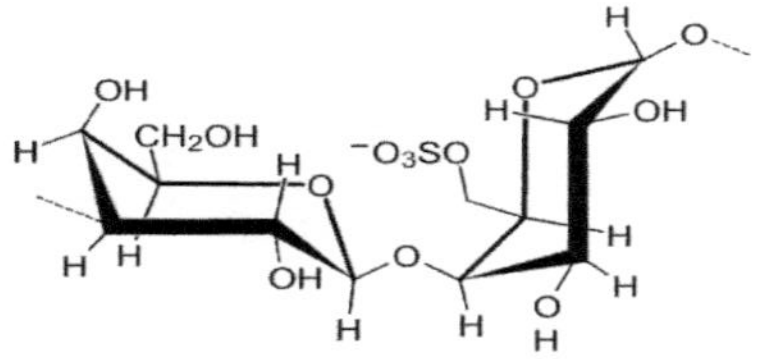	Chitosan 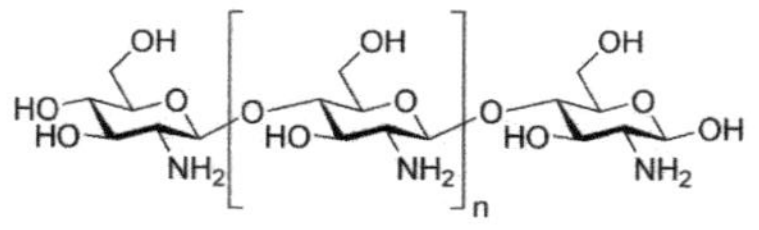
	Starch (amylopectin) 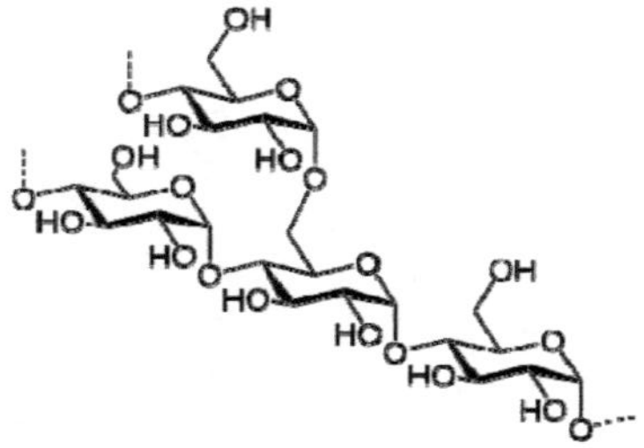	Dextran 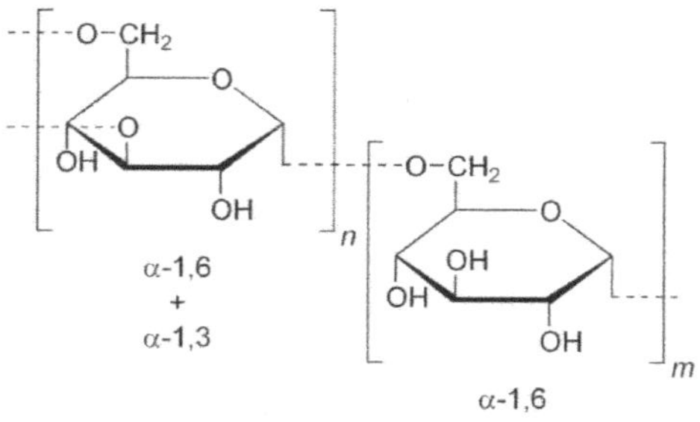	

Table 12.3 *Contd...*

Name of polymers	Examples of the specific polymers with their structure		
	Natural polymers		
polyhydroxyal kanoates	poly(3-hydroxybutyrate) 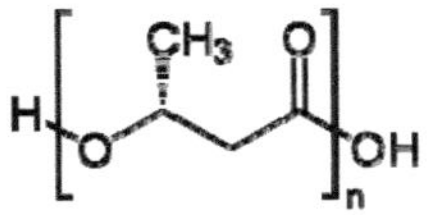	poly(3-hydroxybutyrate-co-hydroxyvalerate) 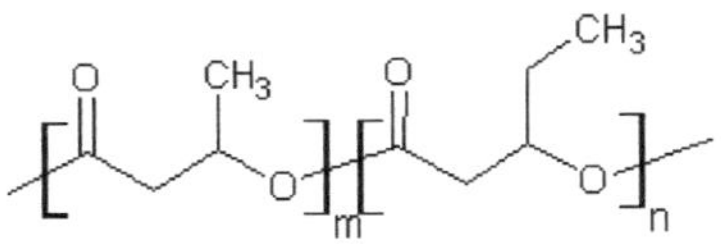	Hyaluronic acid 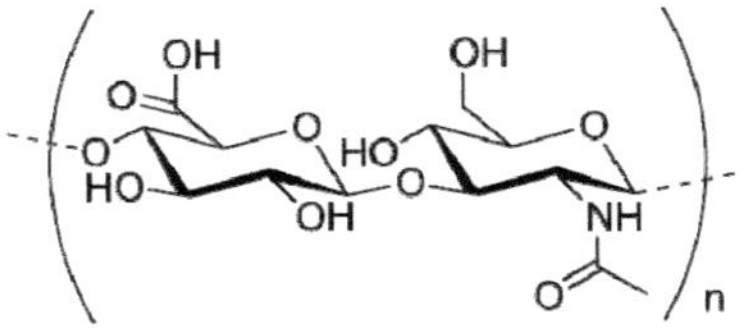
	Alginate 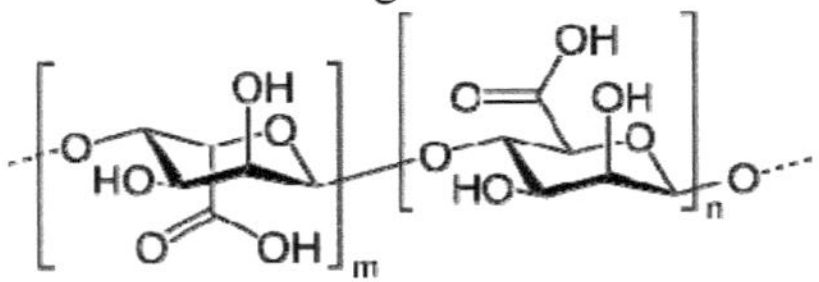		
	Synthetic polymers		
Non bio-degradable	Acrolein, 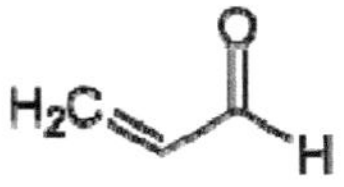	Glycidyl methacrylate 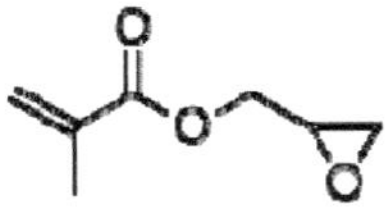	Polymethyl methacrylate, 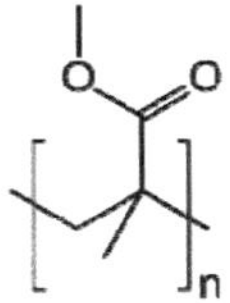

Table 12.3 *Contd...*

<table>
<tr><th>Name of polymers</th><th colspan="3">Examples of the specific polymers with their structure</th></tr>
<tr><td></td><td colspan="3">Epoxy polymers
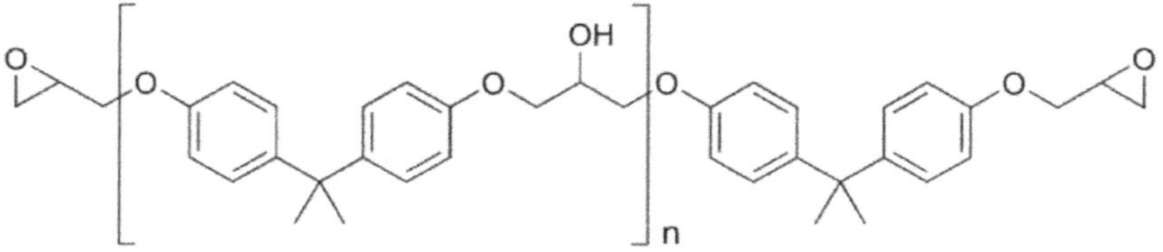</td></tr>
<tr><td rowspan="2">Biodegradable</td><td>Polyalkyl cyano acrylates
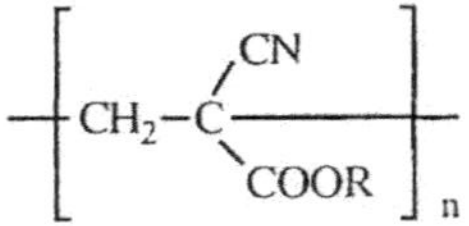</td><td>Poly anhydride
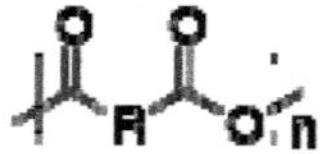</td><td>Poly(glycolide)
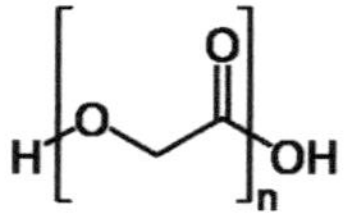</td></tr>
<tr><td>Poly(D,L-lactide)
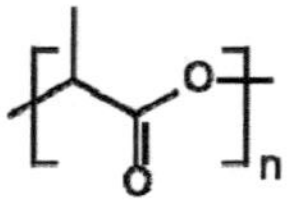</td><td>Poly(D,L-lactide-co-glycolide)
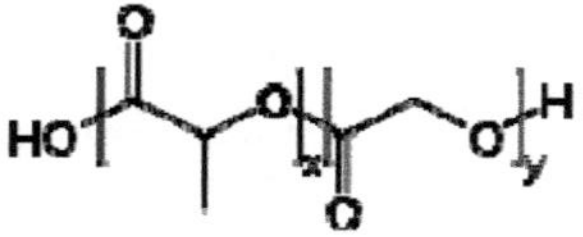</td><td>Poly(caprolactone)
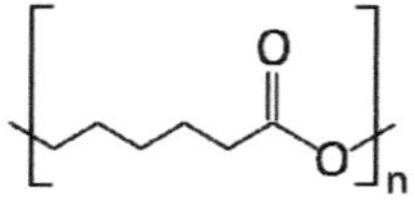</td></tr>
</table>

Table 12.3 *Contd...*

Name of polymers	Examples of the specific polymers with their structure		
Miscellaneous	Methacrylates 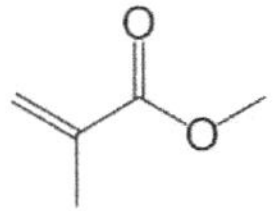	Poly(vinyl chloride) 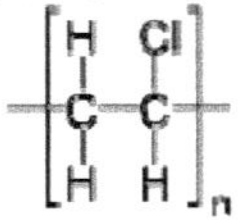	Silanes 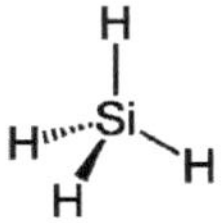
	Polyurethanes 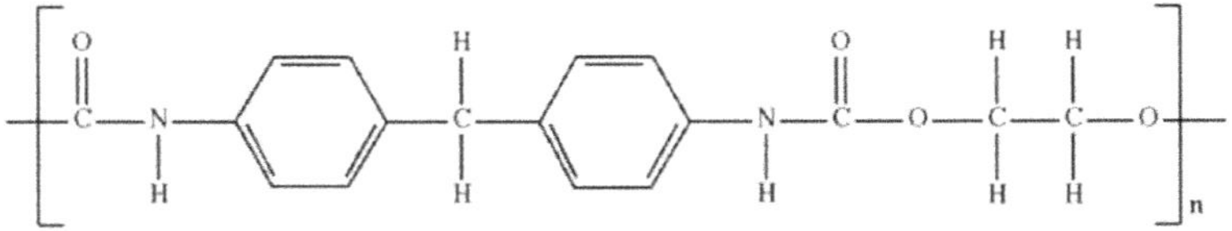		
	Poly(ortho esters) 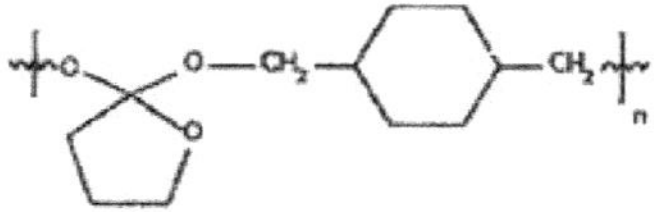	Poly(phosphoesters) 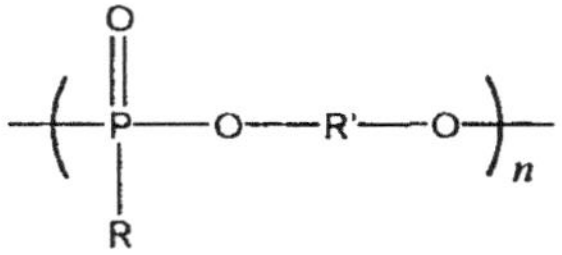	
	Polycarbonate 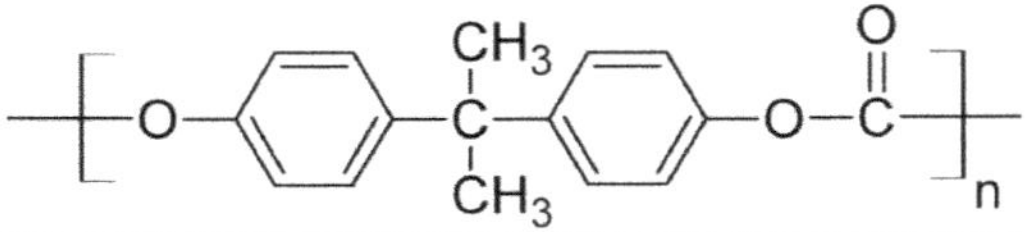		

Table 12.3 *Contd...*

Name of polymers	Examples of the specific polymers with their structure		
Semi-synthetic polymers			
Modified starch	Hydroxyethyl starch 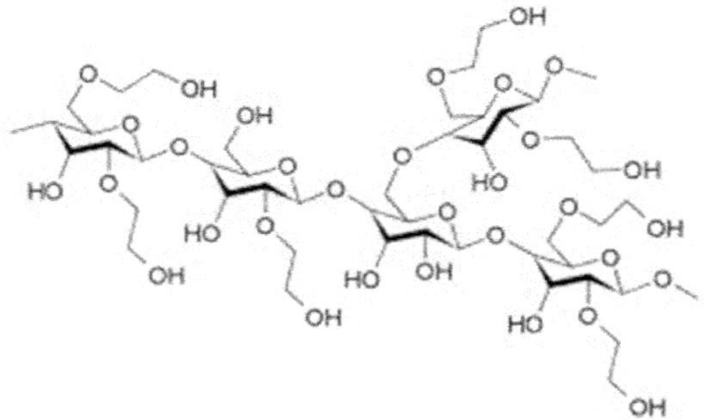	Poly (acryl) starch, Poly (acryl) dextran	
Others	Polyalkylcyanoacrylates 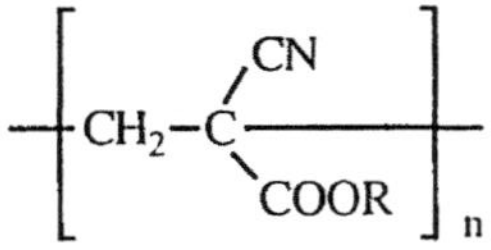	Polyamide 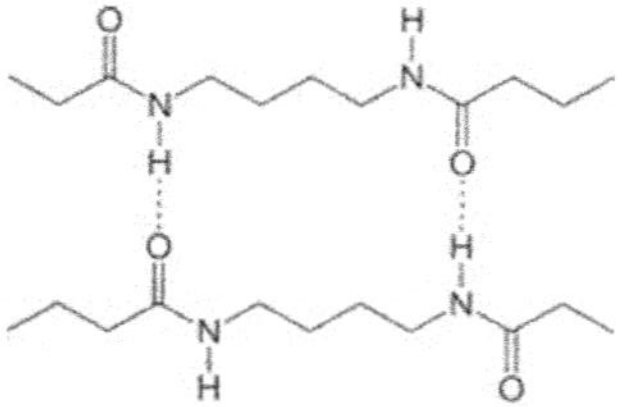	Polyphosphazene 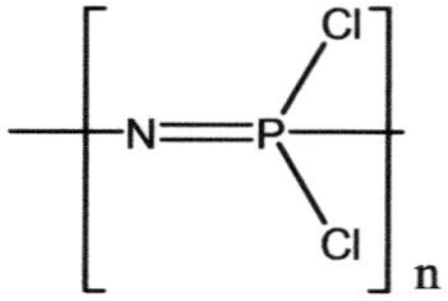
	Pseudo-polyamino acids		

12.2.2 Solvents

In the formulation of microspheres, solvents have a critical role. As the microspheres need a fluid environment to be formed the solvents are essential component in the development of microspheres. There are two phases viz. continuous phase and the dispersed phase in the formulation process. Continuous phase may be aqueous solvent like water, or any other oil and the dispersed phase may be an organic solvent. The desirable properties for the organic solvents are (i) high polymer solubility, (ii) high volatility, (iii) poor solubility in the continuous phase, (iv) low boiling point and (v) non-toxic/ low toxicity (Hamishehkar *et al.,* 2009). The most commonly used solvents are methylene chloride, ethyl acetate, and ethyl formate. High volatility, low boiling point, and low miscibility with water are the features that make methylene chloride as the most preferred solvent for PLGA microsphere preparation by solvent evaporation technique. Some reports on the carcinogenicity of methylene chloride have been testified. Butyl acetate and methylethyl ketone are also other solvents used in this technique. As per USP classification these solvents are categorized as either class 2 or class 3 solvents. Apart from these solvents many fixed oils such as corn oil, soya bean oil, light liquid paraffin etc., are also used. Selection of the aqueous or non-aqueous phase as continuous or dispersed phase depends on the solubility of the API. Ethyl acetate is another potential solvent used in microsphere formulation. Microspheres with a larger particle size than those prepared with methylene chloride but with no significant difference in drug loading was reported by Jeong *et al.,* (2003). Other solvents like acetone, ethanol, chloroform, hexane etc., are also employed as either co-solvent or non-solvent in microspheres production. Addition of non-solvent is a special process in the formulation of microspheres and hence selection of suitable non-solvent needs much attention. Formulation of proteins or peptides into microspheres is now a very hot topic in drug delivery and the solvent used not only determines the encapsulation efficiency but also affects protein stability. Last but most essential concern of solvent is the toxicity as it may adversely affect the patient/user, personnel in manufacturing area and also the approval of the microparticle product by regulatory authorities. As a precautionary measure industries avoid the use of harmful solvents, conduct training and awareness program for worker/operators in manufacturing area and also adopt strategies such as lyophilization or elevated temperature drying of the microparticles, to reduce the amount of residual solvent to an acceptable level.

12.2.3 Cross Linking Agents

Cross linking agents are used in some of the microparticles formulation technology. Most widely used cross linking agents are glutaraldehyde, formaldehyde, genipin (natural), calcium chloride, zinc sulphate, and dextran (Chan *et al.,* 2002). Calcium cations are frequently used to cross-link alginate polymers which are linier polymers of α-l-guluronic acid and β-d-mannuronic acid. These cations bind preferentially to the poly-guluronic acid units of alginate in a planar two-dimensional fashion, producing the "egg-box" structure. Natural polymer chitosan is usually cross linked with glutaraldehyde and the diffusion of drug from this polymeric matrix/capsule can be modulated by cross linking the polymer (Jameela and Jayakrishnan, 1995). Mechanism involved in the cross linking process is not clear. Glutaraldehyde is chemically a linear, 5-carbon di-aldehyde and physically it is a clear, colorless to pale straw-colored, pungent, oily liquid that is soluble in all proportions in water and alcohol, as well as in organic solvents. It reacts rapidly with amine groups at around neutral pH and generates thermally and chemically stable cross links. It can react with a number of functional groups of proteins, such as amine, thiol, phenol, and imidazole because of the presence of the most reactive amino acid side-chains (nucleophiles). In 1970s the crosslinking ability of glutaraldehyde was reported for the first time in the development of microspheres containing immunological and therapeutic agents. The tremendous fixative properties of glutaraldehyde was used for the preparation of microspheres from gelatin or alginate. It is noticeable that gelatin is water soluble and as such not suitable for sustained/controlled drug delivery systems, hence cross linking procedure is adopted that cause formation of insoluble networks within the microsphere wall leading to late dissolution.

Genipin (an aglycone obtained from an iridoid glycoside "geniposide" present in fruit of *Gardenia jasminoides*) is a natural and non-toxic cross-linking reagent which has been used for microparticles formulation. Genipin has very strong cross linking properties for proteins, collagen, gelatin, as well as chitosan. Yuan *et al.,* (2007) have explored the cross linking capacity of genipin by developing chitosan microspheres. They concluded that drug release rates from chitosan microspheres could be controlled and extended by controlling the degree of cross-linking with Genipin.

12.2.4 Stabilizers

The role of stabilizer in microparticles is imperative as it contributes in the formation of stable microspheres. When the protein-peptide API or any other sensitive API is to be formulated into microparticles the stabilizer protects these drugs from any chance of degradation. Polyols, carbohydrates, and amino acids are commonly used as stabilizers in parenteral microsphere formulations containing protein as API. Protein folding is the main point of concern for formulation scientist in any manufacturing process involved in formulation of microparticles that can be eradicated by the use of stabilizer, which maintains the structural orientation of water molecules around the protein molecule. Trehalose and mannitol are also used as stabilizer for proteins in the micro-particulate formulations (Meinel *et al.,* 2001). Till now we have seen the stabilization of the API, but in some instances the formulation process as such needs to be stabilized. For example in case of emulsification solvent evaporation methods, the stabilization of the emulsion (simple W/O, O/W or multiple W/O/W, O/W/O) is required for successful development of microparticles and surfactants are employed for this purpose. Non-ionic surfactants, poloxamer are used as surface active agents which reduce the surface tension and help in formation of microparticles (Ma and Song, 2007). Polyvinyl alcohol is also used as a stabilizer in the formulation of PLGA microparticles (Galeska *et al.,* 2005).

12.2.5 Active Pharmaceutical Ingredients (Core Material)

Theoretically the API or core materials (material to be entrapped) may be solid, liquid or gas, but in regular practice mainly solid and liquid materials are only used in the microencapsulation techniques in the pharmaceutical field. It has been estimated that up to 40% of new chemical entities show poor solubility. A majority of drug molecules also fall in BCS class II and IV category with poor bioavailability. The facets of delivering protein-peptides and large bio-macromolecules are real challenges in drug delivery. Encapsulation technology is an answer to such challenges. The quantity of the core material depends on the dose as well as well the desired release characteristics. Loading efficiency is an important parameter in this regard. In case of hydrophobic drugs the increase in the loading efficiency above 50% may alter the drug release properties but does not significantly increase the particle size and distribution (Mao *et al.,* 2008). Similarly in case of the hydrophilic drugs also the concentration of the core material influences the drug loading, size and size distribution. For the protein-peptide API, it's very difficult to choose the manufacturing procedure as these items are very much sensitive to heat, pH and even solvents. Usually stabilizers are employed to protect these types of API as core material in the microparticles. Hence it's very much crucial to choose the polymeric materials in the development of a suitable microparticles. The physicochemical properties of the core material must be taken seriously in selecting the polymers and other excipient of the microparticles formulation. In the category of ionizable drugs the pH dependency of the solubility needs to be carefully characterized. The effect of excipients, e.g., tween or span (which are often used in release buffers), on the drug solubility should also be determined. Drug polymorphism is an important phenomenon as it may show differences in physicochemical properties including melting point, solubility, density, dissolution rate, chemical reactivity, optical and electrical properties as well as vapor pressure. These changes may affect the performance of formulations in terms of bioavailability, stability, toxicity etc. The conversion of API to another form (polymorphs) cannot be ruled out during microencapsulation, storage, or under drug release conditions. Thus, solid drug as thermodynamically most stable polymorph must be preferred for pharmaceutical development. Similarly, formation of true or metastable molecular dispersions is possible during microencapsulation and the second form may be crystallized during storage which might severely affect the release properties of the formulation. Therefore it is, better to characterize the state of the drug inside the formulation by thermal analysis. Overall these points are to be taken in to consideration during the formulation of microparticles as these determine the fate of API and its therapeutic effect.

12.3 Preformulation Aspects in Microparticles

Preformulation studies are the prerequisite for the development of any formulation or dosage form. These studies essentially involve the physicochemical characterization as well as the compatibility studies of the API and excipients. A well designed preformulation study reduces the chances of failure in the formulation and development. Apart from formulation design and development, adequate and accurate data of the physicochemical parameters studied in preformulation are also helpful in the clinical investigation. As such preformulation is a vast topic of research, but we will have a very brief overview of the preformulation studies conducted for microparticles research in the following section.

12.3.1 Physicochemical Characteristics of API and Excipients

Different physicochemical properties of the API and excipients used in the formulation of microparticles such as solubility, melting point, partition co-efficient, stability at different pH, ionization constant, photosensitivity, crystalline/amorphous state etc., are to be characterized before formulation (Ahsan *et al.,* 2002). The solubility of the drug suggests in selecting the polymer as well as the solvents to be employed. Based in these properties, the requirement of microparticles in term of drug release, targeting and loading can be achieved. Melting point is a characteristic feature of purity and state of matter. The amorphous/crystalline nature of polymer and API is determined by melting point examination. Conversion of crystallinity to amorphous and vice-versa during manufacturing process may alter the solubility and dissolution of API. The stability of API at various pH conditions may be evaluated before formulation. This is very crucial in special formulation such as pH responsive microparticles. The physicochemical properties can be obtained from literature if the API and excipients are already existing. In case newer API or excipient, especially polymers not reported/used before, it is mandatory to determine these physicochemical characteristics. Another important aspect in the preformulation is the development of a suitable analytical method for the estimation of the API in the formulation/biological samples. The analytical method development further relays on these physicochemical parameters. So, as a final note, molecular-physical properties, analytical method, crystallographic characteristics, identification of polymorphs/ solvatomorphs, and solubilization methods should be available before formation of microparticles (Martins *et al.,* 2007).

12.3.2 Inter-Excipients and Drug-Excipients Compatibility

Formulation development process has to report the most important information regarding the chemical compatibility of the drug substances and the excipients used in the formulation. It cannot be denied that a drug-excipient reaction might produce a new impurity or degradant of undesired properties. Analytical methodology must be developed for the qualitative and quantitative detection of impurity species in the formulation. Thin-layer chromatography, high-pressure liquid chromatography, and gas chromatography are the popular methods employed for this purpose. The most advanced liquid chromatography-mass spectrometry and gas chromatography-mass spectrometry are analytical techniques used in pharmaceutical industries for the above mentioned purpose. Apart from the chromatographic methods, the other spectroscopy methods like UV-VIS, FTIR and NMR are also employed for the characterization of the chemical instability of the excipients as well as API-excipients mixture (Fu *et al.,* 1999; Zhang *et al.,* 2004).

Drug-excipient interactions are not confined to only chemical alteration, but very often change in physical characteristics may also be observed. Rather, it has been found that the chemical instability is led by the physical interaction between API-excipients or even excipients themselves. The basic tools used in the study of physical interaction in preformulation studies are X-ray diffraction (crystallography), differential scanning calorimetry (DSC) and thermo-gravimatric analysis (TGA) (thermally induced phase transitions), UV/VIS diffuse reflectance (alteration in color), and vibrational spectroscopy (FTIR) (alteration in functional groups). All of the above mentioned studies can be employed for microparticles in their preformulation investigation. The details of methodologies of these techniques are available in specialized texts and the readers are encouraged to go through those literature for more information (Adeyeye and Brittain, 2008; Gibson, 2001; Steele, 2004).

12.4 Microparticles Preparation Techniques

Microparticles are manufactured by different methods which can be categorized broadly as polymerization, emulsification, coacervation-phase separation and spray drying/congealing. Further these methods are classified into diverse sub-methods. Selection of raw materials and manufacturing methods are very much crucial in the development of microspheres. Before considering these, the formulation scientist has to look upon the drug-polymer compatibility, required-charge, shape, size and size distribution, drug release characteristics, biodegradability and biocompatibility. Apart from these pharmaceutical requirements, many other points must be considered such as the base formulation (solid, liquid or semisolid) where the microparticles are to be incorporated, the purpose of microparticles (internal/external application), any restriction on use of materials from specific origin (ingredients from animal, plant or microbial source) etc. It is also noticeable that the mechanisms include in the development of microparticles are phase separation, precipitation, interfacial polymerization or polycondensation, cross linking, and gelation. The following section will describe different methods of microparticles formulation in details.

12.4.1 Interfacial Polymerization

In the interfacial polymerization techniques the monomers (dispersed in solvent with opposite solubility) are employed for polymerization and formation of microparticles. Although the preparation of all microparticles needs use of polymers but this is different from other methods that formation of polymers occur *in situ*. This process involves utilization of monomers and initiator in a dispersed medium in such a way that polymerization of growing polymer is forced to form spherical particles. Two different ways are possible in the formation of microparticles which include (i) spherical droplets formed by oil-soluble organic monomers dispersed in aqueous media (oil in water, O/W) or (ii) spherical droplets formed by water-soluble monomers dissolved in water and dispersed in an organic medium. These dispersed monomers are polymerized by three different methods (i) dispersion, (ii) suspension and (iii) emulsion techniques (Freiberg and Zhu, 2004).

12.4.1.1 Dispersion Polymerization

Dispersion polymerization is the simple technique of polymerization method. In this method the monomers, initiator and the stabilizer are taken in a single organic solvent or mixture of solvents (single phase). The bioactive materials may be incorporated in the dispersion medium. In the presence of the initiator and the experimental condition (heat and stirring) the reaction starts and the process continues until nano-sized particles are formed. As the initiator is soluble in the monomer, polymerization takes place inside the monomer droplets. These smaller particles aggregate to form a comparatively larger particle and also attach to the developing oligomer to further increase the size up to 1-20 μm. The polymer formed are insoluble in the organic solvent, and remain well dispersed which is further facilitated by the stabilizer. After formation, the polymeric microparticles (insoluble in organic solvent) can be separated from the dispersion medium by filtration. Fig. 12.4 gives the schematic presentation of the dispersion polymerization technique.

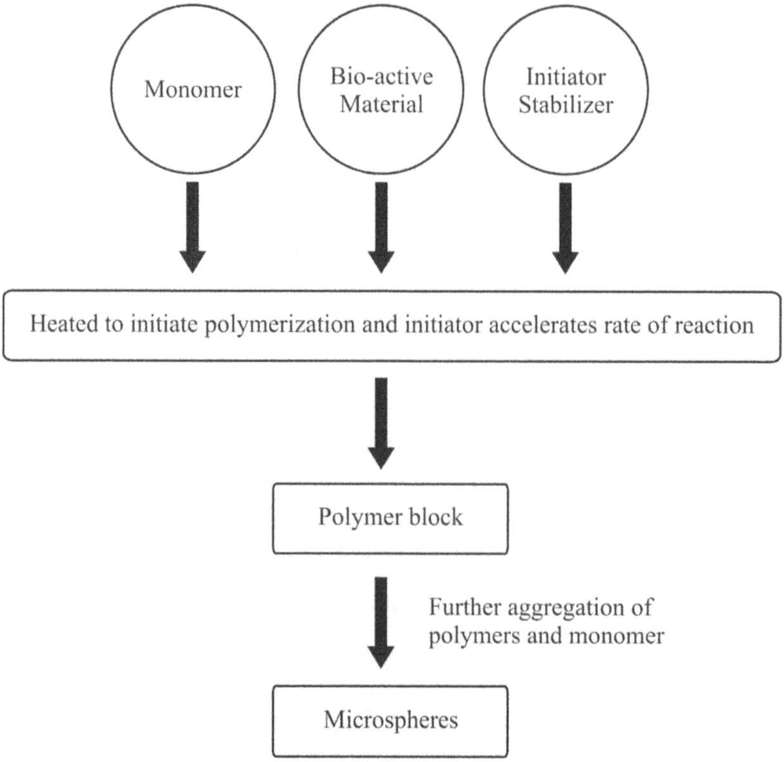

Fig. 12.4 Dispersion polymerization.

12.4.1.2 Emulsion Polymerization

Emulsion polymerization is one of the widely used polymerization techniques where the monomer (hydrocarbon based) is dispersed in aqueous media and a water soluble initiator is added to the medium. Suitable surfactant(s) are used for the formation of micelles which occurs above the critical micelle concentration (CMC) in the aqueous medium. In the formed micelles the monomers initiate polymerization and formation of the polymeric particles. Anionic stabilizers are used which form micelles with the hydrophobic monomer aggregates. Above the CMC the oligomers diffuse into the micelles and react with the entrapped monomers. This happens because the initiator is soluble in the continuous medium (aqueous phase) and insoluble in the non-aqueous part of the system. The bioactive material may either be encapsulated in the microparticles or even adsorbed on the surface of the particles. Fig. 12.5 gives a flow diagram of narrated technique.

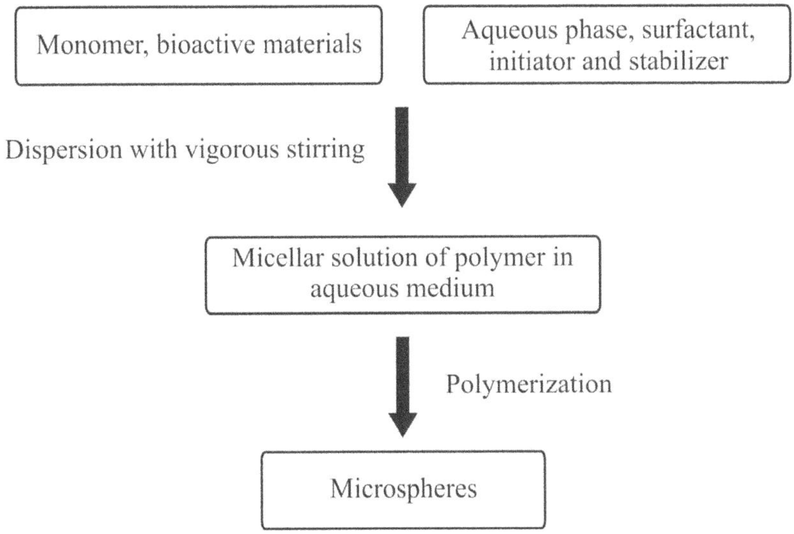

Fig. 12.5 Emulsion polymerization.

12.4.1.3 Suspension Polymerization

In the suspension polymerization technique the monomer and the initiator are solubilized in a suitable solvent or solvent mixture (aqueous solvent). A suspension medium (solvent) is taken in which the monomer and the initiator are insoluble. The monomer solution is added in the suspending medium and constant stirring and heat is supplied for the commencement of the reaction. Stabilizer is also added which might be any low molecular weight polymer or surfactant. Droplets of the solvent are formed in the suspension and the polymer aggregates are formed within the solvent droplet. As the monomer and the formed polymers are insoluble in the suspension medium, they tend to develop a size and shape of the solvent droplets (spherical shape) leading to the formation of polymeric microparticles. The usual particle size ranges from 50-500 μm. Suspension polymerization is schematically shown in Fig. 12.6.

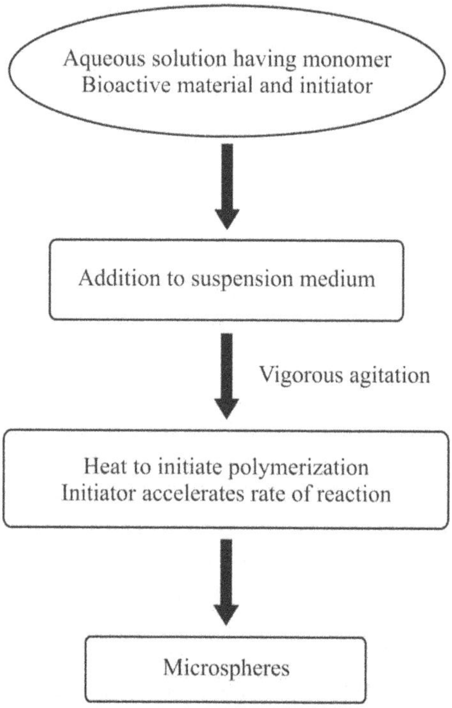

Fig. 12.6 Suspension polymerization.

12.4.2 Emulsion Solvent Evaporation

Emulsification followed by solvent evaporation or solvent extraction technique is one of the methods of microparticle preparation. It differs from the interfacial polymerization in that it employs the polymer (preformed) instead of monomers. Both the water soluble and insoluble drugs can be accommodated inside microparticles by this technique. There are three basic steps viz. (i) emulsification of polymers with solvent droplet incorporated with drug, (ii) evaporation of the solvent leading to microparticle formulation and (iii) washing, filtration and separation of microparticles. Two classical methods are usually adopted in the emulsification techniques viz. (i) single emulsification and (ii) double emulsification.

12.4.2.1 Single Emulsion

In the single emulsion technique the drug (water insoluble) and the polymer are dissolved in an organic solvent. The aqueous (continuous;

non-solvent) phase is prepared by mixing a suitable emulsifier and stabilizer. The organic phase is added to the aqueous phase with constant stirring and if required heat is applied to the system. The emulsification takes place and droplets of organic solvent are formed containing polymer and drug. After the emulsification process is over, the solvent evaporation is done by stirring process. As the solvent evaporates the polymer starts taking shape of droplets encapsulating the drug within itself. Finally the formed microparticles are washed, filtered and separated and may be lyophilized. Fig. 12.7 gives a layout of single emulsion method.

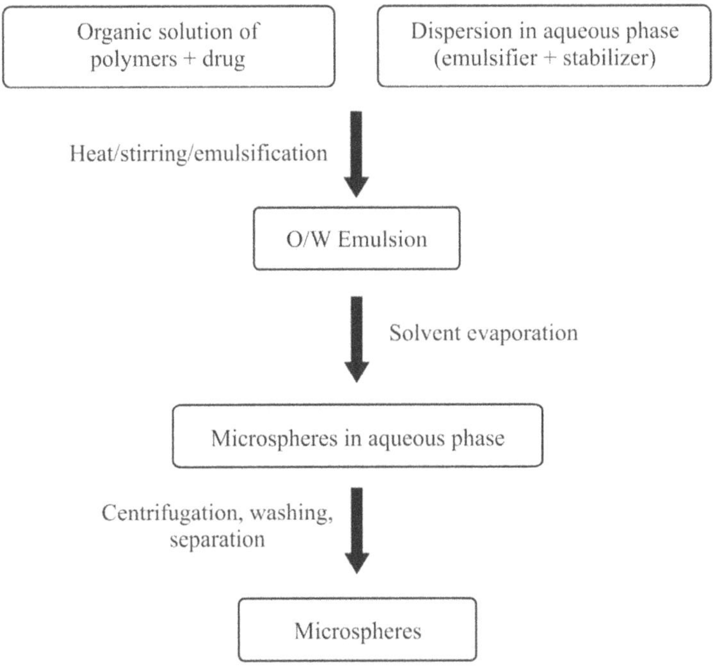

Fig. 12.7 Single emulsion method.

12.4.2.2 Double Emulsion

Double emulsification technique is suitable for water soluble drugs. The mechanism of the microparticles formation is same here but instead of O/W a W/O/W multiple emulsion is formed. Water soluble drug is emulsified in an organic solvent (with polymer) to form W/O emulsion.

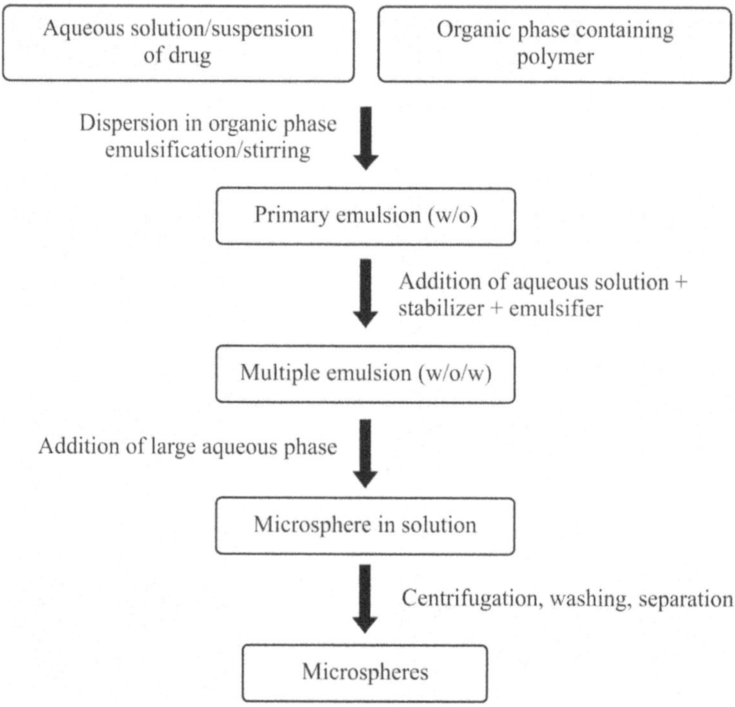

Fig. 12.8 Double emulsion method.

In the next step the W/O primary emulsion is dispersed in the continuous aqueous phase to form a W/O/W multiple emulsion. Rest all process is same as that of single emulsion method. Fig. 12.8 illustrates the scheme of preparation of microparticles by double emulsion method.

12.4.3 Coacervation Phase Separation

Coacervation phase separation is one of the most feasible methods in preparing microparticles. In this case three phases interact with each other and finally phase separation occurs leading to formation of microparticles. The three phases employed in this method include phase-1 consisting of drug in suitable solvent and polymer in suitable solvent serves as phase-2. Phase-3 is responsible for the phase separation which can be done either by addition of salt or non-solvent or by polymer-polymer interaction, incompatible polymer addition or by temperature change. First the phase-1 is added to the phase-2 and vigorously agitated to develop a W/O emulsion. The water soluble drug can be accommodated in the phase-1 whereas water insoluble drug can be mixed in the phase-2. Addition of phase-3 leads to the phase separation in the above formed W/O emulsion. Soft coacervate droplets are formed entrapping the drug of phase-1. After this the coacervate droplets are transferred to large volume of hardening agent (organic solvent other than used as phase-3). The hardening agent should be able to wash out the phase-3 materials and also should be volatile so that it can be removed to get the pure microparticles. Fig. 12.9 illustrates a systematic approach of formulation of microparticles by coacervation phase separation method. As mentioned above the phase separation may be achieved by any of the methods described below.

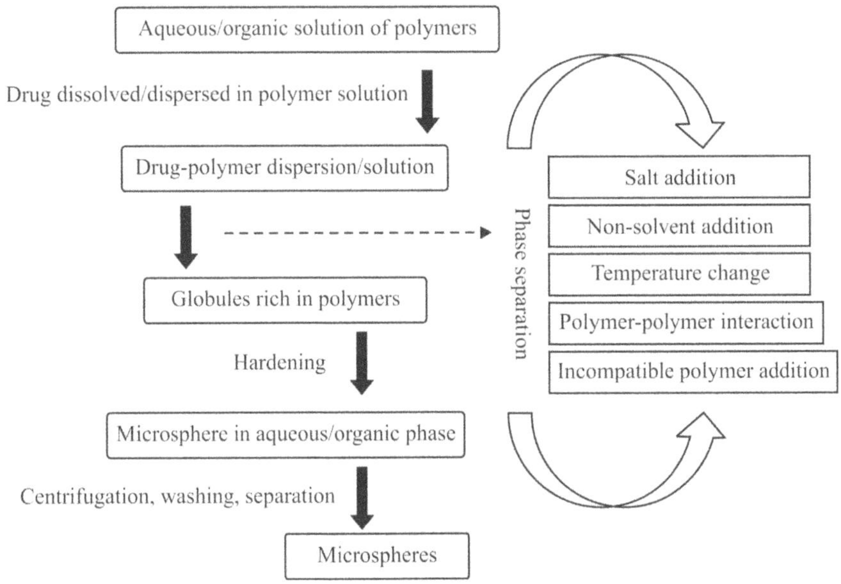

Fig. 12.9 Coacervation phase separation method.

12.4.3.1 Salt Addition

Various inorganic salts can be added to the aqueous solution of water soluble polymers to induce phase separation. Encapsulation of vitamin with gelatin polymer by the addition of sodium sulfate, formulation of poly-[di(carboxylatophenoxy)phosphazene] (PCPP) microparticles upon addition of sodium chloride are the example of the phase separation by salt addition method (Andrianov *et al.*, 1998). However, any incompatibility of the drug molecule to the salt must be ascertained before applying this approach of microparticle preparation. The further step of hardening of the polymer layer is done by the same methods as mentioned above. Fig. 12.10 gives the example in a schematic manner.

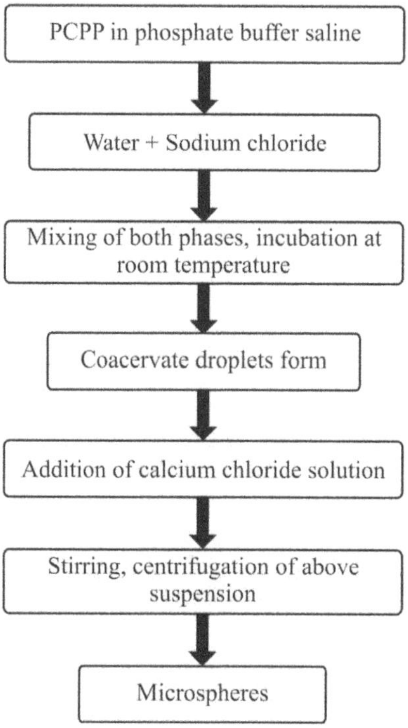

Fig. 12.10 Salt addition.

12.4.3.2 Non-Solvent Addition

In this method a non-solvent is used as phase-3 for the phase separation process. The non-solvent is added to the W/O emulsion and the phase-2 (polymer solvent) is separated out from the mixture leading to the formation of coacervate particles of polymer and drug. The non-solvent must have good solubility with the phase-2 solvent whereas it must not have solubility with either drug or polymer. Phase-2 solvent is extracted out from the mixture by the non-solvent and the coacervate particles are subjected to hardening by exposing the same to large volume of organic hardening agent. Example of non-solvent addition method is illustrated in Fig. 12.11 where silicon oil is used as a non-solvent to cause phase separation and formation of PLGA microparticles containing BSA.

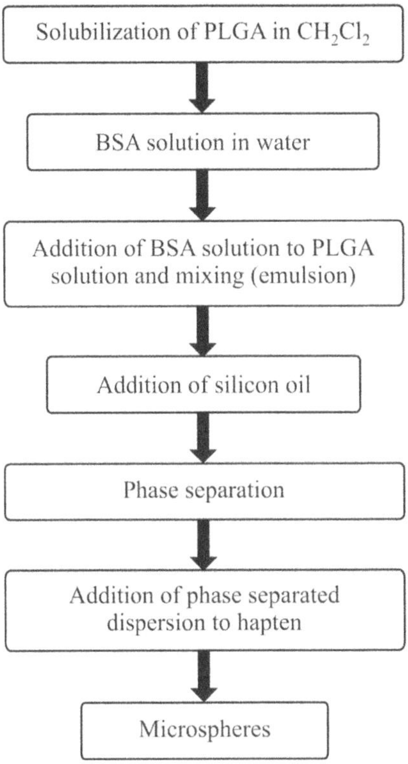

Fig. 12.11 Non-solvent addition.

12.4.3.3 Temperature Change

Change in the temperature is employed to impart phase separation and consequently formation of microparticles. Certain polymers are insoluble in some organic solvent at room temperature but with the increase in temperature the solubility increases and at the boiling point a homogeneous mixture is formed. At this stage drug is dispersed finely in the polymeric mixture and properly mixed. After this, the temperature is reduced and the mixture is allowed to cool down up to room temperature. As per the inherent characteristics the solubility of polymer in the solvent reduced and this leads to phase separation. Further the formed coacervate droplets are subjected to hardening as previously mentioned and microparticles are collected after proper washing. Fig. 12.12 demonstrates an example for the development of microparticles by temperature change method where ethyl cellulose (insoluble in cyclohexane at room temperature) is solubilized in cyclohexane at high temperature and drug is incorporated. Further by reducing the temperature microparticles are formed encapsulating the drug.

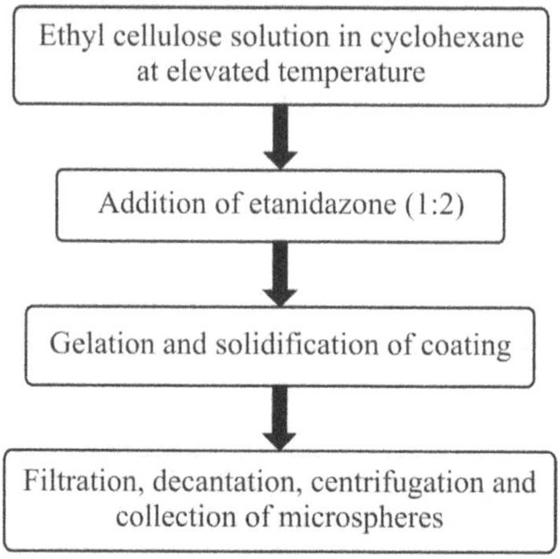

Fig. 12.12 Temperature change method of coacervation phase separation.

12.4.3.4 Polymer-Polymer Interaction

Polymer-polymer interaction is one of the techniques used in coacervation phase separation method of microparticle formulation. The inherent characteristics interaction of polymers of oppositely charged groups is employed here as the means of phase separation. As a consequence of polymer-polymer interaction a complex is formed which causes phase separation in the mixture and further leads to development of soft coacervate particles. An example of this category of phase separation is interaction of gelatin and gum arabic. At acidic pH (around 4.5) gelatin possess a positive charge whereas gum arabic has negative charge. When mixed together at required temperature, these two polymers interact with each other and form a complex which causes phase separation. It further leads to the development of soft coacervates which are processed for gaining rigidity. Similarly some other polymers exhibiting charge at specific pH, can be reacted with each other to form complex and further phase separation of the developed complex leads to formation of coacervates. These coacervates are hardened by appropriate method and microspheres are separated by stirring and centrifugation.

12.4.3.5 Incompatible Polymer Addition

As the name indicates, this process of phase separation is achieved by the addition of a polymer that is incompatible with the other polymer which already exists in the system. Polymer-1 is dissolved in an organic solvent up to a certain concentration. The drug which is insoluble in the solvent is added to the polymeric solution. Then polymer-2 is added to the system which has comparatively higher solubility in the organic solvent at the same time polymer-2 is incompatible with polymer-1. This phenomena cause phase separation and formation of coacervate droplets which are subjected to other steps as mentioned in the previous methods for the purpose of providing rigidity to the particles.

12.4.4 Spray Drying and Congealing

Spray drying and congealing are industrially feasible methods for the preparation of microparticles. In spray drying technique the polymer is dissolved in a volatile organic solvent followed by addition of drug either in form of solution or suspension by high velocity homogenization. The mixture is atomized to convert into tiny droplets which are exposed to stream of hot air. Hot air exposure provides latent heat of vaporization leading to solvent evaporation and formation of the microparticles. The next crucial step in spray drying method is the separation of the formed microparticles. Spray dryer is the instrument that uses this atomization technique and is available in laboratory, pilot as well as industrial scale production. A diagrammatic representation of a laboratory spray dryer is shown in Fig. 12.13. Various process parameters such as volume of solvent containing polymer, viscosity of polymeric mixture, diameter of spraying nozzle, temperature of inlet and outlet air, flow rate of solvent and air affect the preparation of microparticles. Agglomeration of the microparticles among themselves and to the wall of the spray dryer is one of the major concerns in this method. Recent advancement in spray drying technique has solved this problem up to a considerable extent by applying solution of mannitol to the preparation process. A mannitol coating on the microparticles avoids agglomeration. This process is done by a novel double nozzle spray drier. Spray drying technique is one of the successful commercial techniques and used widely in many pharmaceutical and cosmetic industries. Parlodel® (LAR Sandoz, Switzerland) the first commercialized injectable microspheres composed of PLGA and containing bromocriptine as API was produced by spray drying. A flowchart depicting spray drying technique is shown below in Fig. 12.14. Spray congealing technique works in the same way and the only difference is that solidification of coacervates (polymeric particles) occurs by thermally congealing a molten polymeric material or by addition of non-solvent (Hu *et al.*, 2013; Lachman L. *et al.*, 1990).

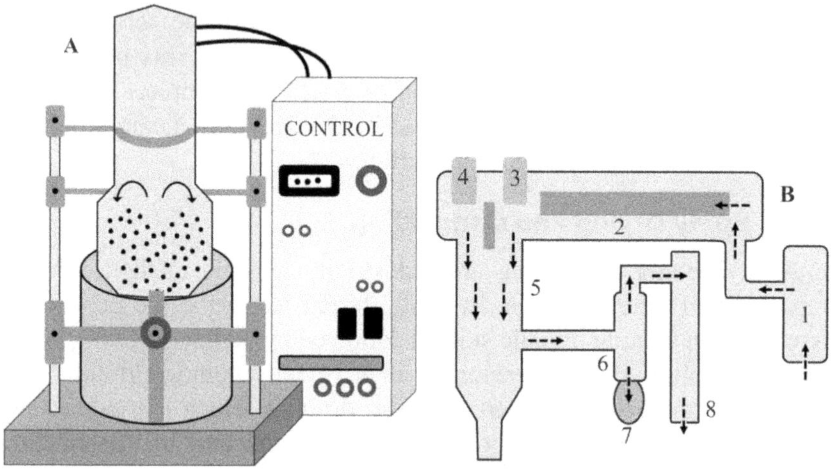

Fig. 12.13 Diagrammatic representation of (a) Laboratory spray dryer, (b) Scheme showing block diagram of spray dryer. 1. Air inlet and filtration, 2. Air heater, 3. Compressed air, 4. Sample spray nozzle, 5. Desiccation chamber, 6. Cyclone separator, 7. Microparticles collector 8. Air outlet.

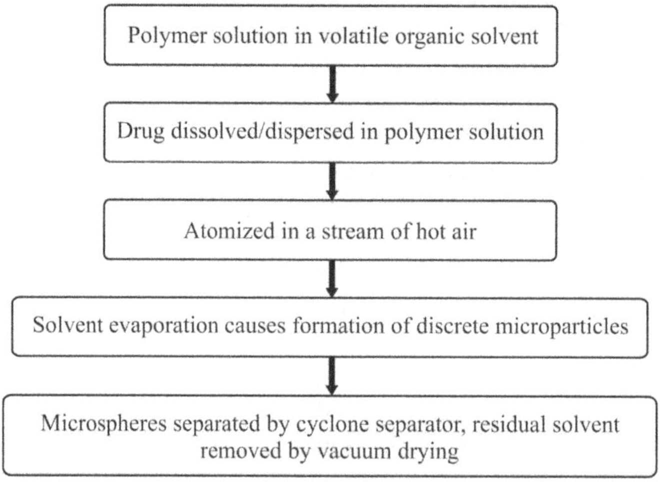

Fig. 12.14 Steps in spray drying technique.

12.4.5 Advanced Methods

The above discussed methods are classical methods in microparticle formulation. Apart from these methods various other techniques are also reported. Some of these are improved version of the classical methods whereas others are novel methods. Among all these some methods are successful at the industrial stage and others are only feasible at the laboratory scale. In this part we will discuss advanced/novel methods of microparticle formulation.

12.4.5.1 Extrusion Method

In the extrusion method the polymeric blend along with the drug and other excipients are extruded through a very fine orifice. One of such techniques is Shirasu porous glass technique where a polymer solution is passed through a glass membrane of uniform pore size. This leads to the formation of spherical microparticles which are further subjected to various rigidization techniques to get good quality microparticles. Various polymeric microparticles such as PLA, PLGA, gelatin and chitosan microspheres are formulated by this method. However, some authors reported formation of asymmetrical microparticles by these methods (Varde and Pack, 2004).

12.4.5.2 Supercritical Fluid Method

Microparticles have been prepared by super critical fluid such as supercritical carbon dioxide (SCO_2). The low critical point i.e., 31.1 °C at 73.8 bar makes SCO_2 a striking processing medium for heat labile drugs. The mechanism of using SCO_2 in preparing microparticles is that SCO_2 liquefies some polymers at temperature significantly below their glass transition temperature by acting as a molecular lubricant. At the required pressure conditions liquefied polymers encapsulate the drug and is depressurized through a nozzle which causes evaporation of SCO_2 leaving microparticles of polymer with drug. This method has various advantages that it does not use any organic solvents and it's a single step method with very less consumption of SCO_2. The SCO_2 can be used as solvent, reaction medium or anti-solvent in manufacturing of microparticles. This technique has been employed to develop microparticles with small molecules as well as macromolecules viz. paclitaxel, human growth hormone, insulin, etc.

12.4.5.3 Ink-/liquid-jet Technology

A variety of microparticles such as conventional (normal), core-shell, double walled and hollow microparticles are prepared by ink-/liquid-jet technology. The piezoelectric or acoustic excitation technique coupled with the emulsion-solvent evaporation method is employed in the ink-/

liquid-jet technology. In this technique a specialized device is designed with multiple (2/3) nozzles along with an acoustic excitation device. In this device polymer solution/dispersion containing drug is flowed through the inner nozzle, while a carrier stream (aqueous phase) is flowed around the polymeric phase by outer nozzle. The liquid stream is acoustically excited using an ultrasonic transducer controlled by a frequency generator which causes in the production of the microparticles (Mao *et al.,* 2012b).

MicroFab Technologies, Inc. Texas, USA has developed SphereJet™ system, an ink-jet based microsphere production methods. This technique combines drop-on-demand, pressure assisted drop-on-demand, and continuous ink-jet drop formation and uses solvent extraction/evaporation method of microsphere manufacturing. Drop generation rates of up to 50 kHz and drop diameters of 20 to 100 μm can be achieved by this novel techniques.

12.4.5.4 Microsieve Technology

Microsieve technology is one among the advanced methods in manufacturing microparticles. Microsieves are used in this technique which are silicone-based membranes with uniform pore size. A special technique namely photolithographic technique is used for this purpose. An organic solvent containing polymeric mixture and drug is forcefully introduced through this microsieves into an aqueous solution leading to formation of micro-emulsion. The next step is to remove the solvent by evaporation which causes the development of microparticles. The separation and drying of microparticles is done by the standard procedures. Microparticles of various sizes are produced by this method (Mao *et al.,* 2012b).

12.4.5.5 Microfluidics Technique

Microfluidics technique uses the microfluidic channels which are made up of polydimethylsiloxane and soft lithograph are sealed against an oxidized glass slide. The organic phase containing drug and polymer as well as the aqueous phase are introduced into the microfluidic device with constant flow rate. The flow of both the phases is regulated in such a way that, organic phase comes through a central channel and aqueous phase comes through 2 channels, above and below the central channel. At the junction of these three channels the emulsification occurs and fine droplets of polymer containing drug are formed. These droplets get converted in to microparticles after evaporation of the organic phase. The developed microparticles are washed properly and filtered. Various polymeric microparticles are formed by this technique (Mao *et al.*, 2012b).

12.4.5.6 Electrospray Technique

The principle behind Electrospray technique is to utilize a high electrostatic force that is created within a liquid in an electric field to break the liquid into fine charged droplets. The electrospray device has three important parts including a pump for handling liquid at desired rate, a tip with high electric potential and a collector kept near to the tip. The polymeric solution/dispersion containing drug is pumped in to the tip at a very controlled rate and an electrostatic force of specified strength is applied which leads to the formation of a very fine micro-emulsion. The organic phase is evaporated out and microparticles are formed which are further washed and separated. Electrospray technique is employed to develop microspheres of different size range and also microspheres with a core-shell structure.

12.5 Characterization of Microspheres

Microparticles are characterized for various *in vitro* and *in vivo* parameters. As these are microparticles, determination of size, shape, and size-distribution are important parameters to be analyzed. The internal structural-characteristics as well the surface morphology are also vital parameters in microparticles and their performance. Apart from these parameters, the pharmaceutical characterization for drug including drug loading, encapsulation efficiency, content uniformity, zeta potential, burst release, *in vitro* release kinetics, floatability, syringeability/injectability, water/residual solvent contents are investigated for the developed microparticles. The *in vitro/in vivo* toxicity, *in vivo* activity are other evaluation criteria that might differ as per the incorporated API. In some instances the *ex vivo* studies are also carried out, where the drug is intended for transdermal/topical application. Stability studies are final but very crucial studies for a micro-particulate product to be a successful formulation.

12.5.1 Size, Shape, Charge and Surface Morphology

The size of microparticles ranges from 1-1000 μm and can be characterized by automated laser diffraction technology. The samples are diluted as required and subjected to analysis by the laser analyzer. Mean particle size, frequency distribution profile and polydispersibility index are usually the analyzed output that can be interpreted for the developed microparticles. This method is very efficient and less cumbersome than any other method. Optical microscopy is also employed for determining the size of microspheres larger than 10 μm. Imaging analysis facilities (imaging and analysis software) are very much helpful in determining the size distribution of microspheres. The advantages of this method are direct visualization of the size and shape as well as the state of aggregation. The charge of microparticles must be analyzed as it indicates the dispersion of the micron size particles in a medium. The surface charge of microspheres decides the degree of aggregation upon storage or even reconstitution, which further leads to alteration in the stability, syringeability of microspheres. Zeta potential is measured for microparticles and it indicates the electrostatic interactions. It is measured by micro-electrophoretic techniques where the movement of particles is measured under the influence of a known electric field. Alternatively electrophoretic light scattering techniques can be used for measuring the zeta potential of microspheres.

The shape of the microparticles can be analyzed by electron/confocal microscopic techniques such as scanning electron microscopy (SEM) and transmission electron microscopy (TEM). SEM and TEM are the most widely used technologies for qualitative analysis of the microparticles. These techniques can give the picture of the surface properties (smooth, rough, irregular, porous) and internal structure, whereas more advanced techniques such as High-resolution TEM can give the size of particle by point to point resolution (Engel and Colliex, 1993; Klein *et al.,* 2012). The quantitative analysis of internal structures are also possible by mercury intrusion porosimetry. Another strong microscopic tool is confocal laser scanning microscopy which facilitate in obtaining high-resolution optical pictures with depth discernment. It indicates the uniformity of drug distribution on the microspheres formulated under different conditions with three-dimensional images. Atomic force microscope is also employed for the study of surface characteristics as well as the internal core structure of microparticles. Different 3-D and 2-D height images, topographical features of a microsphere can be analyzed by this microscopy. Any surface modification like coating or functionalization with specialized molecules can be visualized and analyzed by these highly efficient microscopic techniques.

12.5.2 Flow Properties

Good flowing characteristic is required in the manufacturing of pharmaceutical products at bulk scale. Especially in the manufacturing of tablets, capsules or any other dosage form where unit operation of flow is required, the raw materials must have good flow properties. Microparticles as one of the materials to be used in the manufacturing of pharmaceutical dosage form (tablets, capsules, parenteral products etc.) must have adequate flowability. The flow characteristics of microparticles can be determined by the simple experiments like measurement of angle of repose, Hausner's ratio and Carr's index (Zhao *et al.,* 2008). Because of the spherical shape, microspheres are expected to have good flow, but in some instances, the adhesive nature of the polymers used in the formulation may cause in poor flow as well as adhesion. Different strategies can be employed to increase the flow properties of microspheres such as adequate drying, use of non-adhesive and non-hygroscopic materials, and use of glidant/lubricant/anti adherent especially in formulation of solid dosage forms.

12.5.3 Thermal Analysis

Thermal analysis of the microparticles is done in order to investigate the physical status of the drug in the encapsulated form and also the characteristics of polymer after being formulated in to the microparticles. These studies can be done immediately after formulation (real time detection) of microparticle as well as over its life time. The API undergoes different conditions and treatments in the formulation process and may alter any of its physicochemical/biological properties. DSC can be employed to check the solid state chemistry as well as physicochemical properties of the drug such as melting point. Any alteration or disappearance in the melting point peak may indicate the change of crystal structure of the API. Apart from the analysis of API, thermal analysis of polymer viz. glass transition temperature can be assessed by using DSC (Sandor *et al.,* 2002). Thermo-gravimatric analysis may also be used to investigate phase transitions, desolvation, decomposition sublimation, absorption, adsorption, and desorption behavior of the polymeric microparticles. Recent advancement in the thermal analysis is the introduction of DSC-FTIR (Differential Scanning Calorimetry and Fourier-Transform Infrared Micro-Spectroscopy) which is an emerging tool in the analysis of solid state chemistry of different dosage forms.

12.5.4 Encapsulation Efficiency (EE)

Microparticles are the carriers which hold API either in the central core or in a dispersed state. EE is the actual amount of drug entrapped in the microparticles in comparison to the total amount of drug added in the formulation. It can be denoted by the following formula

$$EE = \frac{D_E}{D_A} \times 100$$

Where, D_E = amount of drug encapsulated in microparticles

D_A = total amount of drug added

For estimation of EE, the un-encapsulated or free drug is separated from the microparticles by multiple washing. The microparticles free from un-entrapped drug are lysed and drug content is determined using suitable analytical technique (Avula *et al.,* 2013). Higher EE of drug is required for an ideal microparticles formulation and it depends on multiple factors such as method of preparation, quality and quantity of polymers, process variables viz. temperature, pH, stirring speed and time etc.

12.5.5 *In vitro* Drug Release

Drug release from microparticles may be from the surface, through pores, diffusion from swollen microparticles, by erosion, or bulk degradation. It's interesting and very much important to study the drug release behavior as it determines the bioavailability of drug. The IP/USP dissolution apparatus or any modified apparatus (magnetic stirrer, orbital shaker etc.) are used for the *in vitro* drug release studies of microparticles (Avula *et al.,* 2013). Researchers adopt different methods for this study. The microspheres are directly added to the dissolution media (PBS of required pH), may be filled in the baskets (USP-type-1 dissolution apparatus) or can be incorporated into a dialysis tube and kept inside the dissolution media. The experiment is run with specified speed and temperature for a specific time (as decided by the type of formulation i.e., sustained release, floating, immediate release followed by sustained release etc.) by maintaining the sink condition. Aliquots of required volume are collected at pre-specified time period and analyzed by a suitable analytical method. Alternatively microspheres loaded with API are suspended in dissolution medium in screw-capped tubes and placed in an orbital shaker (uniform shaking at certain RPM) maintained at 37 ± 1 °C. Tubes are removed out at pre-decided time interval and subjected to centrifugation. Then supernatant is removed and the remaining microspheres are re-suspended in fresh dissolution media and placed back in the shaker. The supernatant containing the drug is analyzed by a suitable analytical method. Some researchers advocate the employment of ceacal content in order to mimic the gastric environment in a more appropriate manner. Chaurasia *et al.*, (2008) have reported the *in vitro* drug release of methotrexate microspheres in PBS containing rat ceacal content. The drug release data obtained is subjected to different release kinetic models such as zero, first order, Higuchi's, korsmeyer peppas and other suitable mode to investigate the mechanism of *in vitro* drug release.

12.5.6 *Ex vivo* Drug Permeation

Microparticles intended for transdermal or topical applications are approved by FDA and are commercially available. One of the examples is Tretinoin gel (USP), a porous microspheres formulated with methyl methacrylate/glycol dimethacrylate crosspolymer for topical treatment of acne vulgaris. Several such microparticles for transdermal/topical applications are reported by researchers worldwide. Before performing the *in vivo* activity the developed microparticles are examined for *ex vivo* drug permeation. This study is either performed with Franz diffusion cell, Keshri Chain diffusion apparatus or flow through diffusion cells. Fig. 12.15 exhibits the *ex vivo* permeation studies of microparticles. The skin of animal (rat, goat or pork) is fixed at the junction of the donor and the receptor compartment of Franz diffusion cell. The microparticles (raw or in any dosage form such as gel/cream) is put on the skin surface. Required dissolution medium is filled in the respective compartment and temperature is maintained at 37 ± 1 °C. The dissolution medium is stirred with the help of a magnetic stirrer. The API permeated in the dissolution medium through the biological membrane (skin) is collected through the sampling probe and subjected to evaluation by a suitable analytical technique. As like the *in vitro* drug release studies, these drug permeation data are subjected to different drug permeation kinetics and the mechanism of drug permeation is studied. Jain *et al.,* (2004) have used Franz diffusion to study the permeation of salbutamol from mucoadhesive microspheres for nasal delivery.

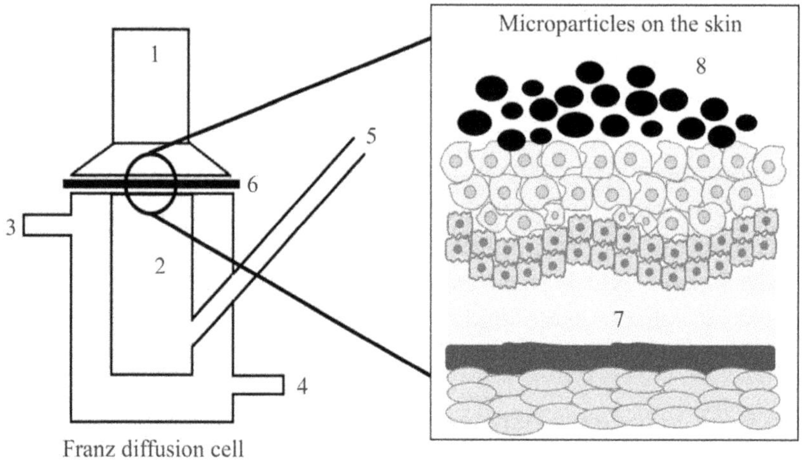

Fig. 12.15 Diagrammatic representation of *ex vivo* (skin) permeation study of microsphere in Franz diffusion cells. 1. Donor compartment, 2. Receptor compartment, 3. Water inlet, 4. Water outlet (to maintain temperature), 5. Sampling probe, 6. Skin/mucosal membrane, 7. Ultra structure of skin, 8. Microspheres over the skin surface.

12.5.7 *In vitro* Toxicity

The formulated microparticles may have some toxic effect on the live organisms/cells because of various reasons. It is the responsibility of the manufacturer/formulation professionals to ensure the non-toxic potential of the microparticles. As per the regulatory compliances (animal cruelty act 1960) microparticles formulations should qualify the *in vitro* safety, before *in vivo* (pre-clinical/ clinical) experimentation. Hence, comer-cially available *in vitro* cell lines [human renal proximal tubule epithelial cells (HRPTE), TR146, LLC-PK1, OK, NRK-52E and HK-2] for both animal as well as human are employed to investigate the *in vitro* toxicity studies. Now-a-days it has become a regular practice for industries and academia to inspect the toxicity profile of developed formulation. Suitable cell culture procedure is adopted and the developed microparticles are subjected to toxicity studies. The free drug (API), API loaded-microparticles, placebo (microparticle without API) and any reference standard are compared for the toxicity profile. The most popular assay procedure employed to evaluate cellular process is the MTT (3-(4, 5-dimethylthiazol-2-yl)-2,5-diphenyltetrazolium bromide, a yellow tetrazole) assay. This assay is based on the concept that tetrazolium dye is reduced to purple colored formazan which is dependent on NAD(P)H-dependent oxido-reductase enzymes largely in the cytosolic compartment of cells. This color solution is measured by spectrophotomeric/colorimetric methods at 570 nm. Reduction of MTT dye increases (increase formation of formazan and consequently color) with cellular metabolic activity due to elevated NAD (P) H flux and *vice versa*. Asthana et al. (2013) have reported MTT assay for cytotoxicity studies in *in vitro* J774A cell lines. Percent viability of cells is calculated and only if the developed microparticles qualify this test, it is further promoted to *in vivo* experimentation. The mechanism of MTT assay is shown below in Fig. 12.16.

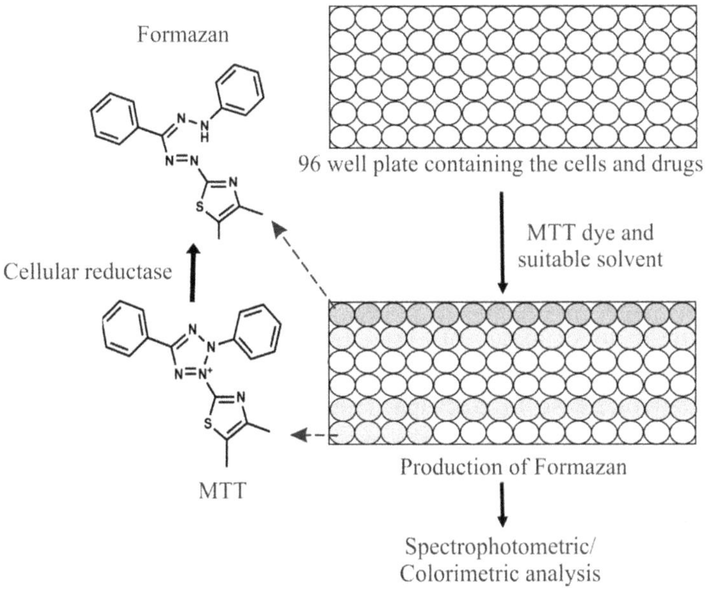

Fig. 12.16 An outline of mechanism of MTT assay in *in vitro* cell toxicity studies

12.5.8 Specific Analysis based on Type of Microparticles

Till now we have seen the generalized characterization parameters of microparticles, but as itemized in the section 1.2 (types of microparticles), there are specific types of microparticles such as magnetic, pH/thermo-responsive, floating, mucoadhesive microparticles etc. Apart from the generalized characterization, these specific microparticles need to be characterized for some categorical parameters. For the mucoadhesive microparticles, the test for mucoadhesive force/ strength is performed. These tests can be done by the classical methods of modified physical balance apparatus as done for mucoadhesive films/patches. Jain *et al.,* (2004) have described a classical method for mucoadhesive test of microparticles using goat intestinal mucosa and glass slide. They have stated that the cross-linked chitosan microspheres showed very good mucoadhesion which was found to reduce on increasing the drug concentration. Advanced techniques such as texture analyzer may also be used for these tests. Mucoadhesive microparticles are used in the delivery of drugs through buccal route as well as gastro retentive delivery. Similarly, for the floating microspheres, the bouncy test must be performed. The time required for the microspheres to float on the surface of dissolution fluid and the density of the same should be evaluated (Pawar *et al.,* 2012). pH responsive microparticles have come up as a successful delivery system in microparticles technology. These microparticles are very much promising in the tumor (acidic) environment. Tumor tissues have comparatively more acidic environment because of lactic acid production by acidic intracellular organelles. In this acidic microenvironments, amphiphilic copolymers holding pH-responsive histidine and sulfonamide moieties present a sharp pH-dependent micellization/demicellization transition, resulting in the demicellization leading to rapid drug release at target tumor tissues. This release behavior is characterized for the pH responsive microparticles by exposing these to different pH condition (*in vitro* and *in vivo*). The gamma scinitigraphy technique is also applied for this purpose to follow the degradation/release of microparticles in different locations *in vivo.* For magnetic microparticles, it is expected that maximum amount of microparticles will be accumulated to the place as directed by externally applied magnetic field. The magnetic microparticles are attached to florescent compounds and administered *in vivo.* The motion and location of the microparticles can be examined using fluorescence microscope. Recently Gui *et al.,* (2013) have encapsulated a magnetic and fluorescent meso-porous silica into thermo-sensitive chitosan microspheres for cell imaging and controlled drug release *in vitro.* This multi-functional microspheres exhibited encouraging application especially as thermo/pH-sensitive drug carriers for *in vivo* therapy.

12.5.9 *In vivo* Imaging of Microparticles

Microparticle location and movement can be traced out *in vivo* after administration of the radiolabeled microparticles. The first job is to label the microparticles with radioactive marker such as Technetium (^{99m}Tc), Yttrium (^{86}Y), Cerium (^{141}Ce), Iodine (^{131}I) etc. Different protocols are available for the labelling of microparticles to the radioactive groups. After labeling, the microparticles (suspension) are administered to the animal by the pre-specified route. The *in vivo* transit behavior of radiolabeled microparticles can be studied by directly subjecting the animal to imaging by a gamma camera. At pre-decided time interval images are captured and analyzed for the movement of radiolabeled microparticles. In order to check the bio-distribution, the animal is sacrificed and vital organs like liver, spleen, kidney, thyroid gland, stomach and intestine etc. (as per requirement) are isolated and radioactive counts of organs are recorded using gamma camera. The following Fig. 12.17 shows the artistic representation of the gamma scintigraphic images of microparticles in rabbits/rats.

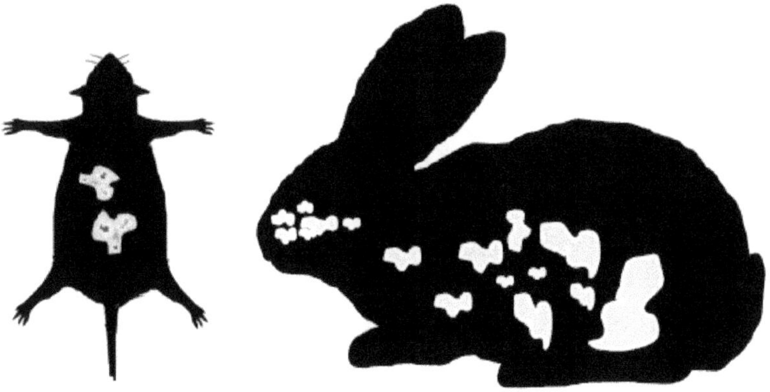

Fig. 12.17 Gamma scintigraphic images of microparticles in rat (in stomach) and rabbit in body *via* nasal route.

12.5.10 Stability Studies

The microparticles must be in a stable form throughout its self-life. The purpose of stability testing of microparticles is to gather information on the quality of drug product over time under the influence of a variety of environmental factors such as temperature, humidity and light. Stability testing also suggests the appropriate storage conditions and re-test periods for microparticles. Rather, to investigate and determine the self-life of microparticles either as such or in dosage form, the stability evaluation is performed. There are specific protocols for the stability evaluation of the conventional and novel drug delivery systems. ICH is the worldwide accepted body and the protocol fixed by ICH is followed for stability evaluation of new drugs or drug products. In the stability evaluation, microparticles are subjected to the different accelerated and conventional stability testing procedures. The intrinsic stability of the drug molecule is evaluated in the stress testing and it suggests the degradation pathways, degradation products as well as the stability indicating capability of the analytical procedures employed. The first step in the stability testing is the selection of batches which must be a random selection and evaluation data of at least three batches are required. The storage conditions should be (i) 25 ± 2 °C/ 60% ± 5% RH for 12 months in long term testing and (ii) 40 ± 2 °C/75% ± 5% RH for 6 months in accelerated testing conditions. Certain parameters such as size, shape, charge, drug content, surface morphology etc. (parameters likely to change during storage and expected to influence quality, safety and/or efficacy) are studied in the stability analysis. Any 'significant change' observed in the accelerated stability testing of microparticles are further subjected to an intermediate condition e.g., 30 ± 2 °C/60 ± 5% RH. 'Significant change' at the accelerated condition as per ICH guidelines is defined as:

1. A five percent potency loss from the initial assay value of a batch
2. Any specified degradant exceeding its specification limit
3. The product exceeding its pH limits
4. Dissolution exceeding the specification limits
5. Failure to meet specifications for appearance and physical properties e.g., color, phase separation, re-suspendibility, delivery per actuation, caking, hardness, etc.

The long term testing will be performed for a sufficient time beyond 12 months to cover shelf life at appropriate test periods. The testing frequency should be adequate to establish the stability characteristics of the drug product and is normally at every three months over the first year, every six months over the second year and then annually.

12.5.11 *In vivo* Studies

In vivo pre-clinical studies are basically performed to investigate the (i) therapeutic effect (ii) bio-distribution and pharmacokinetics and (iii) toxicity profile of the developed formulations. Animal models (rabbit, rat, mice, guinea pig etc.) are used in the pre-clinical investigation. The microspheres of intended activity (anticancer/antidiabetic/antileishmanial or any other action) are administered to the animal in the proposed dosage form as per the officially approved protocols [Organization for Economic Co-operation and Development (OECD), Food and Drug Administration (FDA), International Conference on Harmonization (ICH)] (Martínez *et al.,* 2011) (Stumpf, 2007). The therapeutic effect is examined by suitable methods/protocols and is disease/problem specific. Bio-distribution of the drug may be studied by blood, urine or any other suitable biological samples. A suitable analytical technique (LCMS, GCMS, and HPLC etc.) is required for the quantification of drug in these biological samples. In the *in vivo* toxicity studies, the effect of API/microparticles on the vital organs like liver, kidney, spleen and any specific tissues etc. are examined. Histo-pathological and biomarkers (cytokines; TNF-α, IL-12, IL-4, IL-10 and TGF-β) alteration/changes are examined as the evaluation parameters for toxicity studies.

12.5.12 *In vitro-In vivo* Correlation (IVIVC)

The pharmaceutical formulation has to clear the *in vitro* drug release test before being subjected to stability and *in vivo* studies. For the conventional formulations (tablet, capsules etc.) there are well documented protocols (regulatory/pharmacopeial procedure) for the *in vitro* drug release tests but in case of sustained/controlled release formulations, no standard drug release test methods are available. The microparticles formulations showing promising result in the *in vitro* drug release test are subjected to *in vivo* performance evaluation but many times poor correlation is observed in these evaluations. A competent *in vitro* test with *in vivo* relevance is very much useful for pharmaceutical industries in saving money and time. Many pharmaceutical companies aim to obtain the bio-waiver by using the IVIVC instead of the cumbersome bio-studies. Two (or more) formulations with different drug release rates are employed for IVIVC and a level A-IVIVC (point-to-point correlation) is necessary for the *in vitro* drug release method to be used as an alternate for bioequivalence studies. It has been found very difficult to get a good IVIVC in case of any novel drug delivery products like microparticles. The reasons being; biological fluid viscosity (barrier) interfering drug diffusion, enzymatic degradation of microparticles (polymers), degradation product of microparticles leading to autocatalysis of polymer, immunogenic/inflammatory reaction of microparticles etc. Regulatory guidelines have been set by FDA for IVIVC as different (five) levels viz. Level A, Level B, Level C and multiple level C and level D.

1. **Level A**: It gives a point-to-point correlation between *in vitro* and *in vivo* drug release profiles.
2. **Level B**: It utilizes statistical moment analysis in comparing a mean *in vitro* dissolution time to either a mean *in vivo* dissolution or residence time.
3. **Level C**: It establishes a single point relationship between a dissolution parameter such as time required for 50% dissolution and a pharmacokinetic parameter e.g., C_{max}/AUC.

4. **A multiple level C**: It relates multiple dissolution time points to one or more pharmacokinetic parameters such as C_{max} or AUC.
5. **Level D**: It is a rank order correlation for IVIVC.

Rawat *et al.,* (2012) has investigated IVIVC of Risperdal® Consta® (commercial risperidone microspheres; a long acting injection). They had de-convoluted the clinical *in vivo* plasma profile data (as reported by the innovator) for comparison with the *in vitro* release profiles. In their study they found the *in vivo* profile was faster initially and then slower after approximately 30 days in comparison to the real time *in vitro* profile. The reasons attributed to such behavior were owing to variations in the *in vivo* conditions (small interstitial volume, low pH and immune response). In the same study Rawat and co-worker reported a linear IVIVC with correlation coefficients of 0.97 and 0.99 at accelerated temperature (accelerated *in vitro* tests) i.e., 50 °C and 54.5 °C respectively. Conclusively, they have demonstrated that the accelerated *in vitro* tests performed showed the potential to be used for *in vivo* performance prediction as well as for quality control purposes.

12.6 Sterilization of Microparticles

Microparticles are intended for various applications and many routes of drug administration are employed for this purpose. In case of parenteral and ocular products sterilization is a major step and products containing microparticles of these categories need to be sterilized before coming to the market for commercialization. For the conventional products moist heat sterilization is the preferred process as this is easier than other sterilization process. But in case of heat sensitive drugs as well as novel formulation such as microparticles, nanoparticles, liposomes, dendrimers etc., heat sterilization is not suitable because it may disrupt the drug as well as polymers used in the formulation. So the other sterilization techniques viz. filtration, radiation and chemical sterilization are applied. Chemical sterilization has its own disadvantages of being reactive with the drugs and excipients, at the same time filtration (through 0.22 µm filter pore) sterilization cannot be used for microparticles. The only option left is radiation sterilization and gamma-irradiation has been widely used for this purpose (Puthli and Vavia, 2008). However, other requirements for parenteral product manufacturing e.g., maintenance of various classes (100, 10,000 and 1, 00,000) clean room as per cGMP are must for formulation and processing of microparticles for parenteral purposes. It has also been reported that irradiation of the formulation products sometimes cause degradation of drug as well as other excipients (especially biodegradable polymers).

12.7 Factors Influencing Microparticle Formulation-Development and Characteristics

Various methods used in formulation of microparticles are already discussed in this chapter. A number of excipients are used in the formulation of microparticles. These excipients may be either functional or inactive and in some instances some excipients are only used to facilitate the microparticles formulation process. So it is obvious that these preparation process, excipients (additives), API and also the experimental conditions would have impact on the formulation-development and performance of microparticles. It is also noticeable that the scale of manufacturing plays crucial role in the formulation and characteristics of microparticles. In this section of this chapter the readers will be introduced in to the effect of some of the important parameters affecting the overall performance of microparticles.

12.7.1 Method of Preparation

The method of formulation has a greater impact on the overall performance of microparticles. Various process parameters such as fluid flow, heat and mass transfer impart major effects on the formation of microparticles. In addition to these factors, stirring conditions, vessel and nozzle geometry, feed conditions, process like spray drying/freezing, and supercritical fluid techniques etc., play determining role in the development of microparticles (Benita, 2005). These parameters are of immense impact at the industrial measure and multinational companies have their own technology transfer department, which is solely responsible in shooting out problems encountered in the laboratory-pilot/commercial scale-up program.

Emulsion technique is one of the most feasible techniques of microparticles formulation, and the solubility of the drug in the aqueous media, appropriate concentration of surfactants, temperature, polymer-phase ratio are the important parameters that need to be determined in the initial phase of every encapsulation study. The agitation speed may cause variation in the size of microparticles and it has been reported that high agitation causes formation of smaller microparticles which might be attributed to the formation of fine droplets of polymer encapsulating the drug. In some instances it has also been seen that a very high agitation have resulted in low loading and reason might be the efflux of drug from the polymer capsule during formulation. Solvent volatility is another important aspect in the emulsification-solvent evaporation technique. For methylene chloride the rate-limiting stage in a laboratory (beaker) method is revealed to be the liquid-side transport, whereas the ethyl acetate evaporation is also restricted by the unstirred gas layer, and flushing the headspace of the beaker with another gas, (N_2), is observed to proficiently rise the solvent removal in the second case. Conversely, for industrial applications in closed vessels a frequent replacement of the gas phase by intensively flushing the liquid surface has been suggested to be necessary for appropriate solvent evaporation.

The use of ultrasound for emulsification might cause degradation of drugs and polymers, especially those that contain hydrolyzable bonds such as esters. Accumulation of some polymer (PLA/PLGA) degradation products inside the microparticles (under release conditions) results in an acidic microclimate that also may affect hydrolyzable bonds in the drug molecule. In the emulsification-solvent evaporation technique, it has been observed that a very high drug loading, (e.g., 50% progesterone or 70% testosterone propionate in PLA microparticles), has led to crystallization of the drug during the solvent removal, which consequently resulted in perforation of the particle wall by drug needles. This phenomena may alter the size and shape of microparticles as well as drug release characteristic (Wischke and Schwendeman, 2008).

Spray drying and congealing is one of the widely used methods in microparticles formulation at industrial scale. Here the feed size and properties (viscosity, uniformity and concentration of core materials), coating materials, solvent and its characteristics, exposure time remain the main parameters in the formation of good quality microparticles. The process of aromatization and also the latent heat of vaporization of the solvent are the key factors in the bulk scale production. By this microencapsulation method, issue of large volumes of solvent-contaminated water phase that result from emulsion-based encapsulation methods can be resolved. Moreover, larger batch size can be effectively produced with spray drying method in comparison to the emulsion-solvent evaporation method.

In the coacervation-phase separation method, the microparticles are formed by various approaches viz. salt addition, non-solvent addition, in-compatible polymer addition or temperature change. All these methods are very much specific and microparticles formulation is affected by selection of parameters involved in the process. The type of salt, non-solvent and its effect on the solubility of API, nature of incompatible polymer etc. determine the shape and size as well as the encapsulation efficiency of API. As these steps determine the microparticle formation, any fluctuation in their concentration or properties result into change in the characteristics of microparticles.

12.7.2 Pharmaceutical Excipients, API and Other Raw Materials

Microparticles basically contain the API, pharmaceutical excipients and some other raw materials. Raw materials include the ingredients (solvents and chemicals) which are used in the formulation but finally removed from the microparticles. These basic three components have major role in the development as well as characteristics of developed microparticles.

Let us first understand the effect of API in the microparticles. API is the chief part of microparticles, and its physicochemical properties controls the type of microparticles (micro-spheres/-capsules) to be formulated. The biological half-life ($t_{1/2}$), absorption window, molecular weight, dissociation constant, pH stability, solubility and most importantly the dose are major points to be taken into consideration. Solubility and $t_{1/2}$ of API decide the type and quantity of polymer to be used in order to get the desired release. Sometimes it is recommended that a combination of polymers (hydrophilic and hydrophobic) can be used to get required drug release. Further, based on the nature of API and polymers other solvents, non-solvents and methods of microparticles are chosen for formulation. Floating microspheres may be formulated for API beneficial to be released in stomach by using excipients such as sodium bicarbonate and polymer. This method is based on the mechanism that, upon contact with water such system releases carbon dioxide and becomes porous and floats in the gastric fluid and releases drug in the stomach (Bhadouriya *et al.,* 2012). Likewise several other strategies are adopted to develop microparticles based on nature of API. Literature reveals the effect of quantity of drug on the size, shape, distribution as well as drug release characteristics. Mao *et al.,* (2008) have reported that an increase in drug (hydrophobic) loading (> 45%) negatively influences the drug release of microspheres, whereas no significant effect on the other *in vitro* characteristic has been seen. The mechanism of such behavior may be attributed to the fact that, increase in content of hydrophobic drug might have caused in phase separation between the drug and polymer and favored formation of hydrophobic drug aggregates leading to slower drug dissolution and release. High molecular weight protein molecules can be released through pores during polymer degradation of microparticles, at the contrary, smaller protein molecules can diffuse through pores primarily present in the microparticle polymer matrix. Amine drugs can catalyze degradation of the most widely used polymers PLA/PLGA polyester and if weak bases or acids are to be encapsulated, the presence of any drug-induced polymer degradation should be evaluated. So in a nut-shell it is the characteristics of the API that influence the behavior of microparticles in many aspects.

Pharmaceutical excipients are the building blocks of microparticles. These excipients include polymer, cross linking agent, stabilizers as discussed in the earlier section of this chapter. Polymer plays a central role in the formulation as well as the basic characteristic of microparticles. The selection of polymers solely depends on the physicochemical properties of API and desired drug release profile. An interesting example of the effect of polymer is reported in the literature which states that the particle size and encapsulation efficiency of microspheres decreased slightly when the polymer containing free carboxyl groups compared to those formed with the polymer containing ester end groups. The degradation of microparticles in the dissolution medium is a function of molecular weight of polymers. An erratic degradation and the consequent drug release behavior (slow or fast release or even dual/two-stage release) is due to the alterations in glass transition temperatures and crystallinity of polymers with different molecular weight. The size and shape of microparticles of PLGA with different molecular weights are significantly dissimilar. Literature is flooded with numerous reports on the effect of polymers on the modulation of size, shape and drug release of microparticles. The state of polymers i.e., amorphous/crystalline also determines the drug release as well as other parameters. The amorphous character causes absorption of more water than crystalline polymers leading to faster release rates compared to crystalline polymers or polymers with a high proportion of crystalline regions (Conway *et al.,* 1997). Another proposed mechanism of delayed release of drug from crystalline polymer is the increase in the diffusional path length. Polylactic acid represents polymer with a high proportion of crystalline regions, and polyglycolic acid represents high proportion of amorphous regions.

Other raw materials include the surfactants used in the emulsion polymerization or simple emulsion methods of microparticle formulation. Emulsifiers/surfactants have effect on the size of microparticles. During the emulsification process, the packing arrangement of emulsifiers controls the size of droplets formed and consequently the size of microparticles. Inappropriate packing arrangement of emulsifier (wrong selection) can lead to formation of larger poly-dispersed unstable particles.

12.7.3 Temperature

The microparticles are exposed to different temperature conditions either during the preparation or storage. Temperature during microparticle formulation may alter the EE and drug release. An interesting outcome of studies on effect of temperature on EE revealed that approximately 50% of EE was obtained at 4 and 38 °C whereas only 19% at 22 and 29 °C (Yang *et al.,* 2000). Such anomalous domino effect indicates involvement of different mechanisms in the encapsulation process at varying temperature. It is anticipated that at lower temperature, augmented immiscibility concerning the microparticles and water results in a hastily forming outer sphere wall, thus entrapping the drug in a faster manner early in the evaporation process. In contrast, an increased rate of solvent evaporation at higher temperature, results in a rapidly hardening sphere wall and quicker trapping of drug.

The size of microparticles are also changed with different temperature during formulation process. It is well-known that the viscosity of solution is a function of temperature. Researchers have reported that at lower temperatures, excipient-drug solution pose higher viscosity and forms larger microparticles. Similarly in the solvent evaporation method, at higher temperature quick solvent evaporation occurs and cause formation of larger microparticles.

12.7.4 pH of Solvents

The formulation of microparticles are done in a manufacturing vehicle medium, which is the continuous phase. The solubility of drug may be dependent on the pH, in other words, an altered spectrum of solubility is seen with different pH conditions. In such cases, if the solubility of the drug is favorable in the pH condition of the continuous phase, then the drug may be dissolved in the same medium resulting in low drug encapsulation. It is thus important to check the pH dependent solubility of the drug, which may influence the drug loading in microparticles. Caution must be displayed in order to protect the drug in the altered pH conditions of finished product during storage. It has been demonstrated that low pH microenvironment due to degrading polymer matrix can cause alteration in the physicochemical as well as pharmacological/ toxicological potential of API which are susceptible to acid catalytic degradation such as proteins, bio-macromolecules, steroids etc. The nature of polymers in the formulation of microparticle has a significant role and these polymers are again dependent on pH for their optimum performance. For instance, the de-acetylated subunit of chitosan has a primary amine group (pKa; 6.5), making it soluble in acidic media but insoluble at neutral and alkaline pH which necessitates that formulating microparticles with chitosan, the pH of polymer solution must be critically controlled.

12.8 Scale up in Microparticles

Scale up techniques are the way through which the formulation-research worked out in the laboratory can be realized at the industrial scale. After all, at the end of the day it is about the feasibility of the developed formulation for commercialization and without this every attempt is of no use for businesses or public health. Very often it has been seen that many drug delivery systems are developed with extravagant techniques and excipients (excipients that are not recognized by regulatory agencies), but have no space for up-gradation into bulk manufacturing level. So, the ground reality is to conceptualize the use of feasible and realistic techniques as well as use of the approved excipients. Basic techniques mean those unit operations (steps in the manufacturing of a drug-product) which are successfully being employed in the pharmaceutical industries for the development of bulk scale products. By utilizing these techniques any newly developed drug-product can be scaled up to the industrial measure. As we have discussed, the unit operation like sonication, ultra-centrifuge can be utilized very easily in the laboratory scale for the development of microparticles, but these methods are relatively not feasible in the industrial scale in the current industrial setup. Similarly, evaporation (unit operation) by rotavapor instrument in the development of micelles/liposomes is one of the very convenient techniques in the laboratory scale but many times cannot be scaled up to the bulk scale. Instead of using these techniques, utilization of the industrially feasible methods viz. spray drying, coacervation, lyophilization, homogenization, hot melt extrusion, emulsification-solvent evaporations can be taken in to consideration before developing the microparticles. However research must be undertaken in making the small/laboratory scale techniques (ultra-sonication, evaporation by rotavapor, ultra-centrifuge etc.) to be feasible at industrial level and a multidisciplinary approach in this regard is required. In the bulk production reproducibility of formulations/ products is very much important and depends upon delicate phases of the production process. In the industrial scale it is rarely the case that production occurs as a simple multiple of component masses or volumes, vessel geometries, mixing, or filtration conditions as in laboratory scale. Pharmaceutical companies have developed scaled-up processes for microsphere manufacturing and are available in the market as successful products.

The use of optimization techniques and factorial design is very much decisive in the industrial scale. These techniques not only reduce the failure chances but also meet the regulatory requirement in filing a new drug product. In the development of microparticles at the industrial scale, the multinational companies (MNCs) protect information about scale-up and all the obligatory information on equipment and manufacturing constraint as in-house ''know how''. Pharmaceutical industries employ dimensional analysis to manage the variations in manufacturing of the microparticles. Four similarity factors viz. geometric, dynamic, thermal and chemical factors are the backbone of dimensional analysis during microparticle scale up. In the geometric similarity the fluid motion in a vessel is made similar, while dynamic similarity deals with the ratios of forces moving masses viz. pressure, gravitational, and centrifugal forces. The other two factors i.e., thermal and chemical similarity deliberate heat transfer in the process and the variation in chemical composition as a function of time, respectively.

12.9 Pharmaceutical Applications

Microparticles have a wide range of applications. Both in the pharmaceutical (biomedical) as well as personal care products microparticles are playing a significant role. A number of MNCs are employing the microencapsulation techniques in their product development campaign. Some of the major players (MNC products) are Pfizer (Telstar®; Triptorelin pamoate microspheres), Janssen Pharmaceuticals (Risperdal® Consta®; Risperidone microspheres), Novartis (Sandostatin LAR® Depot; Octreotide acetate microparticles), Exact (Exact®; benzoyl peroxide microspheres), OraPharma (Arestin®; Minocycline hydrochloride microspheres), P&G (Vicks Breathe Right®; pressure-released microparticulate menthol), Clorox (Spic and Span®; encapsulated enzyme) and Avon (Skin-so-Soft®; hand lotion, mineral oil capsule). A lot many microparticles products are under clinical trial and are expected to be in the market in near future. A huge number of research publications and patents are available in the scientific data bases advocating the successful application of microparticles. Microparticulate technologies cover the delivery of biopharmaceuticals, protein-peptides, and vascular tissues in the field of orthopedics, diabetes, tuberculosis, cancers and immunology, vaccines, gene therapy, stem cell research, as well as development of biomedical devices. In the following section readers will have a journey on the different aspects (practical and theoretical) of application of microparticle in different fields.

12.9.1 Sustained, Controlled and Targeted Drug Delivery

Microparticles are primarily formulated with polymers to achieve sustained and/or controlled release drug delivery system. Although microparticles are also formulated with the metallic ingredients, but these are yet to get success for therapeutic use in human. Metallic microparticles are especially reported in literature as drug targeting tools rather than sustained or controlled delivery. One of the prerequisite for sustained/controlled delivery is short biological half-life of drug molecules, which making the molecules eligible to be delivered in a sustained manner for a long period. Also there are many more intentions for the development of sustained and controlled delivery systems of drugs such as prolonged therapy, patient compliance, localized action as well as minimization of dose. Hence drug molecules having any physiological shortcomings such as low solubility, low permeability, less biological half-life, high first pass metabolism, non-selectivity leading to unwanted adverse effect etc., can be accommodated as sustained/controlled or targeted drug delivery systems in order to enhance therapeutic effect. On the contrary targeted drug delivery is somewhat different from the sustained/controlled delivery system. Here, in this case drug molecule is fabricated with a delivery system in such a manner that it can reach a specific region of body in its intact form. Drug targeting may be for organs, tissues, cells or even sub-cellular components. Microparticles are basically devised for organ and tissue targeting. Many functionalized polymers such as mucoadhesive, pH resistant and thermo-sensitive polymers are used in this purpose.

Pulsatile drug delivery of microparticles also comes under sustained/controlled delivery system. It is an established fact that certain diseases such as asthma, cardiac arrest, arthritis, ulcer etc., have a specific pattern as far as their attack/occurrence is being concerned. This is a function of the circadian rhythm of the body, which regulates the activation or inhibition of certain biological phenomena leading to these diseases. Even recently it has been found that blood flow to tumor tissue and cancer growth have a chrono-biological behavior. These facts bring about the necessity of a time-programmed therapeutic system which ensures the required quantity of drug at the site of action at the right time.

Microcapsules (reservoir type) are of specific use in the pulsatile drug delivery system. These microcapsule pulsatile delivery systems are coated with a polymer layer, which dissolves or erodes after a specified lag period, following the release of drug from the reservoir core. The lag time prior to drug release is controlled by the thickness and the viscosity grade of the polymer layer on the microcapsules. Spansule is one of the examples of this category of micro-particulate delivery system. The spansules are so prepared that an initial dose is released promptly and the remaining medication is released gradually over a prolonged period of time. The gradually released medication is usually the microparticles which have varying polymer coating leading to the pulsatile release of drug. The diagrammatic view of spansule and its internal structure is represented in Fig. 12.18.

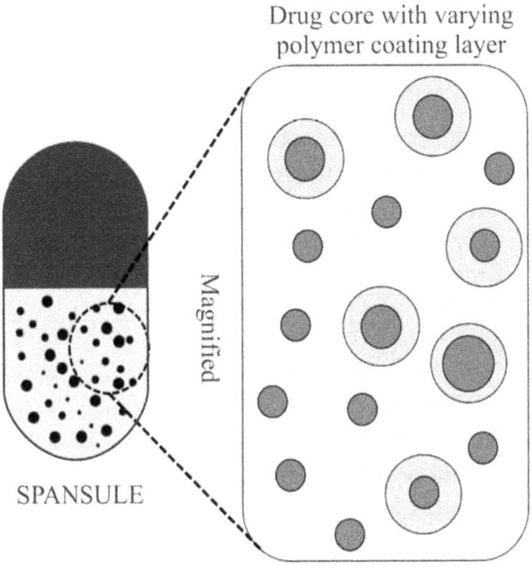

Fig. 12.18 Diagrammatic representation of spansule and its internal structure showing microcapsules with varying thickness of polymer coating surrounding the drug core.

12.9.2 Topical and Transdermal Drug Delivery

Microparticles have been attempted to be delivered by topical route. Apart from the pharmaceutical uses, coated titanium dioxide microparticles are commonly used as UV filter substances in commercial sunscreen products. de Jalón *et al.,* (2001) have developed PLGA-microparticles and investigated their fate on topical delivery. They have used rhodamine as a fluorescent probe and the PLGA-microparticles loaded with rhodamine were studied for skin distribution by horizontal and vertical slicing of frozen skin. They have found that the PLGA-microparticles could penetrate through the stratum corneum and reach the epidermis but could not reach to the receptor compartment of the diffusion cells. Many drug molecules such as acyclovir, cidofovir, quercetin, gentamicin etc., have been developed in to microspheres and their therapeutic effects were found to be comparatively better than the conventional formulations. The basic objective of the topical delivery is to sustain the release of the drug at the target site. Many antiacne formulations are also developed targeting the *Propionibacterium acne* through the microsphere drug delivery. Tretinoin gel, (USP) is a porous microsphere formulation in aqueous gel available in market for topical treatment of acne. For transdermal delivery, the microparticles are incorporated either into any semisolid conventional dosage forms like creams, gels and ointments or can be delivered by the transdermal films or patches.

12.9.3 Nasal and Pulmonary Drug Delivery

Readers must be clear with the difference in the delivery of drug through the nasal cavity and pulmonary route. There is a difference in the nasal and pulmonary delivery of drugs, the previous being the localization of drugs in the nasal route and absorption by the nasal mucosal blood capillary system, whereas the latter is the delivery of drug to the respiratory tract (inhalation therapy). Bioadhesive microspheres for nasal delivery of drugs are developed with albumin, starch and dextran, which upon contact with water get swelled and stay for a long time in the nasal cavity, leading to increase in drug absorption. Various microspheres for nasal delivery are available viz. Sephadex®, DEAE-Sephadex® (dextran crossed link with epichlorohydrine; 10-180 μm), and Spherex® (degradable starch microspheres; 10-180 μm). The drug absorption is hypothesized to be increased from nasal route by increasing contact time, and also due to increase in the gap between the tight junctions of the epithelial cells. Experimentally (*in vitro*) it has been found that when the microspheres absorb water from the mucus and swell, the epithelial cells get dehydrated leading to development of gap between cells. This process is reversible and do not adversely affect the human body. Insulin has been found to be absorbed rapidly *via* microspheres through nasal route and also caused lowering of blood glucose level in animals. Degradable starch microspheres are found to improve therapeutic efficacy of desmopressin, gentamicin, human growth hormone and metoclopramide upon nasal delivery. It has also been seen that in some instances there is nasal mucosal immune response upon delivery of microparticles and hence the irritability and inflammatory response of the ingredients used in microparticles must be analyzed before formulation and development. Jain *et al.,* (2004) have developed mucoadhesive chitosan microspheres containing salbutamol by emulsion solvent evaporation method. Cross-linked chitosan microspheres showed very good mucoadhesion, which was decreased on increasing the drug and citric acid concentration. *In vivo* performance of mucoadhesive microspheres exhibited extended and controlled release of salbutamol as compared to conventional oral dosage form. Till now, the success of nasal drug delivery of many drugs including proteins and peptides are seen in animal models, however these are yet to be confirmed in the human.

As mentioned above the pulmonary route of drug administration deals with the delivery of drug to the respiratory system and the mode of drug administration is inhalation. The therapeutic target may be trachea, bronchus or even bronchiole. In order to get maximum efficiency for deposition in the lung, the particles should be critically controlled in a size range of 1-10 μm. Particles larger than 10 μm may be deposited in the throat whereas if the particles are smaller than 1 μm these may be exhaled out during normal breathing. Some researchers advocate the use of mass median aerodynamic diameter (MMAD) which is the diameter of a hypothetical sphere of unit density having the same terminal settling velocity as the particle in question (here in this case it is the microparticles), regardless of the particle's geometric size, shape and density. Researchers assume that MMAD of 1-5 μm is considered to be satisfactory for microparticles targeted to lung. Inhalable microparticles are developed for a number of diseases including hypertension, asthma, diabetes, tuberculosis, and other diseases associated with lung infections. A large numbers of drugs viz. rifampicin, heparin, insulin, nitric oxide, ciprofloxacin, isoniazid etc., have been entrapped in microparticles and found to be therapeutically effective than the conventional delivery systems. Insulin has been extensively studied for pulmonary delivery and the first breakthrough came in January 2006, when the U.S. FDA approved the first inhalable insulin formulation "Exubera" developed by Pfizer. It was formulated in a powder dosage form containing recombinant human insulin, which was intended to be delivered through an inhaler into the lungs. Exubera was available as blisters of 1 mg (3 IU insulin) or 3 mg (8 IU insulin) and the formulation was composed of homogeneous powder formulation containing insulin, sodium citrate (dihydrate), mannitol, glycine, and sodium hydroxide. The average particle diameter of the powder formulation was < 5 μm. In October, 2007, Pfizer discontinued manufacturing and withdrawn Exubera from the market. Reason for the same was assigned to be non-acceptance of the product by patients as well as physicians. As such no toxic effects of Exubera were reported but it was associated with some other issues of concern which might be the reasons for its failure. Major issues among these were (1) dose accuracy (insulin is prescribed in international units by subcutaneous route but Exubera was prescribed in "mg" and there was no linear relations in the conversion of "mg" to international units), (2) the inhaler was too big and not handy, (3) higher dose administration was time consuming process (subcutaneous injection can be instantly administered), (4) selection of a specific insulin dose was not possible (possible in insulin injection), and (5) higher cost than traditional formulation.

12.9.4 Oral Drug Delivery

Microparticles can be delivered in tablets, capsules, powders and liquid dosage forms *via* oral route as per the intended therapeutic action. After the oral administration, the microparticles get exposed to gastric followed by intestinal fluids and based on the nature of polymers (acid resistant/degradable polymers employed for preparation of microparticles) the drug gets released either in the stomach or in the intestine. The release of drug from polymer matrix/reservoir depends on many factors viz. permeability/solubility of GI fluids into polymers, morphology/dimension of the microparticles, mechanism of hydrolysis, nature of additives etc. Uptake mechanisms, site of the absorption as well as the magnitude of particle taken up from the GI tract have been investigated by researchers but a common conclusion could not be drawn because of the anatomical and physiological complexity. Although it is observed that the absorption of intact microparticles occurs mainly in the Peyer's patches, but the same cannot be ruled out from the non- Peyer's patches area of the GI tract. Both the transcellular and paracellular pathways are responsible for absorption but the previous is found to be predominant.

A brief knowledge of the GI tract anatomy and physiology is useful in understanding the absorption of microparticles. Fig. 12.19(a) and (b) exhibit the diagrammatic presentation of GI tract showing the Peyer's patches and lymphatic uptake of microparticle by M cell in the Peyer patches. As it can be seen in the diagram, an epithelium lining is present on the GI tract containing the enterocytes (absorptive cells) and mucus secreting cells (goblet cells). These cells are very tightly attached and act as the barrier layer of GI tract. There is a special area in this barrier layer (enterocytes) which contains the specialized follicle associated epithelium. In this enterocyte layers of the GI tract, lymphoid follicles are found in a scattered manner. These lymphoid follicles form a cluster structure which is known as Peyer's patches (named after the Swiss anatomist Johann Conrad Peyer). Distribution of these Peyer's patches differs in species and individuals as per age. Peyer's patches are shielded by a distinct epithelium layer containing specialized microfold cells (M cells). These M cells can uptake antigen (microparticles) directly from the lumen by endocytosis/phagocytosis and transport them to intraepithelial macrophages and lymphocytes, which then migrate to lymph nodes. Researchers have found that these area (Peyer's patches) are the most common place for particle uptake.

In the *in vitro* cell studies it has been found that starch particles are able to open the tight junctions of Caco-2 cells (heterogeneous human epithelial colorectal adenocarcinoma cells, morphologically and functionally similar to enterocytes of small intestine). This further facilitates the absorption of the larger particles across the epithelial barrier. Some authors have found that particles are also taken up by the non-Peyer's patches tissues of GI tract and the uptake is size dependent. Some studies in animals (rabbits and rats) demonstrate that particles smaller than 5 μm could be transported into lymph whereas particles larger than 5 μm remain in the Peyer's patches. Many drug molecules are developed and evaluated for oral drug delivery and some of them are discussed herein. Hyaluronic microsphere with the better oral bioavailability of poorly water-soluble cyclosporin A (CsA) is developed using a spray-drying technique. Solubility and dissolution rate of CsA is increased about 17- and 2-fold respectively compared to CsA powder.

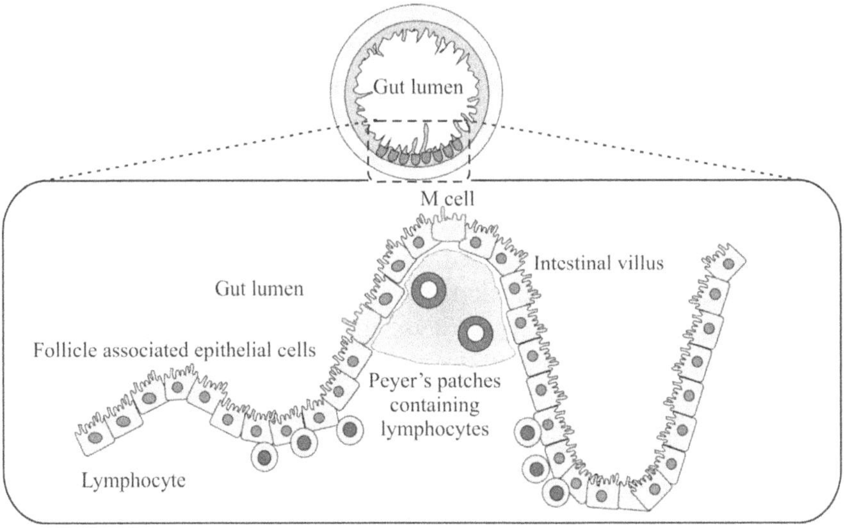

(a)

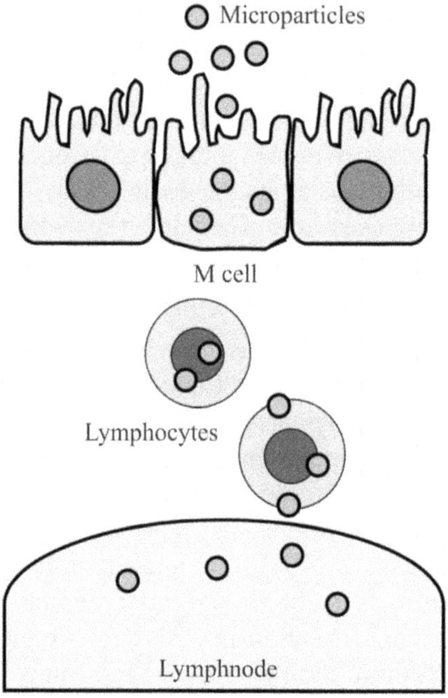

(b)

Fig. 12.19 (a) Diagrammatic representation of GI tract showing the Peyer's patches and M-cells (b) Diagrammatic representation of lymphatic uptake of microparticles by M-cell in Peyer's patches.

The CsA-microsphere and Sandimmun neoral sol® is found to show considerably higher blood levels compared with CsA powder alone. Oral calcitonin (CT; a cyclic polypeptide of 32 amino acids) is developed for the treatment of hypercalcemia by avoiding the existing injectable formulation. The pH sensitive microparticles of calcitonin is developed by the double emulsion technique with Eudragit for colon targeting. The colonic microsphere delivery of CT exhibited a distinct increase of the pharmacological effect compared to free CT. Recently protein and peptides are tried to be developed as microparticles delivery system. Many research works are reported on the microparticulate delivery of insulin. Insulin-loaded chitosan microspheres are developed by emulsion cross-linking method. The optimized microsphere prepared with 3% chitosan exhibited mean particle size of 29.5 μm, and insulin encapsulation efficiency of 71.6 ± 1.3%. *In vivo* studies in Wistar albino rats revealed a substantial reduction in blood glucose level after administration of the chitosan microsphere formulation, in comparison to a subcutaneous insulin injection. Developed chitosan microspheres were found to sustain protein release better than conventional insulin formulation. There is a long list of such scientific reports showing oral delivery of microparticles is a better way in manipulating the pharmacokinetic and dynamics of many drug molecules. The development of novel polymers having desired surface characteristics to increase the particle affinity for the GI tract epithelium surface is a hot topic of research in the current time. Fate of microparticles upon oral administration is still under debate and progress in molecular-biology will uncover the hidden actualities.

12.9.5 Parenteral Drug Delivery

Parenteral routes mainly include IV, IM and SC routes and microparticles are conveniently administered *via* these routes. There are more numbers of products available in market as parenteral products than oral products. Some of the marketed formulations are depicted in Table 12.1. Lupron Depot®, Nutropin Depot®, Optison, Risperdal® and Consta® are some of the representing products current available as parenteral marketed formulations. Many chemotherapeutic drugs, proteins, vaccines and gene delivery products are developed as microparticulate systems which are discussed separately in detail.

Biodegradability and biocompatibility are two major questions in the formulation and development of microparticulate parenteral products. Foreign body reaction to the microparticles as well as the tissue-material (polymers/excipients) interactions are the issues of concern for formulation scientists and a comprehensive understanding of the biodegradation and compatibility is highly needed in successfully developing a safe and effective microparticulate drug delivery system. Chemical composition, mechanism of hydrolysis, molecular weight of polymers, porosity, size shape and site of implantation/administration determine the fate of microparticles for biodegradation.

Recently D'Souza *et al.,* have reported parenteral delivery system of Risperidone that would provide initial and extended drug release and thereby avoid the need for co-administration of oral tablets (D'Souza *et al.,* 2013). They developed three PLGA based microsphere formulations that encapsulated Risperidone utilizing the solvent extraction/evaporation method. After optimizing *in vitro* and *in vivo* parameters they conclude that a microsphere dosage form of Risperidone can be formulated with an optimum particle size and drug loading to provide an initial bolus followed by maintenance levels, thereby eliminating combination therapy and improving patient compliance.

In their studies Voigt *et al.*, demonstrated a physically stable non-aqueous *in situ* forming microparticle emulsion capable of forming biodegradable microparticles upon injection (Voigt *et al.*, 2012). The microparticle emulsion consisted of a biocompatible organic PLGA solution dispersed in a continuous oil phase prepared in a two-syringe/connector system prior to administration. The injectability of the stabilized formulation was improved by about 30% compared to PLGA solution. The injectability improvement allows a faster administration or enables the use of thinner needles and hence reduced patient discomfort. Mao *et al.*, have discussed the polymeric microspheres prepared as parenteral drug delivery system for sustained release of therapeutic agents *via* subcutaneous or intramuscular injection (Mao *et al.*, 2012a).

12.9.6 Ocular Drug Delivery

Microparticles are developed as ocular delivery systems for various drug molecules for treatment of many ocular diseases/disorders. Ocular disorders viz. proliferative vitreoretinopathy, endophthalmitis, recurrent uveitis, acute retinal necrosis and cytomegalovirus retinitis are major causes of blindness globally and require frequent intravitreous injections to achieve intraocular drug levels within the therapeutic range. Microparticles provide sustained/controlled release of medicaments and offer a better way of treatment. Due to biocompatible and biodegradable nature, PLA, PLGA and copolymers of lactic and glycolic acids are commonly employed for preparation of microparticles for ocular delivery.

Depending on the microsphere size, injections of microspheres suspensions are usually made using 27-gauge, 26-gauge, 25-gauge and 18-gauge needles as well as a micro-injector connected to a glass micropipette (tip diameter 40 mm). The microspheres are usually suspended in physiological solution (phosphate buffer solution/balanced salt solution; pH 7.4) and are administered to the eye. Sterilization is extremely important for microparticulate drug delivery systems intended for ocular administration. The preferred sterilization mode is irradiation dose of 25 KGy (2.5 Mrad) which is accepted for sterilizing pharmaceutical as per cGMP regulations (Herrero-Vanrell and Refojo, 2001).

Liu and group have developed alginate microsphere-collagen composite hydrogel for ocular drug delivery and implantation (Liu *et al.*, 2008). The composite hydrogel supported human corneal epithelial cell growth and had adequate mechanical strength and excellent optical clarity. They suggested it to be used as therapeutic lens for drug delivery and/or use as corneal substitute for transplantation into patients with corneal diseases. Shinde *et al.,* have prepared and characterized chitosan-alginate microspheres for ocular delivery of azelastine using modified ionotropic gelation technique (Shinde *et al.,* 2014). The developed microparticles exhibited a particle size range suitable for ocular delivery. *In vitro* release and *in vivo* efficacy studies revealed that the microspheres were effective in prolonging the drug's presence in cul de sac with improved therapeutic efficacy.

PLGA microspheres for the ocular delivery of a peptide drug, vancomycin using emulsification/spray-drying technique was reported by Gavini *et al.,* (Gavini *et al.,* 2004). *In vivo* studies were performed by evaluating the pharmacokinetic profile of drug in the aqueous humor of rabbits after topical administration of microspheres (aqueous suspensions). Higher and prolonged drug concentrations as well as increased AUC values (2-fold) with respect to an aqueous solution of the drug were observed.

12.9.7 Protein and Gene Delivery

Since last couple of decades delivery of protein-peptides have exhaustively been studied by researchers globally. Both the pharmaceutical industries and academia are trying to get effective and stable products containing these ingredients as API. Serious challenges are faced by the formulation scientists in developing the delivery system of these drugs because of their larger and complex molecular orientation. Physicochemical properties such as solubility and permeability are other issues of concern. At such situation the added hindrance in this regard is the protection of proteins against inactivation by the gastrointestinal tract barriers, pH and proteolytic degradation. Enhanced bioavailability, half-life and reduced number of therapeutic doses are the key aspects of protein delivery.

A number of protein microparticulate systems are under clinical trials such as (i) basic fibroblast growth factor (bFGF) as gelatin hydrogel microspheres (clinical Phase I-IIa), for the treatment of critical limb ischemia by IM injection of microspheres, (ii) Locteron™; poly(ether-ester) microsphere (Phase-I) of recombinant interferon-alpha-2b for hepatitis C treatment. Apart from these, a number of research reports are available in scientific text on the delivery of protein by microparticles. Encapsulation of bone morphogenetic protein 2 in gelatin microspheres for local delivery, prepared by the emulsion method followed by crosslinking with genipin has been reported. Sustained release of vascular endothelial growth factor from alginate microparticles formed by ionic crosslinking is described by researchers. Reports are available on insulin delivery systems, such as, insulin-loaded alginate-chitosan microspheres by membrane emulsification technique.

The advancement of drug delivery science does not rest with achievement of protein delivery only, rather it accelerates into the development of more advanced delivery system. One of the growing fields in drug delivery is utilization of genetic materials such as plasmid deoxyribo-nucleic acid (pDNA), antisense oligonucleotides and antigens into target cells. The purpose in delivering these ingredients is to improve or alter the protein expression. But the major interruption in delivery of these nucleic acids are their properties viz. negative charge, hydrophilicity and vulnerability to degradation in the biological fluids.

Biodegradable microparticles have been developed for local delivery of gene therapeutics. PLGA microparticles were prepared to deliver oxytocin receptor antisense oligo-deoxynucleotides for social recognition inhibition in mice. PLGA microparticles have also been used to deliver plasmid-encoding interleukin-10 (IL-10) to alleviate neuropathic pain. Chitosan microparticles were equipped to deliver pigment epithelium-derived factor plasmid for treatment of osteosarcoma in mice and it was found to reduce bone degradation (osteolysis). Poly-(ethyleneimine) is employed as a cationic molecules in fabrication of microspheres, in delivering genetic materials such as DNA, RNA, or oligonucleotide (negatively charged). Employment of cationic excipients in microspheres can result in condensing of genetic materials by electrostatic interaction. Endolysosomal degradation of genetic materials is inhibited by these cationic molecules via proton sponge mechanism and facilitates the effective gene therapy without degradation of genes.

12.9.8 Vaccine Delivery

Vaccination is the back bone of healthcare system of a nation. Greater success in this field of medical research will ensure a good health for human being. The main hurdles in the development of vaccine formulations for human use are antigen stability, storage and release matters. Microspheres for vaccine delivery have been reported broadly for a variety of antigens such as protein, peptide, DNA, toxin and viruses.

Microspheres offer an additional intrinsic adjuvant effect to induce humoral and cellular immune responses which is shown to be superior to conventional adjuvants like aluminum salts. Many microparticles formulation are under clinical trial and expected to be in the market after positive results in the clinical investigation. PLGA microparticles containing ZYC300, a plasmid DNA of CYP1B1 (universal tumor antigen over expressed in human tumors) have been studied in human clinical trials (Phase-I) for cancer treatment. The treatment was found to be safe, without significant adverse effects such as autoimmunity. PLGA microparticles encapsulated plasmid DNA vaccine was administered intramuscularly to treat human papilloma virus associated high-grade cervical dysplasia.

Ajdary *et al.,* (2007) have developed alginate microparticles containing Bacille Calmette Guerin (BCG) and vaccinated BALB/c mice orally. They found a significantly higher proliferative, delayed-type hypersensitivity responses and g-interferon production, lower bacterial count and better immune responses in comparison with the free BCG. In case of oral vaccine delivery the access of these vaccines to the proper site for immune response must be considered. The vaccine should reach the M-cells of Peyer's patches in the gut and avoid the hostile acidic pH condition of the stomach. Sometimes immune response is not induced because of inadequate availability and uptake of vaccine to the Peyer's patches. Microparticles have been investigated to show that the uptake by M-cells is considerably boosted and degradation of drug in the GI tract is prevented.

12.9.9 Enzyme and Growth Factor Delivery

Enzymes are very much sensitive to pH and very often degraded by the gastric acid or even intestinal alkaline pH. The delivery of enzymes are therefore very challenging especially through oral route. At such situation protection of the enzyme by drug delivery tools is necessary in delivering to target site in appropriate quantity.

Delivery of enzymes by microparticles is reported in scientific literature. Glucocerebrosidase is an enzyme, highly unstable in solution under physiological conditions and is used in the treatment of Gaucher disease (genetic disease in which lipid accumulates in cells and certain organs). Ribeiro *et al.,* (2004) have reported the microspheres of glucocerebrosidase which is composed of calcium titanium phosphate-alginate and hydroxyapatite-alginate. They incorporated enzyme in the ceramic-alginate matrix as either pre-adsorbed onto the ceramic particles or dispersed in the polymeric matrix. The enzyme release was found to be different by these approaches.

Prolidase (naturally occurring enzyme involved in protein catabolism) deficiency causes autosomal recessive inherited disorder, leading to imino-peptiduria and pleiotropic clinical features (ulcerations of the skin, mental retardation, recurrent infections, hepatosplenomegaly etc.). PLGA-prolidase loaded microparticulate systems have been prepared utilizing the w/o/w double emulsion solvent evaporation method. After *in vitro* and *ex vivo* evaluation authors have claimed that the formulation can be employed as a parenteral depot drug delivery system.

Growth factors either stimulate or inhibit the growth of cells by regulating the cell signaling. It influences direct cell proliferation, differentiation, migration and angiogenesis in tissues. These growth factor can be administered into the body but rapid degradation both through intravenous or oral route is the major hindrance in their application. Drug delivery technology serves an answer to these problems. Vascular endothelial growth factor (VEGF) (a potent angiogenic regulator, facilitating formation of blood vessels) was attempted to be delivered by the novel drug delivery systems. VEGF is very much prone to chemical degradation such as de-amidation, diketo-piperazine and oxidation, at the same time it has a very short half-life. Sharp high level of VEGF in blood causes unwanted side effects. So it needs to be protected and released in a sustained manner. Wu *et al.,* (2012) have developed the microspheres of chitosan-polycaprolactone with high (80%) encapsulation efficiency. These microspheres were accomplished of retaining sustained VEGF-release in a nearly linear manner over a period of time longer than four weeks and did not involve a significant initial burst.

12.9.10 Radio Diagnostics

Microparticles of various size can be radiolabeled and studied by suitable imaging techniques for diagnosis of different disease conditions. These are termed as the radiopharmaceuticals and come under nuclear medicine. The widely used imaging technique is single photon emission computed tomography technique, which can give clear images of labeled microparticles. Microparticles of different polymeric materials and radio isotopes are used to target various sites in the body. Albumin microparticles labeled with ^{99m}Tc are used for lung imaging (10-90 μm) under the trade name Draximage (Pharmalucence, USA). ^{99m}Tc-sulphur microparticles (Pharmalucence, Billerica, MA) are employed for a variety of uses viz. liver and spleen imaging, bone marrow and lymph imaging, GI blood loss and gastric emptying studies. Other examples include ^{90}Y labeled resin microspheres (25-35 μm) used in radio-embolization of liver tumor under the trade name SIR-Spheres® (SIRTex, United States), microparticles for the same purpose under the trade name TheraSphere® (MDS Nordion, United States), ^{32}P-chromic phosphate colloid (2 μm) is used for the treatment of peritoneal or pleural effusions caused by metastatic disease, under the trade name Phosphocol P^{32} (Mallinckrodt Inc., USA).

12.9.11 Miscellaneous Applications

Major applications of the microparticles in healthcare sector are narrated above but it does not limit the uses and application of microparticles. There are various other applications of the microparticles such as vaginal, cosmetic, bone generation/grafting, periodontal and colon delivery. A polymer-lipid based mucoadhesive microspheres for vaginal delivery of econazole nitrate was developed by spray-congealing technique by Albertini *et al.,* (2009). Authors claimed that microparticles had inhibition effect on the *Candida albicans* growth and can be employed as an effective treatment for vaginal candidiasis, with additional advantages of reduced administration frequency. Solid lipid microspheres of octyl methoxy cinnamate (UV light absorber) was prepared by Yener and co-worker to achieve controlled release, decrease penetration from skin and improve its photostability. The microspheres were found to be effective in the desired action and suggested by authors to be employed as skin care product (Yener *et al.,* 2003). A new technologically improved microencapsulated sunscreens has been developed by Anselmi and co-workers (Anselmi *et al.,* 2002). They have characterized the developed microparticles and reported superior UV-radiation stability, low toxicity, and better tolerability. The microparticles were easy to manufacture and exhibited promising effect. Microparticles of pseudo-ceramide were developed for imparting barrier function to skin. The developed microparticles were evaluated *in vivo* for potential to reduce trans-epidermal water loss of impaired murine skins. The researchers concluded that the developed pseudo-ceramide-based microparticles could be used for barrier recovery as dermatology/cosmetics products. Porous biomedical composite microspheres have been developed for cell delivering scaffold in bone regeneration by Shin and co-workers (Shin *et al.,* 2010). This has been found that the developed microparticles of hydroxyapatite-polycaprolactone were effective in proliferating bone marrow mesenchymal stem cells of rat. This has shown new hopes in bone tissue regeneration by application of microparticulate systems. Microparticles are also used in the periodontal diseases. In one of their research Mundargi and his team have formulated biodegradable microspheres based on PLGA and polycaprolactone for controlled delivery of doxycycline in the treatment of human periodontal pocket (Mundargi *et al.,* 2007). The optimized formulation after *in vitro* and pre-clinical investigation was examined *in vivo* in thirty sites of human periodontal pockets. The results were found to be very much promising and authors suggested it to be employed as a successful therapy in human periodontal complications. Microparticles has also been explored for many more applications in various diseases.

12.10 Future Prospectives

Performing research to find new microencapsulation techniques or to improve existing techniques for newly discovered active molecules are in constant progress because of the limitations of the current pharmacopoeial requirement. The new active molecules found with the help of advances in biotechnology and therapeutic science are more often peptides or proteins, which are very active in small doses, sensitive to heat or organic solvents, available only in small quantities, potent and very expensive. Design and delivery of these novel therapeutics to achieve safe and effective therapy will be the future scope for micro-particulate drug delivery systems. Customized polymers with the added attributes of being biodegradable, biocompatible as well as bioadhesive for specific cells or mucosa will be the futuristic needs in drug delivery, which could also function as enzyme inhibitors for the successful delivery of proteins and peptides. A multi-disciplinary approach will therefore be required to overcome these challenges and to employ microparticles as a cutting edge technology for site targeted controlled release drug delivery of new as well as existing drugs. Despite considerable research efforts and impressive progress made in recent years, the question of feasibility of injectable microspheres as protein/peptide or vaccine delivery system remains a topic of debate. After all, the scale up and stability disputes associated in bringing these microsphere techniques into pipelines of pharmaceutical industries may be a challenging task to be accepted as well as to be resolved.

References

Adeyeye M.C, and Brittain H.G (2008). Preformulation in solid dosage form development (Informa Healthcare New York).

Adler-Moore J, and Proffitt R.T (2002). AmBisome: liposomal formulation, structure, mechanism of action and pre-clinical experience. *Journal of Antimicrobial Chemotherapy* **49:** 21-30.

Ahsan F, Rivas I.P, Khan M.A, and Torres Suárez A.I (2002). Targeting to macrophages: role of physicochemical properties of particulate carriers-liposomes and microspheres-on the phagocytosis by macrophages. *Journal of Controlled Release* **79:** 29-40.

Ajdary S, Dobakhti F, Taghikhani M, Riazi-Rad F, Rafiei S, and Rafiee-Tehrani M (2007). Oral administration of BCG encapsulated in alginate microspheres induces strong Th1 response in BALB/c mice. *Vaccine* **25:** 4595-4601.

Albertini B, Passerini N, Di Sabatino M, Vitali B, Brigidi P, and Rodriguez L (2009). Polymer-lipid based mucoadhesive microspheres prepared by spray-congealing for the vaginal delivery of econazole nitrate. *European Journal of Pharmaceutical Sciences : Official Journal of the European Federation for Pharmaceutical Sciences* **36:** 591-601.

AndrianovA.K, Chen J, and Payne L.G (1998). Preparation of hydrogel microspheres by coacervation of aqueous polyphosphazene solutions. *Biomaterials* **19:** 109-115.

Anselmi C, Centini M, Rossi C, Ricci M, Rastrelli A, Andreassi M, Buonocore A, and La Rosa C (2002). New microencapsulated sunscreens: technology and comparative evaluation. *International Journal of Pharmaceutics* **242:** 207-211.

Asthana S, Jaiswal A.K, Gupta P.K, Pawar V.K, Dube A, and Chourasia M.K (2013). Immunoadjuvant chemotherapy of visceral leishmaniasis in hamsters using amphotericin B-encapsulated nanoemulsion template-based chitosan nanocapsules. *Antimicrobial Agents and Chemotherapy* **57:** 1714-1722.

Avula M.N, Rao A.N, McGill L.D, Grainger D.W, and Solzbacher F (2013). Modulation of the foreign body response to implanted sensor models through device-based delivery of the tyrosine kinase inhibitor, masitinib. *Biomaterials* **34:** 9737-9746.

Benita S (2005). Microencapsulation: methods and industrial applications (CRC Press).

Bhadouriya P, Kumar M, and Pathak K (2012). Floating microspheres: to prolong the gastric retention time in stomach. *Current Drug Delivery* **9:** 315-324.

Campos E, Branquinho J, Carreira A.S, Carvalho A, Coimbra P, Ferreira P, and H Gil M (2013). Designing polymeric microparticles for biomedical and industrial applications. *European Polymer Journal* **49(8):** 2005-2021.

Chan L, Jin Y, and Heng P (2002). Cross-linking mechanisms of calcium and zinc in production of alginate microspheres. *International Journal of Pharmaceutics* **242:** 255-258.

Chang T.M (1964). Semipermeable microcapsules. *Science* **146:** 524-525.

Chaurasia M, Chourasia M, Jain N.K, Jain A, Soni V, Gupta Y, and Jain S (2008). Methotrexate bearing calcium pectinate microspheres: a platform to achieve colon-specific drug release. *Current Drug Delivery* **5:** 215-219.

Chen H, Pan S, Xiong Y, Peng C, Pang X, Li L, Xiong Y, and Xu W (2012). Preparation of thermo-responsive superhydrophobic TiO2/poly(N-isopropylacrylamide) microspheres. *Applied Surface Science* **258:** 9505-9509.

Conway B.R, Eyles J.E, and Alpar H.O (1997). A comparative study on the immune responses to antigens in PLA and PHB microspheres. *Journal of Controlled Release* **49:** 1-9.

Curcio M, Gianfranco Spizzirri U, Iemma F, Puoci F, Cirillo G, Parisi O.I, and Picci N (2010). Grafted thermo-responsive gelatin microspheres as delivery systems in triggered drug release. *European Journal of Pharmaceutics and Biopharmaceutics* **76:** 48-55.

D'Souza S, Faraj J, and Deluca P (2013). Microsphere delivery of Risperidone as an alternative to combination therapy. *European Journal of Pharmaceutics and Biopharmaceutics : Official Journal of Arbeitsgemeinschaft fur Pharmazeutische Verfahrenstechnik eV* **85:** 631-639.

de Jalón E.G, Blanco-Prieto M.J, Ygartua P, and Santoyo S (2001). PLGA microparticles: possible vehicles for topical drug delivery. *International Journal of Pharmaceutics* **226:** 181-184.

Drews J (2000). Drug discovery: a historical perspective. *Science* **287:** 1960-1964.

Engel A, and Colliex C (1993). Application of scanning transmission electron microscopy to the study of biological structure. *Current Opinion in Biotechnology* **4:** 403-411.

Folkman J, and Long D.M (1964). The Use of Silicone Rubber as a Carrier for Prolonged Drug Therapy. *The Journal of Surgical Research* **4:** 139-142.

Freiberg S, and Zhu X.X (2004). Polymer microspheres for controlled drug release. *International Journal of Pharmaceutics* **282:** 1-18.

Fu K, Griebenow K, Hsieh L, Klibanov A.M, and Langera R (1999). FTIR characterization of the secondary structure of proteins encapsulated within PLGA microspheres. *Journal of Controlled Release* **58:** 357-366.

Galbiati A, Rocca B.M.d, Tabolacci C, Beninati S, Desideri A, and Paradossi G (2011). PVA engineered microcapsules for targeted delivery of camptothecin to HeLa cells. *Materials Science and Engineering: C* **31:** 1653-1659.

Galeska I, Kim T.-K, Patil S.D, Bhardwaj U, Chatttopadhyay D, Papadimitrakopoulos F, and Burgess D.J (2005). Controlled release of dexamethasone from PLGA microspheres embedded within polyacid-containing PVA hydrogels. *The AAPS Journal* **7:** E231-E240.

Gavini E, Chetoni P, Cossu M, Alvarez M.G, Saettone M.F, and Giunchedi P (2004). PLGA microspheres for the ocular delivery of a peptide drug, vancomycin using emulsification/spray-drying as the preparation method: *in vitro/in vivo* studies. *European Journal of Pharmaceutics and Biopharmaceutics : Official Journal of Arbeitsgemeinschaft fur Pharmazeutische Verfahrenstechnik eV* **57:** 207-212.

Gibson M (2001). Pharmaceutical preformulation and formulation: a practical guide from candidate drug selection to commercial dosage form (Interpharm Press).

Grinberg O, Hayun M, Sredni B, and Gedanken A (2007). Characterization and activity of sonochemically-prepared BSA microspheres containing Taxol - An anticancer drug. *Ultrasonics Sonochemistry* **14:** 661-666.

Gui R, Wang Y, and Sun J (2013). Encapsulating magnetic and fluorescent mesoporous silica into thermosensitive chitosan microspheres for cell imaging and controlled drug release *in vitro*. *Colloids and Surfaces B: Biointerfaces* **113C:** 1-9.

Hamishehkar H, Emami J, Najafabadi A.R, Gilani K, Minaiyan M, Mahdavi H, and Nokhodchi A (2009). The effect of formulation variables on the characteristics of insulin-loaded poly(lactic-co-glycolic acid) microspheres prepared by a single phase oil in oil solvent evaporation method. *Colloids and Surfaces B, Biointerfaces* **74:** 340-349.

Hasçiçek C, Gönül N, and Erk N (2003). Mucoadhesive microspheres containing gentamicin sulfate for nasal administration: preparation and *in vitro* characterization. *Il Farmaco* **58:** 11-16.

Herrero-Vanrell R, and Refojo M.F (2001). Biodegradable microspheres for vitreoretinal drug delivery. *Adv Drug Deliv Rev* **52:** 5-16.

Holliday W.M, Berdrick M, Bell S.A, and Kiritsis G.C (1970). Sustained relief analgesic compositions, U. Patent, ed. (US).

Hu L, Zhang H, and Song W (2013). An overview of preparation and evaluation sustained-release injectable microspheres. *Journal of Microencapsulation* **30:** 369-382.

Jain S, Chourasia M, Jain A, Jain R, and Shrivastava A (2004). Development and characterization of mucoadhesive microspheres bearing salbutamol for nasal delivery. *Drug Delivery* **11:** 113-122.

Jalil R, and Nixon J.R (1990). Biodegradable poly(lactic acid) and poly(lactide-co-glycolide) microcapsules: problems associated with preparative techniques and release properties. *Journal of Microencapsulation* **7:** 297-325.

Jameela S.R, and Jayakrishnan A (1995). Glutaraldehyde cross-linked chitosan microspheres as a long acting biodegradable drug delivery vehicle: studies on the *in vitro* release of mitoxantrone and *in vivo* degradation of microspheres in rat muscle. *Biomaterials* **16:** 769-775.

Jeong Y.I, Song J.G, Kang S.S, Ryu H.H, Lee Y.H, Choi C, Shin B.A, Kim K.K, Ahn K.Y, and Jung S (2003). Preparation of poly(DL-lactide-co-glycolide) microspheres encapsulating all-trans retinoic acid. *Int J Pharm* **259:** 79-91.

Kawaguchi H (2000). Functional polymer microspheres. *Progress in Polymer Science* **25:** 1171-1210.

Kim H, Park H, Lee J, Kim T.H, Lee E.S, Oh K.T, Lee K.C, and Youn Y.S (2011). Highly porous large poly(lactic-co-glycolic acid) microspheres adsorbed with palmityl-acylated exendin-4 as a long-acting inhalation system for treating diabetes. *Biomaterials* **32:** 1685-1693.

Klein T, Buhr E, and Georg Frase C (2012). Chapter 6 - TSEM: A Review of Scanning Electron Microscopy in Transmission Mode and Its Applications. In Advances in Imaging and Electron Physics, W.H. Peter, ed. (Elsevier), pp. 297-356.

Lachman L, Libermen H, and J, K. (1990). The Theory and practice of industrial Pharmacy. In (Varghese publishing house), pp. 366.

Li F, Li X, and Li B (2011). Preparation of magnetic polylactic acid microspheres and investigation of its releasing property for loading curcumin. *Journal of Magnetism and Magnetic Materials* **323:** 2770-2775.

Lipinski C.A, Lombardo F, Dominy B.W, and Feeney P.J (1997). Experimental and computational approaches to estimate solubility and permeability in drug discovery and development settings. *Advanced Drug Delivery Reviews* **23:** 3-25.

Lipovetskaya Y (2010). Microspheres: technologies and global markets (Wellesley: BCC Research).

Liu W, Griffith M, and Li F (2008). Alginate microsphere-collagen composite hydrogel for ocular drug delivery and implantation. *Journal of Materials Science Materials in Medicine* **19:** 3365-3371.

Liu X.Y, Zheng S.W, Hong R.Y, Wang Y.Q, and Feng W.G (2014). Preparation of magnetic poly(styrene-co-acrylic acid) microspheres with adsorption of protein. *Colloids and Surfaces A: Physicochemical and Engineering Aspects* **443:** 425-431.

Ma G, and Song C (2007). PCL/poloxamer 188 blend microsphere for paclitaxel delivery: Influence of poloxamer 188 on morphology and drug release. *Journal of Applied Polymer Science* **104:** 1895-1899.

Ma N, Xu L, Wang Q, Zhang X, Zhang W, Li Y, Jin L, and Li S (2008). Development and evaluation of new sustained-release floating microspheres. *International Journal of Pharmaceutics* **358:** 82-90.

Mao S, Guo C, Shi Y, and Li, L.C (2012a). Recent advances in polymeric microspheres for parenteral drug delivery-part 1. *Expert Opinion on Drug Delivery* **9:** 1161-1176.

Mao S, Guo C, Shi Y, and Li, L.C (2012b). Recent advances in polymeric microspheres for parenteral drug delivery-part 2. *Expert Opinion on Drug Delivery* **9:** 1209-1223.

Mao S, Shi Y, Li L, Xu J, Schaper A, and Kissel T (2008). Effects of process and formulation parameters on characteristics and internal morphology of poly (D, L-lactide-co-glycolide) microspheres formed by the solvent evaporation method. *European Journal of Pharmaceutics and Biopharmaceutics* **68:** 214-223.

Mao S, Xu J, Cai C, Germershaus O, Schaper A, and Kissel T (2007). Effect of WOW process parameters on morphology and burst release of FITC-dextran loaded PLGA microspheres. *Int J Pharm* **334:** 137-148.

Martínez C.E, Pamies D, Sogorb M.A, and Vilanova E (2011). Chapter 10 - OECD guidelines and validated methods for *in vivo* testing of reproductive toxicity. In Reproductive and Developmental Toxicology, C.G. Ramesh, ed. (San Diego: Academic Press), pp. 123-133.

Martins S, Sarmento B, Souto E.B, and Ferreira D.C (2007). Insulin-loaded alginate microspheres for oral delivery-effect of polysaccharide reinforcement on physicochemical properties and release profile. *Carbohydrate Polymers* **69:** 725-731.

Mathiowitz E, Jacob J.S, Jong Y.S, Carino G.P, Chickering D.E, Chaturvedi P, Santos C.A, Vijayaraghavan K, Montgomery S, and Bassett M (1997). Biologically erodable microspheres as potential oral drug delivery systems. *Nature* **386:** 410-414.

Meinel L, Illi O.E, Zapf J, Malfanti M, Peter Merkle H, and Gander B (2001). Stabilizing insulin-like growth factor-I in poly (D, L-lactide-co-glycolide) microspheres. *Journal of Controlled Release* **70:** 193-202.

Muller R.H, Jacobs C, and Kayser O (2001). Nanosuspensions as particulate drug formulations in therapy. Rationale for development and what we can expect for the future. *Adv Drug Deliv Rev* **47:** 3-19.

Mundargi R.C, Srirangarajan S, Agnihotri S.A, Patil S.A, Ravindra S, Setty S.B, and Aminabhavi T.M (2007). Development and evaluation of novel biodegradable microspheres based on poly(d,l-lactide-co-glycolide) and poly(ε-caprolactone) for controlled delivery of doxycycline in the treatment of human periodontal pocket: *In vitro* and *in vivo* studies. *Journal of Controlled Release* **119:** 59-68.

Muthu M.S, Kulkarni S.A, Raju A, and Feng S.-S (2012). Theranostic liposomes of TPGS coating for targeted co-delivery of docetaxel and quantum dots. *Biomaterials* **33:** 3494-3501.

Owens III D.E, and Peppas N.A (2006). Opsonization, biodistribution, and pharmacokinetics of polymeric nanoparticles. *International Journal of Pharmaceutics* **307:** 93-102.

Pawar V.K, Kansal S, Asthana S, and Chourasia M.K (2012). Industrial perspective of gastroretentive drug delivery systems:

physicochemical, biopharmaceutical, technological and regulatory consideration. *Expert Opinion on Drug Delivery* **9:** 551-565.

Pham T, Loiseau P, and Barratt G (2013). Strategies for the design of orally bioavailable antileishmanial treatments. *International Journal of Pharmaceutics* **454(1):** 539-552.

Puthli S, and Vavia P (2008). Gamma irradiated micro system for long-term parenteral contraception: An alternative to synthetic polymers. *Eur J Pharm Sci* **35:** 307-317.

Rawat A, Bhardwaj U, and Burgess D.J (2012). Comparison of *in vitro-in vivo* release of Risperdal® Consta® microspheres. *Int J Pharm* **434:** 115-121.

Ribeiro C.C, Barrias C.C, and Barbosa M.A (2004). Calcium phosphate-alginate microspheres as enzyme delivery matrices. *Biomaterials* **25:** 4363-4373.

Rowe R.C, Sheskey P.J, Quinn M.E, and Press P (2009). Handbook of pharmaceutical excipients, Vol 6 (Pharmaceutical press London).

Sandor M, Bailey N.A, and Mathiowitz E (2002). Characterization of polyanhydride microsphere degradation by DSC. *Polymer* **43:** 279-288.

Saravanan M, and Anupama B (2011). Development and evaluation of ethylcellulose floating microspheres loaded with ranitidine hydrochloride by novel solvent evaporation-matrix erosion method. *Carbohydrate Polymers* **85:** 592-598.

Shang Y, Ding F, Xiao L, Deng H, Du Y, and Shi X (2014). Chitin-based fast responsive pH sensitive microspheres for controlled drug release. *Carbohydrate Polymers* **102:** 413-418.

Shin U.S, Park J.-H, Hong S.-J, Won J.-E, Yu H.-S, and Kim H.-W (2010). Porous biomedical composite microspheres developed for cell delivering scaffold in bone regeneration. *Materials Letters* **64:** 2261-2264.

Shinde U.A, Shete J.N, Nair H.A, and Singh K.H (2014). Design and characterization of chitosan-alginate microspheres for ocular delivery of azelastine. *Pharmaceutical Development and Technology* **19:** 813-823.

Smith A (1986). Evaluation of poly (lactic acid) as a biodegradable drug delivery system for parenteral administration. *International Journal of Pharmaceutics* **30:** 215-220.

Steele G (2004). Preformulation as an Aid to Product Design inEarly Drug Development.

Stumpf W.E (2007). Memo to the FDA and ICH: appeal for *in vivo* drug target identification and target pharmacokinetics: Recommendations for improved procedures and requirements. *Drug Discovery Today* **12:** 594-598.

Tao Y, Lu Y, Sun Y, Gu B, Lu W, and Pan J (2009). Development of mucoadhesive microspheres of acyclovir with enhanced bioavailability. *International Journal of Pharmaceutics* **378:** 30-36.

Varde N.K, and Pack D.W (2004). Microspheres for controlled release drug delivery. *Expert Opinion on Biological Therapy* **4:** 35-51.

Voigt M, Koerber M, and Bodmeier R (2012). Improved physical stability and injectability of non-aqueous in situ PLGA microparticle forming emulsions. *Int J Pharm* **434:** 251-256.

Wade A, and Weller P.J (1994). Handbook of pharmaceutical excipients (Pharmaceutical Press).

Wang F, Liu P, Jiang D, Liu C.B, Zhang F.C, and Chen X (2008). Preparation, Characterization, and *in vitro* Release of Biodegradable Erythromycin-gelatin Microspheres. *Chemical Research in Chinese Universities* **24:** 196-199.

Wang W, Zhou S, Sun L, and Huang C (2010). Controlled delivery of paracetamol and protein at different stages from core-shell biodegradable microspheres. *Carbohydrate Polymers* **79:** 437-444.

Wen H, Guo J, Chang B, and Yang W (2013). pH-responsive composite microspheres based on magnetic mesoporous silica nanoparticle for drug delivery. *European Journal of Pharmaceutics and Biopharmaceutics* **84:** 91-98.

Wischke C, and Schwendeman S.P (2008). Principles of encapsulating hydrophobic drugs in PLA/PLGA microparticles. *International Journal of Pharmaceutics* **364:** 298-327.

Wu H, Liao C, Jiao Q, Wang Z, Cheng W, and Wan Y (2012). Fabrication of core-shell microspheres using alginate and chitosan-polycaprolactone for controlled release of vascular endothelial growth factor. *Reactive and Functional Polymers* **72:** 427-437.

Yan S, Rao S, Zhu J, Wang Z, Zhang Y, Duan Y, Chen X, and Yin J (2012). Nanoporous multilayer poly(l-glutamic acid)/chitosan microcapsules for drug delivery. *International Journal of Pharmaceutics* **427:** 443-451.

Yang Y.Y, Chung T.S, Bai X.L, and Chan W.K (2000). Effect of preparation conditions on morphology and release profiles of biodegradable polymeric microspheres containing protein fabricated by double-emulsion method. *Chemical Engineering Science* **55:** 2223-2236.

Yener G, Incegül T, and Yener N (2003). Importance of using solid lipid microspheres as carriers for UV filters on the example octyl methoxy cinnamate. *International Journal of Pharmaceutics* **258:** 203-207.

Yin R, Han J, Zhang J, and Nie J (2010). Glucose-responsive composite microparticles based on chitosan, concanavalin A and dextran for insulin delivery. *Colloids and Surfaces B, Biointerfaces* **76:** 483-488.

Yuan Y, Chesnutt B.M, Utturkar G, Haggard W.O, Yang Y, Ong J.L, and Bumgardner J.D (2007). The effect of cross-linking of chitosan microspheres with genipin on protein release. *Carbohydrate Polymers* **68:** 561-567.

Zhang C, Ping Q, Ding Y, Cheng Y, and Shen J (2004). Synthesis, characterization, and microsphere formation of galactosylated chitosan. *Journal of Applied Polymer Science* **91:** 659-665.

Zhao M, You Y, Ren Y, Zhang Y, and Tang X (2008). Formulation, characteristics and aerosolization performance of azithromycin DPI prepared by spray-drying. *Powder Technology* **187:** 214-221.

INDEX

C

E

F

G

M

S

V

W

Z

Milton Keynes UK
Ingram Content Group UK Ltd.
UKHW020158061223
433783UK00006B/404